MEDICAL AND NUTRITION EXPERTS WEIGH IN
ON THE GROUNDBREAKING NEW EATING PLAN BASED ON
HARVARD MEDICAL SCHOOL RESEARCH

EAT, DRINK, AND BE HEALTHY
by Walter C. Willett, M.D.

"Dr. Willett describes a way to eat that is both delicious and healthy. Many nutritional scientists will strongly dispute Dr. Willett's contention that our national symbol of healthy eating, the USDA Food Pyramid, is unhealthy. However, very few will deny that the prescription in this book is a good one."

> —Susan Roberts, Ph.D., senior scientist, Energy Metabolism Laboratory, USDA Human Nutrition Research Center at Tufts University

"Finally we can step away from the hype and confusion of fad diets and turn instead to a solidly researched guide we know we can trust. I am grateful to Dr. Willett and his associates for making this information so clear and accessible. Throw away your other volumes; this is all you will need."

> —Mollie Katzen, author of *The Moosewood Cookbook*

"True to the implications of its title, *Eat, Drink, and Be Healthy* provides comprehensive evidence of the links of proper nutrition to better health and extended longevity. Professor Walter C. Willett and his learned colleagues describe new scientific work on the cardiovascular benefits from n-3 fatty acids found in nuts and some oils; on the cancer-fighting substance lycopene, found in tomatoes; on the potential hazards of consuming too much calcium; and on the advisability of taking a standard multivitamin daily. Well written and well reasoned, this book identifies a total diet that affects satiety, meets the body's needs for energy and nutrients, and prevents or delays some specific chronic diseases."

> —Ralph S. Paffenbarger, Jr., M.D., Dr.P.H., Professor of Epidemiology, Emeritus (Active), Stanford University School of Medicine

"Willett has studied real women (not rats) over many years in the Nurses' Health Study and distilled it into a readable guide for healthy living. This is the book on nutrition every woman should read."

> —Susan Love, M.D., author of *Dr. Susan Love's Breast Book* and *Dr. Susan Love's Hormone Book*

"*Eat, Drink, and Be Healthy* is a welcome beacon of clarity among the fog of misleading claims that make up the vast majority of diet books on the market. Dr. Willett's recommendations for healthy eating are based on a sound interpretation of current scientific knowledge, flavored by a joyful appreciation of traditional foodways. Unlike most diet books, he does not emphasize manipulation of one isolated physiological mechanism as a 'cure-all.' Rather, he applies a commonsense interpretation of wide-ranging scientific studies on diet and health. In the process, he challenges widely accepted but poorly supported ideas about nutrition and health, whether they come from the popular press or from federal government committees. The ultimate winners are the readers of this book, who will come away with the tools, guidance, and rationale they need to explore new ways of eating that are delicious, health-promoting, and based on the best of science and tradition."

—Lawrence H. Kushi, Sc.D., Associate Director
for Etiology and Prevention, Kaiser Permanente

CRITICS NATIONWIDE APPLAUD THIS PIONEERING GUIDE

"This excellent and controversial book offers a modified food pyramid that's heavy on fruits, vegetables, and monosaturated oils and nuts. . . . [Dr. Willett] is a heavy hitter in the world of nutrition, so expect his book to exert influence beyond your bookshelf."

—*Detroit Free Press*

"[A] standout health book. . . . Particularly insightful is Willett's revised version of the U.S. Food Guide Pyramid."

—*Chicago Tribune*

"*Eat, Drink, and Be Healthy* wins with easy-to-digest research information and lots of tempting recipes."

—Copley News Service

"Toss out your old diet books, forget the government's famous but flawed food pyramid, and get your hands on *Eat, Drink, and Be Healthy*, by Walter Willett."

—*The Boston Globe*

"[Willett's] new theory threatens to upend the government's food pyramid, [which he says] is outdated and doesn't reflect the latest food research. . . . Willett's criticism may prompt many people to view it more skeptically because of his clout in the nutrition field."

—*USA Today*

*f*P

Eat, Drink, and Be Healthy

The Harvard Medical School Guide to Healthy Eating

A HARVARD MEDICAL SCHOOL BOOK
CO-DEVELOPED WITH THE HARVARD SCHOOL OF PUBLIC HEALTH

Walter C. Willett, M.D., Dr. P.H.

With Patrick J. Skerrett
Contributions by Edward L. Giovannucci, M.D., D.Sc.
Recipes by Maureen Callahan
New Healthy Eating Pyramid illustration by Christopher Bing and Heather Foley

FREE PRESS

NEW YORK • LONDON • TORONTO • SYDNEY

To Gail

This publication contains the opinions and ideas of its author. It is intended to provide helpful and informative material on the subjects addressed in the publication. It is sold with the understanding that the author and publisher are not engaged in rendering medical, health, or any other kind of personal professional services in the book. The reader should consult his or her medical, health, or other competent professional before adopting any of the suggestions in this book or drawing inferences from it.

The author and publisher specifically disclaim all responsibility for any liability, loss, or risk, personal or otherwise, which is incurred as a consequence, directly or indirectly, of the use and application of any of the contents of this book.

*f*P

FREE PRESS
A Division of Simon & Schuster, Inc.
1230 Avenue of the Americas
New York, NY 10020
Copyright © 2001 by the President and Fellows of Harvard College

This Free Press trade paperback edition 2005

FREE PRESS and colophon are registered trademarks of Simon & Schuster, Inc.

For information regarding special discounts for bulk purchases,
please contact Simon & Schuster Special Sales:
1-800-456-6798 or business@simonandschuster.com

DESIGNED BY KEVIN HANEK
Manufactured in the United States of America

10   9   8   7   6   5   4   3

The Library of Congress has cataloged the hardcover edition as follows:
Willett, Walter C.
Eat, drink, and be healthy: the Harvard Medical School guide to healthy eating / Walter C. Willett; written with the assistance of Edward Giovannucci, Maureen Callahan, and Patrick Skerrett.
p.   cm.
"A Harvard Medical School book."
Includes bibliographical references and index.
1. Nutrition—Popular works. I. Giovannucci, Edward. II. Callahan, Maureen. III. Title.
RA784.W635 2001
613.2—dc21   2001020565

ISBN 0-684-86337-5   ISBN-13: 978-0-7432-6642-0 (Pbk)
                       ISBN-10:   0-7432-6642-0 (Pbk)

Contents

Acknowledgments

THE CONCEPTS IN THIS BOOK owe much to the work and ideas of many predecessors, present colleagues, postdoctoral fellows, and doctoral students. In particular, I am grateful for the encouragement, support, and thoughts of my colleagues Ed Giovannucci, Meir Stampfer, Graham Colditz, Bernard Rosner, Laura Sampson, JoAnn Manson, Frank Sacks, David Hunter, Charles Hennekens, Sue Hankinson, Eric Rimm, Frank Hu, and Alberto Aschiero of the Channing Laboratory and Harvard School of Public Health. Frank Speizer provided strong support over many years for the study of diet and disease within the Nurses' Health Study.

The vast majority of the research described in this book, by our own group and by others, would not have been possible without the funding of research grants through the National Institutes of Health. My colleagues and I are most appreciative of the strong public support for health-related research in the United States, and hopefully the information contained in this book will be deemed worthy of this investment.

Many helpful comments were received from Drs. Meir Stampfer, Susan Roberts, Frank Sacks, Eric Rimm, Peter Glausser, and Mollie Katzen, who reviewed all or specific chapters of this book. Dr. Tony Komaroff and Edward Coburn of Harvard Medical School provided important support and encouragement in the development of this update, and Liz Lenart and Debbie Flynn assisted in many aspects of the production. I also want to thank Simon & Schuster and Bill Rosen in particular for their vision of creating a series of high-quality books about health from Harvard Medical School.

At home my wife, Gail, assisted in many experiments in new ways of eating. Our sons Amani, who managed to trade the apples in his lunch for Twinkies at day care, and Kamali, who showed me that a vegetarian diet could mean Coca-Cola, ice cream, and pizza, helped me stay in touch with reality.

Preface

D
URING THE DARK AGES OF DIETARY ADVICE—from which we are just emerging—guidelines for good nutrition were based on guess-work and good intentions. I wrote this book to share with you what solid science is teaching us about the long-term effects of diet on health. The lessons are exciting. They show that a delicious, satisfying diet based on whole grains, healthy oils, fruits, vegetables, and good sources of protein can help you stay heatlthy and active to an old age.

Another reason for writing this book was to challenge the misleading ad-vice embodied in the U.S. Department of Agriculture's ubiquitous Food Guide Pyramid. When the department announced it was considering revising the thirteen-year-old pyramid, my colleagues and I were delighted. I sent the USDA a copy of the first edition of *Eat, Drink, and Be Healthy* and said it was welcome to use the evidence-based Healthy Eating Pyramid my colleagues and I had developed. But politics and business as usual ultimately trumped science, and the USDA's new MyPyramid offers even less guidance on healthy eating than its predecessor.

In this update of *Eat, Drink, and Be Healthy,* I examine the USDA's pyra-mids and show you where they have gone wrong. I also include new informa-tion on weight-loss strategies, trans fats, vitamin D, and other elements of healthy eating that have emerged since this book was first published in 2001.

Over the past twenty-five years, my colleagues and I have been continually surprised by the impact of diet on the risks of a host of chronic diseases. That dietary decisions could significantly affect the chances of heart disease, various cancers, cataracts, and even serious birth defects was not appreciated by the nutrition community until relatively recently. And many aspects of diet that were off the nutrition science radar screen, such as trans fat intake, glycemic load, and low intakes of folic acid and vitamin D, have emerged as important factors in long-term health. You may not be aware of these topics, or perhaps have heard about them only in passing, even though a better understanding can be crucial to attaining long-term health. This book will guide you to make better dietary decisions for yourself and your family.

My current effort to understand the long-term effects of diet on health began in the late 1970s when I realized that people were being given strong advice about what to eat and what to avoid, but that direct evidence to support these recommendations was often weak or nonexistent. A key missing element was data based on detailed dietary intakes from many individuals that could be related to their future development of heart disease, various cancers, and other health problems. Of course, information on medical history, smoking, physical activity, and other lifestyle variables would be needed to isolate the effects of diet. Fortunately, at this time I was already investigating the relation of cigarette smoking to heart disease within the Nurses' Health Study, an ongoing study of over 121,000 women across the United States, and this appeared to be an ideal group in which to investigate the long-term consequences of various diets. The first step was to develop a standardized method of dietary assessment for such a large population; many colleagues were skeptical that this was possible, perhaps appropriately so. Borrowing on work done at Harvard in the 1940s, we developed a series of self-administered dietary questionnaires and were able to document their validity in a series of detailed evaluations. Since 1980 we have been following women in this study with periodic updating of dietary and other information and have also added large cohorts of men and additional women. Although our large prospective studies have provided a unique and powerful flow of information about diet and health, the best understanding of a topic as complex as diet and health should incorporate evidence from all available sources. This book attempts to do this, giving special weight to studies of actual disease risk in humans.

My own interest in food and health actually goes back much further than the studies described above. The Willett family has been involved in dairy farming in Michigan for many generations, so it was only natural that I joined the 4-H club when I was growing up. Vegetable growing was one of my major activities, and I was the Michigan winner of a National Junior Vegetable Growers Association contest. As an undergraduate at Michigan State University, I studied physics and food science, and paid tuition by growing vegetables during the summers. In medical school at the University of Michigan, I had the opportunity to conduct a nutrition survey in a Native American community, my first experience in epidemiologic research and standardized methods of dietary assessment that were later developed for much larger-scale use. For internship and residency, I joined the Harvard Medical Service of Boston City Hospital, where I had the good fortune to meet individuals, many of whom remain colleagues today, who were interested in understanding the environmental and cultural origins of disease, rather than just its treatment. As a result, I enrolled in Harvard School of Public Health, where I studied more about nutrition. After completing a residency in internal medicine, I taught community medicine for three years at the Faculty of Medicine in Dar es Salaam, Tanzania. While there, I studied the relation between parasitic infections and malnutrition in children, and I became even more impressed with the power of epidemiologic approaches to understanding the occurrence of disease and to guide both prevention and treatment. Returning to Boston, I enrolled in a doctoral program in epidemiology at Harvard School of Public Health and began work on the Nurses' Health Study, which had begun one year earlier. Since then, the central theme in my work has been to develop and use epidemiologic approaches to study the relation of diet to the occurrence of disease. This has resulted in a textbook, *Nutritional Epidemiology*, and the publication of over nine hundred scientific articles. As we have seen the results from our research emerge, most of my colleagues and I have taken advantage of this information and substantially modified our activity levels and diet. This book is my attempt to assemble this information in a cohesive manner that is directly accessible to everyone. I hope that this information will lead to healthier, longer, and more interesting lives for others.

In producing this book, I have been joined by Dr. Ed Giovannucci, who has led much of our work on diet and cancer. Patrick J. Skerrett, an experienced science writer, has helped to create a text that departs from our usual terse scientific style. Maureen Callahan, a well-known dietitian and food writer, has added a section on the practical translation of nutritional science to food selection and preparation, and has also contributed many recipes that reflect the evidence presented earlier in the book. Perhaps one of the most important conclusions of our work is that healthy diets—and there is no single healthy diet—do not mean deprivation or monotony. In fact, the opposite is true. The classical midwestern American diet centered on mashed potatoes, roast beef, and gravy—besides being among the world's unhealthiest fares—was terribly dull compared to what I describe in this book. And the recipes included here represent just a sampling of the tremendously varied possibilities for healthy and exciting eating.

CHAPTER ONE

Building a Better Pyramid

Y OU EAT TO LIVE.
It's a simple, obvious truth. You need food for the basics of everyday life—to pump blood, move muscles, think thoughts. But food can also help you live well and live longer. By making the right choices, you can avoid some of the things we think of as the inevitable penalties of getting older. A healthy diet teamed with regular exercise and not smoking can eliminate 80 percent of heart disease and the majority of cancer cases. Making poor choices—eating too much of the wrong kinds of food and too little of the right kinds, or too much food altogether—increases your chances of developing cancer, heart disease, and diabetes. It contributes to digestive disorders and aging-related loss of vision. It may influence Alzheimer's disease. An unhealthy diet during pregnancy can cause some birth defects, and may even influence a baby's health into adulthood and old age.

When it comes to diet, knowing what's good and what's bad isn't easy. The food industry spends billions of dollars a year to influence your choices. Diet gurus promote the latest fads, while the media serves up near daily helpings of often flip-flopping nutrition news. Supermarkets and fast-food restaurants offer advice, as do cereal boxes and a sea of Internet sites.

Where can you turn as a source of reliable information on healthy eating? The U.S. Department of Agriculture (USDA) touts its new food pyramid and "food guidance system" as aids to help you make healthier food choices. In reality, these tools help farmers and food companies more than they will help you.

TURNING TO THE USDA PYRAMID IS A MISTAKE

Through the Food Guide Pyramid, now called MyPyramid (see Figure 1), the USDA presents what it wants you to think of as rock-solid nutrition information that rises above the jungle of misinformation and contradictory claims. What it really offers is wishy-washy, scientifically unfounded advice on an absolutely vital topic—what to eat.

The original Food Guide Pyramid, unveiled in 1992, was built on shaky scientific ground. It included six food groups, each labeled with recommended daily servings. At the foundation sat an admonition to load up on highly refined starches, while the top was crowned with a "Use Sparingly" group that included fats, oils, and sweets. In between were fruits, vegetables, protein, and dairy.

Over the next thirteen years, research from around the globe eroded the Food Guide Pyramid at all levels. Results from scores of large and small studies chipped away at its foundation (carbohydrates), middle (meat and milk), and tip (fats). The USDA never renovated the Pyramid, but left it to crumble under the weight of new scientific evidence.

USDA's new MyPyramid

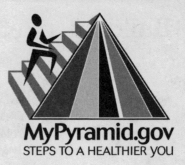

FIG. 1 MyPyramid. In 2005, the USDA unveiled its catchy but information-free replacement for the familiar Food Guide Pyramid.

Taking a cue from television reality shows, the agriculture department gave the Pyramid an extreme makeover in April 2005. It tipped the Pyramid on its side and painted it with a rainbow of brightly colored bands running vertically from the tip to the base. A jaunty stick figure runs up stairs chiseled into the left side. That's it—no labels, no text, not even the equivalent of a nutritional Rosetta stone to help you decipher what it means. For that you need a computer and a connection to the Internet.

The good news about the makeover is that the USDA finally took a wrecking ball to its dangerously outmoded Pyramid. The bad news is that its replacement doesn't offer any real information to help you make healthy choices, and continues to recommend foods that aren't essential to good health and that may even be detrimental in the quantities included in MyPyramid.

At best, MyPyramid stands as a missed opportunity to improve the health of millions of people. At worst, the lack of information and downright misinformation it conveys contribute to overweight, poor health, and unnecessary early deaths.

REBUILDING THE PYRAMID

I wrote this book to show you where the USDA pyramids—old and new—went wrong and why they are wrong. In their place, I offer a better guide to healthful eating based on the best scientific evidence available today. It fixes the fundamental flaws of the USDA's advice and helps you make better choices about what you eat. I also want to give you the latest information on new discoveries that should have profound effects on how and what we eat.

The New Healthy Eating Pyramid (see Figure 2) gathers much of this information into a simple, easy-to-use, and familiar icon. It encourages you to choose most of the foods you eat from the lower sections—whole grains, healthy oils, fruits, vegetables, nuts, and legumes. You don't have to weigh your food or tally up fat grams. There are no complicated food exchange tables to follow. You needn't eat odd combinations of foods or religiously avoid particular foods (except those containing trans fats).

The New Healthy Eating Pyramid isn't a diet designed to help you shed pounds. Instead, it aims to nudge you toward eating mostly familiar foods that have been shown to improve health and reduce the risk of chronic disease. The eating strategies embodied in the pyramid and explained in this book involve

The New Healthy Eating Pyramid

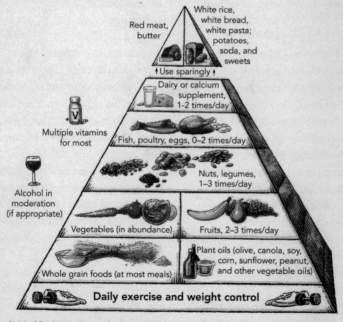

FIG. 2 Healthy Eating Pyramid. This pyramid, based on solid science, offers better guidance for healthy eating than the advice from the USDA.

simple changes you can make one at a time. Because they will make your meals and snacks tastier, and help keep hunger at bay, these changes can also help you lose weight or keep it under control. Best of all, it is a strategy you can stick with for years.

You don't have to take my word for it. After *Eat, Drink, and Be Healthy* was first published in 2001, I received a flood of letters and e-mail messages from readers around the world. Others posted comments in the review sections of online booksellers. Typical of these notes, one reader wrote, "What you get if you follow this book is the satisfaction of feeling you really can, and will, eat this way for the rest of your life and be all the better for it. I lost 30 pounds over six months by eating this way and exercising regularly. It isn't a diet but guidelines on nutrition. Losing weight is just the bonus side effect of being much more healthy."

The Healthy Eating Pyramid isn't a cute idea dolled up in a catchy graphic. It represents evidence distilled from forty years of research conducted at Harvard and around the world. This shouldn't be an important point, but it is. Virtually none of the diets used by millions of Americans—or the USDA pyramids—have been built on this kind of solid evidence.

HOW THE USDA PYRAMID GOT ITS SHAPE

Once upon a time, wrote Rudyard Kipling in his classic children's story "The Elephant's Child," elephants didn't have trunks, only blackish, bulgy noses as big as a boot. That changed when the curious elephant's child ended up in the middle of a terrific tug-of-war, with a crocodile clamped onto its nose and a python wrapped around its legs. That's pretty much how the USDA Pyramid got its structure—yanked this way and that by competing powerful interests, few of which had your health as a central goal.

The thing to keep in mind about the Pyramid is that it comes from the arm of the federal government responsible for promoting American agriculture. It doesn't come from agencies established to monitor and protect our health, like the Institute of Medicine or the National Institutes of Health. And there's the root of the problem—what's good for agricultural interests isn't necessarily good for the people who eat their products.

Serving two masters is tricky business, especially when one of them includes persuasive, connected, and well-funded representatives of the formidable meat, dairy, and sugar industries. The end result of the tug-of-war between the food industry and nutrition science is a set of positive, feel-good, all-inclusive recommendations that distort what could be the single most important tool for improving your health and the health of the nation—guidelines on healthful eating.

FOOD POLITICS

When it (finally) came time to "fix" the Pyramid, lobbying and politics took center stage, while science and the health of the American people took a back seat.

The story begins with the Dietary Guidelines for Americans, a document the USDA says provides "authoritative advice for people two years and older about how good dietary habits can promote health and reduce risk for major chronic diseases." By law, these guidelines must be revised every five years. It is supposed to be a scholarly and scientific process, but is often a free-for-all among lobbyists for agribusinesses, food companies, and special-interest groups.

In 2003, a new executive director was appointed for the center. Curiously, the person chosen for the job was an expert in animal nutrition whose previous jobs had been with the National Livestock and Meat Board, the National Pork Producers Association, and the National Pork Board.

The 2005 revision began as in past years—the USDA selected a committee of thirteen respected nutrition experts from across the country. The committee sifted through the latest research and time-tested knowledge to figure out what we know about the American diet and healthful eating.

But a funny thing happened on the way to the final report. Instead of writing the Dietary Guidelines for Americans 2005, the committee was told to hand over its findings to a second committee charged with translating the science into useful guidelines. That committee was never formed. How the Department of Agriculture developed the final guidelines isn't clear, since the process was so obscure.

This handoff created subtle but important shifts in emphasis in the final guidelines. For example, the committee said that less than 1 percent of our daily calories should come from harmful trans fats, which are found in many prepared foods. What the Dietary Guidelines for Americans ultimately said is that we should keep trans fat intake "as low as possible," a recommendation that is open to interpretation. The committee specified that whole grains should account for *at least* half of daily carbohydrate intake. MyPyramid gives this a gentle but telling twist, "Make half your grains whole," which implies that half should be refined.

For the pyramid redesign, the USDA turned to public relations giant Porter-Novelli, which helped build the first pyramid in 1992. (The company's other current or former clients include McDonald's, The Snack Food Association, Krispy Kreme, Johnnie Walker, and Masterfoods USA, maker of M&Ms.) Porter-Novelli designed MyPyramid, its Web site, and the mini-marketing campaign to promote it.

WHY THIS MATTERS

If the Dietary Guidelines and MyPyramid were merely optional recommendations and diet aids, we might be able to overlook the hijacking of the process used to create them. But the Dietary Guidelines set the standards for all federal nutrition programs. These include food stamps, school lunch programs, and food services for those serving in the armed forces as well as in federal prisons. The Dietary Guidelines and Pyramid also help determine what foods and food products Americans buy. In other words, they influence how billions of dollars are spent each year. No wonder food companies lobby so hard for changes that will benefit them, not the American public.

THE HOLES IN THE USDA PYRAMIDS

Some recommendations on diet and nutrition are misguided because they are based on inadequate or incomplete information. That hasn't been the case for the USDA's pyramids. They are wrong because they brush aside evidence on healthful eating that has been carefully assembled over the past forty years.

Since MyPyramid is mainly a gussied-up version of the old Food Guide Pyramid (see Figure 3), let me explain the original's problems first. Then I will tell you why MyPyramid isn't worth a fraction of the $2.5 million the USDA spent to create it.

Food Guide Pyramid

Here are the Food Guide Pyramid's six most health-damaging faults:
* *All fats are bad.* Wrong—some fats are good for you.

There is no question that two of the four main types of fat contribute to atherosclerosis, the artery-clogging process that leads to heart disease, stroke, and other problems. These are saturated fats, abundant in whole milk or red meat, and trans fats, found in many hard margarines, vegetable shortenings, prepared baked goods, and fried foods in restaurants. But the other main types of fat are good for your heart. These are the monounsaturated and polyunsaturated fats found in olive oil and other vegetable oils, nuts, whole grains, other

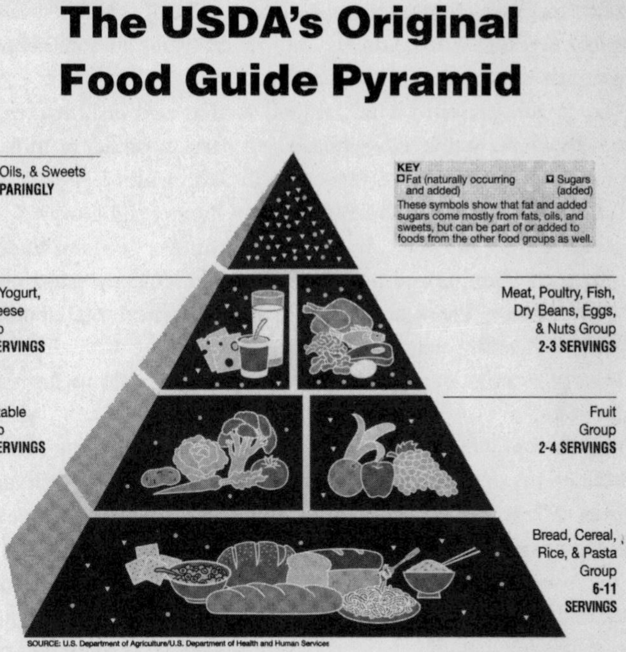

The USDA's Original Food Guide Pyramid

FIG. 3 USDA pyramid, 1992–2005. Despite sweeping changes in the science of healthy eating, this initially flawed pyramid went unchanged for thirteen years.

plant products, and fish. (See chapter 4.) The Food Guide Pyramid's recommendation to use fats "sparingly" helped foster the fat phobia that has led many Americans to throw out the baby with the bathwater.

- *All carbohydrates are good.* Wrong again—some are, some aren't.

The Food Guide Pyramid told us that we should feel good about eating carbohydrates, especially if we ate them in place of fats. For most people, this meant eating white bread, potatoes, pasta, and white rice, the main sources of carbohydrates in the American diet. This simplistic message ignored the fact that some carbohydrates are good for you while others aren't. In fact, eating too much of the wrong kinds of carbohydrates and too little of the right kinds can set you up for the same problems you may be trying to solve, such as overweight and heart disease.

Eating rapidly digested starches, like those in white bread, a baked potato, or white rice, causes a swift, high spike in blood sugar followed by an equally fast fall. This blood sugar roller coaster—and the insulin one that shadows it—triggers the early return of hunger pangs. These starches are also implicated as part of the perilous pathway to heart disease and diabetes. The harmful effects of rapidly digested carbohydrates are especially serious for people who are overweight.

The carbohydrates in whole grains, such as oats or brown rice, in foods made with whole grains, like whole-wheat pasta or bread, or in beans have a slow, low, and steady effect on blood sugar and insulin levels. This helps you feel full longer and keeps you from getting hungry right away. Whole grains and other sources of slowly digested carbohydrates give you important fiber plus plenty of vitamins and minerals. They also protect you against heart disease and diabetes. These are the carbohydrate sources that should form the keystone of a healthy diet.

• *Protein sources are interchangeable.* It's the protein *package* you have to watch out for.

You need protein every day and can get it from a variety of sources. The Food Guide Pyramid served up as equals red meat, poultry, fish, eggs, beans, and nuts. All are indeed excellent sources of protein. But red meat is a poor protein package because of the saturated fat and cholesterol that often tag along. Red meat may also give you too much iron in a form the body absorbs whether it is needed or not. Chicken and turkey give you less saturated fat. The same is true for fish, which delivers some essential unsaturated fats as well. Beans and nuts have some advantages over animal sources of protein. They give you fiber, vitamins, minerals, and healthy unsaturated fats. Like fruits and vegetables, they also provide you with a host of phytochemicals, an ever-expanding collection of plant products that help protect you from a variety of chronic diseases.

• *Dairy products are essential.* You need calcium, not dairy products.

The Food Guide Pyramid called for two to three servings of milk, yogurt, cheese, or other dairy products a day. These foods are good sources of calcium, which is needed to build and protect bones. Exactly how much we need, though, isn't clear.

Osteoporosis, a disease that weakens bones and makes them prone to breaking, affects about ten million older Americans. As part of the fight against it, dairy products have been enlisted to reverse our so-called calcium emergency. It's a message that the hip "got milk?" milk-mustache ads (sponsored by the dairy industry) hammer home to every possible demographic group. Only there isn't a calcium emergency. Americans get more calcium than the residents of almost every other country except Holland and the Scandinavian countries, and still have one of the highest rates of hip fracture in the world.

Other countries with less than half of our average calcium intake have far less osteoporosis. (See chapter 9.) Further complicating the issue are some studies suggesting that drinking or eating a lot of dairy products may increase a woman's chances of developing ovarian cancer or a man's chances of developing advanced prostate cancer.

If you need extra calcium, there are cheaper, easier, and healthier ways to get it than dairy products. (See chapter 9.)

• *Eat your potatoes.* That's okay advice for those who are physically active all day long, but it doesn't work for the rest of us.

Nutritionists and diet books often call potatoes a "perfect food." Eating potatoes on a daily basis may be fine for lean people who exercise a lot or do regular manual labor. But for everyone else, potatoes should be an occasional food eaten in modest amounts, not a daily vegetable. The venerable baked potato increases blood sugar and insulin levels nearly as fast and as high as pure table sugar. French fries do much the same thing, while also typically packing an unhealthy wallop of trans fats. More than two hundred studies have shown that people who eat plenty of fruits and vegetables decrease their chances of having heart attacks or strokes, of developing a variety of cancers, or of suffering from constipation or other digestive problems. The same body of evidence shows that potatoes don't contribute to this benefit.

• *No guidance on weight, exercise, alcohol, and vitamins.* Like the Sphinx, the Food Guide Pyramid was silent on four things you need to know about: the importance of weight control, the necessity of daily exercise, the potential health benefits of a daily alcoholic drink, and what you can gain by taking a daily multivitamin.

MyPyramid

The new pyramid is based on the latest Dietary Guidelines for Americans. This document includes some important advances over previous versions. The 2005 guidelines acknowledge the potential health benefits of unsaturated fats, stress the health benefits of whole grains, and emphasize the importance of controlling weight. Other sections of the new guidelines, though, remain mired in the past. These include the tacit advice that it is okay to consume half your grains as refined starch; the lumping together of red meat, poultry, fish, and beans as interchangeable protein sources; and the recommendation of three daily servings of milk or other dairy products.

The one positive advance of MyPyramid is its stress on exercise and physical activity as an important part of any healthy eating strategy. Sadly, this comes at a time when federal and state budgets continue to cut back on funds for physical activity in schools, and little attention is paid to providing Americans with safe places to exercise.

Other than that, MyPyramid contains . . . nothing. Look at the image on a cereal box and you have no idea what the orange, green, red, blue, and purple stripes mean, and you probably can't see the yellow one. Here's a key: orange for grains, green for vegetables, red for fruits, yellow for oils, blue for dairy, and purple for meat and beans.

MyPyramid dispenses with the simple advice embodied in the old pyramid, which was to eat more from food groups near the bottom of the pyramid and less from those at the top. The use of vertical stripes is a big win for the food industry, which despised the original pyramid design because it presented the food groups at the bottom as good and stigmatized those at the top. The left-to-right design presents all foods as essentially equal. This is in line with the federal government's support for dietary guidance that "promotes the view that all foods can be part of a healthy and balanced diet, and supports personal responsibility to choose a diet conducive to individual energy balance, weight control, and health."* In other words, there is no such thing as a bad food.

MyPyramid advocates three servings of dairy products a day, equates bologna with beans, and implies it's healthful to get half your daily grains in the form of highly refined starch. It doesn't bother to warn you away from foods that play little part in a healthful diet: trans fats, rapidly digested carbohydrates, and added sugars.

MyPyramid is a creature of the World Wide Web (www.mypyramid.gov). To those with Internet access and the time to poke around, it offers layers of information on the striped food groups. It also allows you to "personalize" a pyramid, based on your age, sex, and activity level. This sounds like a good idea, but it isn't.

The personalized pyramids leave out body size, the most important factor in determining how many calories you need each day. Then they serve up diet prescriptions so detailed and precise that even an experienced nutritionist couldn't follow them. Your personalized pyramid might recommend fractions of ounces for servings of meat (no mention of beans or nuts) and fractions of cups of grains and vegetables. The calculations of daily calorie requirements for an individual based on age, sex, and daily activity can easily be off by 500

---

* In a letter from William Steiger, PhD, of the U.S. Department of Health and Human Services to the Director General of the World Health Organization, criticizing a WHO report on diet and nutrition that recommended a limit on sugar intake.

calories. That's enough to cause unwanted weight loss or a gain of 50 pounds over a year or two.

Individuals without Internet access get almost nothing from MyPyramid. By putting virtually all of its nutrition information on the Web, rather than including some of it on the pyramid, the USDA is widening the digital divide and doing little to improve the health and eating habits of those who need the most help.

THE HEALTHY EATING PYRAMID IS BASED ON SCIENCE

You deserve more accurate, more helpful, and less biased information than what's offered by the USDA. I have tried to collect exactly that in the Healthy Eating Pyramid. Without question, I had the advantage of starting with a lot more information than the USDA did when it built its first pyramid. Just as important, I didn't have to negotiate with any special-interest groups when it came time to design this Pyramid.

The Healthy Eating Pyramid isn't set in stone. I don't have all the answers, nor can I predict what nutrition researchers will turn up in the decade ahead. But I can give you a solid sense of state-of-the-art healthy eating today and point out where things are heading. This isn't the only alternative to the USDA's advice. The Asian, Latin, Mediterranean, and vegetarian pyramids promoted by Oldways Preservation and Exchange Trust are also good, evidence-based guides to healthy eating. But the Healthy Eating Pyramid takes advantage of even more extensive research and offers a broader guide that is not based on a specific culture.

In the chapters that follow, I lay out the evidence that shaped this blueprint for healthy eating. I also chart out extra information to help people with special nutritional needs get the most benefit from what they eat. These include pregnant women and people with, or at high risk of, heart disease, diabetes, high cholesterol, high blood pressure, and some other chronic conditions.

For now, though, this summary of the seven healthiest changes you can make in your diet describes how the Healthy Eating Pyramid differs from the USDA's. Topping the list is controlling your weight.

• *Watch your weight.* When it comes to long-term health, keeping your weight from creeping up on you is more important than the exact ratio of fats to carbohydrates or the types and amounts of antioxidants in your food. The lower and more stable your weight, the lower your chances of having or dying from a heart attack, stroke, or other type of cardiovascular disease; of developing high blood pressure, high cholesterol, or diabetes; of being diagnosed with postmenopausal breast cancer, cancer of the endometrium, colon, or kidney; or of being afflicted with some other chronic condition. The advantages aren't just theoretical. A healthy weight makes it easier to keep up with your children, play with a grandchild, be active with friends, or engage in sexual activity. Yes, it is possible to be too thin, as in the case of anorexia nervosa, but otherwise few American adults fall into this category.

• *Eat fewer bad fats and more good fats.* One of the most striking differences of the Healthy Eating Pyramid is the placement of healthy fats in the foundation instead of relegating them to the tiny triangle at the top. The message here is that fats from nuts, seeds, grains, fish, and liquid oils (including olive, canola, soybean, corn, sunflower, peanut, and other vegetable oils) are good for you, especially when you eat them in place of saturated and trans fat.

The all-fat-is-bad message started a huge national experiment, with us as the guinea pigs. As people cut back on fat, they usually eat more carbohydrates. In America today, that means more highly refined or easily digested foods like sugar, white bread, white rice, and potatoes. This switch usually fails to yield the hoped-for weight loss or lower cholesterol levels. Instead, it often leads to weight gain and potentially dangerous changes in cholesterol and other blood fats. The failure of carbohydrates to melt away pounds sparked a national outcry against carbs and led to the enormous popularity of the Atkins, South Beach, and other low-carb diets.

Eating unsaturated fats in place of saturated fats, though, *improves* cholesterol levels across the board and protects you against certain heart rhythm disturbances that can end in sudden death. Good fats won't make you fat as long as you aren't taking in more calories.

The bottom line is this: It is perfectly fine to get more than 30 percent of your daily calories from fats as long as most of those fats are unsaturated. Keep saturated fats to a minimum by eating red meat, whole-milk dairy products, and butter only now and then. And avoid trans fats, since they have no place in a healthful diet.

• *Eat fewer refined-grain carbohydrates and more whole-grain carbohydrates.* The Healthy Eating Pyramid includes two carbohydrate building blocks—whole grains that are slowly digested, in the foundation; and highly refined, rapidly digested carbohydrates, at the very top (along with sodas and sweets).

For almost twenty years, my research team has been one of several groups studying the health effects of foods made from refined and intact grains. The result of this work is compelling. Eating lots of carbohydrates that are quickly digested and absorbed increases levels of blood sugar and insulin, raises levels of triglycerides, and lowers levels of protective HDL cholesterol. Over the long run, these changes lead to cardiovascular disease and diabetes. In contrast, eating whole-grain foods is clearly better for long-term good health and offers protection against diabetes, heart disease, and gastrointestinal problems such as diverticulosis and constipation. Other research around the world points to the same conclusions.

• *Choose healthier sources of proteins.* In the Healthy Eating Pyramid, red meat occupies one half of the pointy "Use Sparingly" tip. I did this to highlight the fact that *something* about red meat—its particular combination of saturated fats or the potentially cancer-causing compounds that form when red meat is grilled or fried—is connected to a variety of chronic diseases. The best sources of protein are beans and nuts, along with fish, poultry, and eggs. The Healthy Eating Pyramid separates vegetable and animal protein sources and makes the latter optional for people who want to follow a vegetarian diet.

• *Eat plenty of vegetables and fruits, but hold the potatoes.* Vegetables and fruits are essential ingredients in almost every cuisine. If you let them play starring roles in your diet, they will reward you with many benefits besides great taste, terrific textures, and welcome variety. A diet rich in fruits and vegetables will lower your blood pressure, decrease your chances of having a heart attack or stroke, protect you against some cancers, guard against constipation and other gastrointestinal problems, and limit the chances of losing your vision as you age. I've plucked potatoes out of the vegetable category and put them in the "Use Sparingly" category because of their dramatic effect on levels of blood sugar and insulin.

• *Use alcohol in moderation.* When the first reports appeared linking moderate alcohol consumption with lower rates of heart disease, many doctors and scientists thought that some other habit shared by drinkers, not the drinking, accounted for the benefit. Today the evidence strongly points to alcohol itself. Based on the best estimates available, one drink a day for women and one or two a day for men cuts the chances of having a heart attack or dying from heart disease by about a third. It also decreases the risk of having a clot-caused (ischemic) stroke. (See chapter 8.)

Alcohol's effects depend on the dose. A little bit can be beneficial. A lot can destroy the liver, lead to various cancers, boost blood pressure, trigger bleeding (hemorrhagic) strokes, progressively weaken the heart muscle, scramble the brain, harm unborn children, and damage lives.

The clear and ever-present dangers of alcohol and alcohol addiction make the recommendation of moderate drinking a social and medical hot potato. While I acknowledge the problems with alcohol, I think it is important to point out its possible benefits for middle-aged and older people.

If you don't drink alcohol, you shouldn't feel compelled to start. You can get similar benefits by beginning to exercise (if you don't already) or boosting the intensity and duration of your physical activity, in addition to following the eating strategy described in this book. But if you are an adult with no history of depression or alcoholism who is at high risk for heart disease, a daily alcoholic drink may help reduce that risk. This is especially true for people with type 2 diabetes or those with low HDL that just won't budge upward with diet and exercise. If you already drink alcohol, keep it moderate.

- *Take a multivitamin for insurance.* Several of the ingredients in a standard multivitamin—especially vitamins B_6 and B_{12}, folic acid, and vitamin D—are essential players in preventing heart disease, cancer, osteoporosis, and other chronic diseases. At about a dime a day, a multivitamin is a cheap and effective genuine "life insurance" policy. It won't make up for the sins of an unhealthy diet, but it fills in the nutritional holes that can plague even the most conscientious eaters. A daily multivitamin is particularly important for people who have trouble absorbing vitamins from their food; for those who can't, or don't, get out in the sun every day; and for people who drink alcohol. (See page 190.)

USDA PYRAMID AND DIETARY GUIDELINES FAIL THE HEALTH TEST

Throughout this book I will talk about "the evidence." I hope I won't sound like an old, scratched record, repeating that there is or is not enough evidence on the benefits or risks of this or that strategy. But the evidence is what matters. Without it, recommendations are little more than opinions and educated guesses that may or may not accomplish what they set out to do.

Did the Food Guide Pyramid accomplish what it was designed to do—help Americans choose diets that would promote health and help ward off major chronic diseases? To answer that question, we need to know how widely it was used and whether the advice translated into better health.

According to the USDA's own estimates, most Americans recognized the old Food Guide Pyramid. Yet fewer than 5 in 100 ate according to its principles.

Assessing the impact of the USDA's diet advice on long-term health posed more of a problem. The Healthy Eating Index devised a few years ago by the department's Center for Nutrition Policy and Promotion provided a way to do this. The index assigns scores of 0 to 10 for each of ten dietary components.

Five are from the Food Guide Pyramid (number of daily servings of grains, vegetables, fruits, meat, and dairy products), and five are from the Dietary Guidelines for Americans (total fat in the diet, percentage of calories from saturated fat, cholesterol intake, sodium intake, and variety of the diet). A score of 100 means an individual perfectly follows the USDA's recommendations, while a score of 0 means he or she totally disregards them.

My colleagues and I used the Healthy Eating Index to test the impact of the USDA's recommendations on health.

We extracted information on eating patterns from questionnaires that 121,000 female nurses and 50,000 male health professionals have been completing every four years for more than a decade. Based on this information, we calculated a Healthy Eating Index score for each individual. Those with the highest scores (who closely followed the government's advice) were just as likely to have developed a major illness or to have died over a twelve-year period as those with the lowest scores. Heart attacks were only slightly less common among those with high scores than they were among those with low scores.

The latest Dietary Guidelines and MyPyramid are too new to have been tested as I write this. However, the lack of any information at all about food choices on MyPyramid means it is unlikely to have an impact on what Americans eat or their long-term health.

The dismal results for the old Food Guide Pyramid shouldn't come as a surprise, since the USDA has consistently ignored the extensive body of evidence linking certain eating patterns with long-term health. Take those results as a warning that following the agriculture department's advice won't help you eat to live well or live longer.

To be fair, we put the Healthy Eating Pyramid to the same test. First we created an Alternate Healthy Eating Index based on our new pyramid. It included indicators such as intake of vegetables, fruits, nuts, cereal fiber, trans fats, and alcohol; multivitamin use; and the ratios of white to red meat and unsaturated fat to saturated fat. Using the same answers from the same nurses and health professionals, we calculated scores for each individual. The results? Women and men with high scores (those who followed the eating strategies embodied in the Healthy Eating Pyramid) had substantially lower risks of developing major chronic diseases, especially heart disease or stroke, than those scoring low on the index.

My colleagues and I were pleased by these results. But we weren't entirely surprised, because each building block of the Healthy Eating Pyramid comes from the finest possible quarry—solid evidence amassed by researchers from around the world. I am confident that the findings from this research, represented in the Healthy Eating Pyramid, can help keep you healthy.

WHAT'S IN THIS BOOK

Between the covers of this book is the latest thinking about diet and health. To give you a quick and easy guide, I distilled as much information as possible into the Healthy Eating Pyramid. But I also wanted you to see the blueprint—the scientific evidence—on which it is based. This is detailed in chapters 3 through 11. Along the way I describe cutting-edge research that may radically alter healthy eating patterns, including new information on slowly digested carbohydrates; on what protein can—and can't—do; on how to put the omega-3 fats found in fish and some plants to work for you; on lycopene, a possible cancer-fighting substance found in tomatoes; on the potential hazards of getting too much calcium, especially from dairy products; and on why it makes sense to take a daily multivitamin.

This book also helps you incorporate this information into your snacks and meals with practical tips on buying healthy foods and eating defensively. It ends with more than sixty tested, tasty recipes that I hope prove to you that healthy eating is not a culinary sacrifice. In fact, it is just the opposite, and can add spice, variety, and pleasure to your meals and your life.

This information isn't meant to take the place of advice you get from your healthcare provider, especially if you have a medical condition that requires a specific diet. Instead, I encourage you to talk with him or her about your diet or share what you've learned from this book to make sure you are on the same wavelength. Unfortunately, the pressures of modern medicine and health care often make it difficult for clinicians to spend time talking about healthy food choices with their patients.

CHAPTER TWO

What Can You Believe About Diet?

RESEARCH ABOUT DIET AND NUTRITION seems to contradict itself with aggravating regularity. You stop using butter and instead start spreading margarine on your toast, only to learn later that margarine can be just as bad for you as butter. After switching to bran muffins for breakfast because high-fiber diets supposedly prevent colon cancer, you hear about a big study showing that fiber doesn't prevent colon cancer. Early research shows that coffee drinking increases the chances of developing pancreatic cancer, while later research shows that coffee drinking is harmless and may even have some benefits. Some studies find that eating fish prevents heart attacks, others don't. These flip-flops are so confusing and so common that a negative report on vitamin E and beta-carotene once goaded *Boston Globe* columnist Ellen Goodman to write, "There seems to be some sort of planned obsolescence now to medical news. Today's cure is tomorrow's poison pellet. Fresh research has a sell-by date that is shorter than the one on the cereal box."

The sheer volume of information doesn't help. Fifty years ago, medical researchers mostly ignored nutrition. For example, the longest study of health in the United States, the legendary and ongoing Framingham Heart Study, collected hardly any data on diet when it was started in 1949. Over the years, though, the trickle of information on diet and health has swelled into a fast-flowing torrent.

It's only natural that people want to know the latest (often confused with the best) results, whether they are looking for ways to fine-tune their diets or for that single magic key—the right food or vitamin or supplement—that will open the door to the longest, healthiest possible life. The media are only too happy to cater to this interest and serve up a steady stew of health news.

The problem is that newspapers, television, the Internet, and other news venues often turn the baby steps of scientific research into "major advances," "breakthroughs," and "possible cures" or highlight the confusing contradictions. This makes getting health news seem like reading pages torn at random from a book.

REPLACING EDUCATED GUESSES WITH EVIDENCE

Another reason for the contradictions is that weighty recommendations about diet were often based on thin evidence. The thinking behind these early recommendations was that since people were going to eat no matter what, guidelines based on intelligent guesses were better than no guidelines at all. That's actually a reasonable approach when there isn't much evidence. Unfortunately, these recommendations never carried warning labels like "Educated Guess, Subject to Change," and after being repeated thousands of times they acquired the ring of truth.

When researchers began learning of the dangers of saturated fat, for example, many recommended that people switch from butter, which is high in saturated fat, to low-saturated-fat margarine. This recommendation made sense, even though there were no studies showing that people who ate margarine instead of butter had fewer heart attacks. Then along came studies showing that margarine eaters didn't fare better in the heart-attack department than butter eaters. To a scientist, this is the normal path of scientific progress—a recommendation based on a good guess is tested and toppled by one based on good science. To the rest of the world, though, it is a frustrating contradiction.

The amount and quality of sound scientific information on diet and health have grown enormously over the past twenty years. That makes today's evidence-based recommendations much more certain and much less likely to need radical changes than those made two decades ago. As the quest for new and better knowledge about diet and health continues, rest assured that even today's recommendations will probably be subject to some fine-tuning.

CONTRADICTIONS ARE INEVITABLE

Medical science has its own special rhythm, one that doesn't fit with the media's need to tell compelling but simple stories. Efforts to present "balanced" stories by quoting opposing views can sometimes confuse things even further.

For nutrition research, the rhythm is more a cha-cha—two steps forward and one step back—than a straight-ahead march. If you look at the day-to-day results reported more like sports scores than scientific research, it's easy to wonder why researchers can't get it right the first time.

They can't because these conflicts and contradictions are the way science works. It happens this way in every field, from archaeology to zoology, nuclear physics to nutrition. Men and women carry out studies and report their results.

Evidence accumulates. Like dropping stones onto an old-fashioned scale, the weight of evidence gradually tips the balance in favor of one idea over another. It is only when this happens that you should make changes in your life.

The size of the stone clearly makes a difference. As we describe on pages 30–33, most studies are like sand grains or small pebbles. Very few are like boulders.

WORKING WITH REAL PEOPLE POSES SPECIAL CHALLENGES

Nutrition research seems to generate more than its share of contradictory results. That's partly because the media pay special attention to nutrition (because of the public's interest), while inorganic chemistry, geology, and many other disciplines escape this daily scrutiny. It's also because nutrition scientists usually can't exert the same kind of control over their research subjects as can chemists or zoologists. Instead they must work with unpredictable, independent, mostly uncontrollable subjects—people.

Here are a few of the challenges that face nutrition researchers:

• People don't eat "human chow" meal after meal after meal. Instead diets change from day to day, week to week, and season to season. What you usually eat now is probably a bit (or maybe a lot) different from what you used to eat two years ago or will eat two years from now. These changes are driven by personal taste, cultural changes, improvements in agriculture and technology, and changes in work and family life. They may also be due to disease or aging.

• Many studies depend on people accurately reporting what they eat, a challenging task. (Try remembering exactly what you ate one day last week.) Despite this difficulty, people are fairly accurate about reporting their longer-term eating pattern. But because they aren't perfect, there's almost always some uncertainty in linking diet and disease.

• The foods you eat each day contain thousands of different natural chemicals, some known and well studied, some known and unstudied, many completely unknown and unmeasurable. So far, we've figured out what only a small percentage of them do in the body. Collecting information on others, and discovering how food compounds interact, is an important job for the future.

• Calculating the nutrients a person gets from the foods she or he eats—how much saturated fat, fiber, vitamin E, and so on—is tricky since it depends on sometimes sketchy information about food composition.

• Almost everyone eats some fat, fiber, sugar, starches, fruits, vegetables, vitamins, and so forth. That means nutrition researchers are faced with the more difficult task of measuring *how much* of something is eaten, not just whether it is part of the diet.

• Heart disease, cancer, diabetes, osteoporosis, cataracts, and other chronic diseases almost always develop over many years. They also have other causes beside diet, including genes, physical activity, smoking, stress, and other factors yet to be identified.

DIFFERENT METHODS FOR DIFFERENT PROBLEMS

To get around these problems, nutrition scientists use a variety of research methods.

• *Randomized trials.* The "gold standard" by which other studies are usually judged is the randomized trial. In these carefully controlled studies, half of a group of volunteers is randomly assigned to the experimental diet or treatment, and the other half is assigned to the standard diet or treatment (the control) or possibly to no treatment at all. After a preset time, the number of people in the control group who have developed the predetermined "endpoint"— death, heart attack, broken hip, and so on—is compared with the number in the experimental group.

For example, say you want to know if vitamin C prevents age-related memory loss. You would round up a large group of volunteers, then randomly assign some to take a daily vitamin C tablet while the others take an identical tablet that contains an inactive ingredient that tastes like vitamin C (a placebo). After ten or twenty years, you would compare the percentage of people in the vitamin C group who have experienced memory loss with the percentage in the placebo group.

This kind of study has plenty of advantages. If it is large enough, the randomization process does a good job of making sure the people in the experimental group are very, very similar to those in the control group in terms of age, health, exercise, and other possibly important factors. So the only thing different between the two groups is the diet or treatment. Unfortunately, randomized trials are often impossible to do when it comes to nutrition. Getting people to fix and eat special meals for a long time is difficult. So is getting people to take a vitamin pill or placebo for maybe a decade or more. Given the large number of volunteers needed, the cost of running a randomized trial can be astronomical. The Women's Health Initiative, which is primarily testing the impact of reducing dietary fat to 20 percent of calories and increasing fruits and vegetables on the development of breast cancer, will cost more than $1 billion and still probably won't yield clear answers on this important question.

- *Cohort studies.* The next best method involves following large groups of what epidemiologists call "free-living humans"—regular people like you—for long periods of time. These cohort studies start with a group of people who often have something in common, like an occupation or place of residence. They are asked about their diets, smoking and drinking habits, education, occupation, medical conditions, and other possibly relevant things. The group is then followed for a period of time, ideally a decade or more, either directly with occasional checkups and mailed questionnaires, or by monitoring death certificates. Once the study has gone on long enough, researchers can examine the accumulated information to test a variety of hypotheses. They could, for example, determine if people in the cohort who eat the most fiber have different rates of colon cancer than those who eat the least fiber, or if those who consume the most folate, an important B vitamin, have lower rates of heart disease than those who consume the least folate. Such long-term studies (see "Cohorts" on page 32) have yielded some of the best insights so far into the link between diet and health. By gathering information at the beginning, before specific diseases have occurred, cohort studies avoid the skewed recall sometimes seen among people who develop a particular disease—and who would like to find an explanation for it. Cohort studies such as the Nurses' Health Study, the Health Professionals Follow-up Study, and others use a carefully tested questionnaire to determine what the participants eat and ask them to fill it out several times over the course of the study. This reduces errors and also lets researchers look at changes in diet over time.

- *Case-control studies.* In this type of study, a researcher gathers information from a group of people who have developed a particular disease (the cases) and a similar group of people who are free of that disease (the controls) and compares the two groups for differences in diet, exercise, or whatever variable he or she is interested in. Case-control studies are effective tools when that variable is clear-cut—say, all-or-nothing things like cigarette smoking or occupation. They don't work as well for diet, when only small differences are likely to be seen from person to person. Case-control studies are also more prone to error and bias than cohort studies. Because case-control studies can be done quickly and inexpensively, they supplied the evidence for many of the early recommendations about diet and health. As information emerges from cohort studies, though, we are finding that the conclusions from case-control studies were often off the mark.

- *Metabolic studies.* These are a kind of short-term randomized trial done with volunteers living in special hospital or clinic wards eating specially pre-

Cohorts

EXAMPLES OF LARGE, PROSPECTIVE COHORT STUDIES

More than thirty cohort studies of diet and health are in progress and will produce a flood of data over the next decade. They include the following:

- *Adventist Health Study:* A six-year study of 27,658 male and female California Seventh-Day Adventists, a group chosen because many members of this religion are vegetarians.

- *EPIC Study:* A collaborative study started in 1993 in nine European countries. In all, 440,000 men and women have been enrolled.

- *Health Professionals Follow-up Study:* A study of 51,529 male health professionals (dentists, veterinarians, pharmacists, optometrists, osteopathic physicians, and podiatrists) who were between the ages of forty and seventy-five in 1986. Like the participants of the Nurses' Health Study, these men have been completing health, diet, and lifestyle updates every other year.

- *Honolulu Heart Study:* A study of 8,006 men of Japanese ancestry between the ages of forty-five and sixty-eight who were living on the island of Oahu, Hawaii, between 1965 and 1968—begun to identify the causes of heart disease and stroke.

- *Iowa Women's Health Study:* A study of 41,836 postmenopausal Iowa women who were between the ages of fifty-five and sixty-nine in 1986—designed to examine the effect of several dietary and other lifestyle patterns on the development of cancer.

- *Multiethnic Cohort Study of Diet and Cancer:* An ambitious study begun in 1993 that includes 215,000 men and women representing five different ethnic groups—whites, African Americans, Japanese Americans, Latinos, and Native Hawaiians.

- *Nurses' Health Study:* A study started in 1976 when 121,700 female registered nurses between the ages of thirty and fifty-five returned completed questionnaires about risk factors for cancer and cardiovascular diseases. Since then, the participants have completed follow-up questionnaires every two years to update information on diet and a variety of health risk factors. Another 116,000 younger nurses were enrolled in the study in 1989. In addition, 15,000 of the children of these nurses are taking part in the Growing Up Today Study.

- *Physicians' Health Study:* In 1982, 22,071 male physicians between the ages of forty and eighty-four began taking either aspirin plus a placebo, beta-carotene plus a placebo, both aspirin and beta-carotene, or both placebos. The aspirin part of the trial was stopped early, after the investigators found a 44 percent decrease in heart attacks among the physicians taking aspirin. The beta-carotene arm showed that this antioxidant had neither benefit nor harm. The Physicians' Health Study has evolved into a cohort study as the physicians continue to answer questionnaires on their habits and health.

pared meals. The controlled conditions make it possible to see how different foods or nutrients affect changes in blood cholesterol or other biochemical markers, but they are too small and don't go on long enough to measure the effect on health. Nor can they measure how real diets affect people living in the far messier and less controlled real world.

DECIPHERING MEDICAL NEWS

Careful journalists try to put new research into perspective. But it's impossible to cram that kind of context into thirty seconds of airtime or 250 words, so you often end up with little more than sound bites or headlines. Other than mastering the fine points of nutrition research, here are a few tips that can help you know what is worth paying attention to:

- *Studies done on people.* How foods, nutrients, and even food additives affect mice, dogs, and monkeys is an important thread in the fabric of nutrition research. But they may have completely different effects on people. Animal studies can pave the way for future research but are rarely the basis for changing one's diet.

- *Studies done in the real world.* Diet studies done in hospitals or special research centers have given us important information on how the body responds to different nutrients and foods. But because they don't look directly at disease risk (only intermediate markers of disease), they can't predict the consequences of different eating habits or strategies on what ultimately matters—your health.

- *Studies that look at real disease endpoints.* Because it takes so long for chronic diseases to develop, many studies use intermediate markers like narrowing of the heart's arteries or changes in bone density as a stand-in for the real disease. These changes don't necessarily translate into real diseases, though. Pay more attention to research that has looked at real health problems like broken bones or heart attacks.

- *Large studies.* In science, the play of chance is a real problem. The larger the study, the smaller the possibility that potentially important differences between two groups can be explained by chance alone. Larger studies are also more likely to spot important connections that would be missed in smaller ones.

- *Consistency of the evidence.* The most persuasive evidence that an effect is real is consistent results from a number of studies done by different researchers at different times, using different methods, and involving different groups of people. A good example of consistent evidence is the link between moderate alcohol use and reduced risk of heart disease. That alcohol may have beneficial effects on the heart has been suspected for more than two thousand years. More than two hundred years ago, William Heberden, the British physician who first described the chest pain known today as angina, wrote that "wine and spiritous liquors—afford considerable relief from angina." Sporadic reports appeared throughout the twentieth century suggesting that drinking alcohol prevented clogged arteries, but so too did reports of the detrimental effects of heavy drinking. Since 1974, though, several dozen case-control and cohort studies from different geographic regions have shown that people who have one or two alcoholic drinks a day are less likely to have a heart attack or die from heart disease than nondrinkers or heavy drinkers. This relation persists even after the results are statistically adjusted for smoking, exercise, and other variables that could differ between drinkers and nondrinkers. These observations have been further bolstered by evidence from laboratory, animal, and metabolic studies showing that alcohol increases levels of HDL (good) cholesterol and also makes blood less likely to clot, both of which would be expected to protect against heart disease. This body of evidence lets us make a firm conclusion that drinking moderate amounts of alcohol reduces the risk of heart disease. (Of course, decisions about drinking should take into account alcohol's full range of risks and benefits. See chapter 8.)

I suggest that you not make big changes in what or how you eat based on a single study. If a result is on the right track, other studies will show the same thing. And it won't matter much in the long run whether you make a change today (like taking a vitamin or increasing the amount of monounsaturated fat in your diet) or six months from now.

In fact, Mark Twain's cynical, laconic view of health information is as good today as it was one hundred years ago: "Be careful about reading health books. You may die of a misprint."

CHAPTER THREE

Healthy Weight

[handwritten annotation: × MEASURE OF = FUTURE HEALTH ×]

M Y AIM IN THIS BOOK is to offer straightforward, no-nonsense advice on nutrition based on the best information available. I'll start right here: If your weight is in the "healthy" range, keep it there. If you are overweight, do your best to avoid adding any more pounds and lose some if you can. This isn't a new idea, it isn't sexy, and it certainly won't land me a spot as the next fad diet guru on *The Oprah Winfrey Show.* But next to whether you smoke, the number that stares up at you from the bathroom scale is the most important measure of your future health. Keeping that number in the healthy range is more important for long-term health than the types and amounts of antioxidants in your food or the exact ratio of fats to carbohydrates. So this chapter will focus mostly on the *amount* of food you eat rather than the type of food. In the rest of the book I will explain what foods to choose for maximum health.

Weight sits like a spider at the center of an intricate, tangled web of health and disease. Three related aspects of weight—how much you weigh in relation to your height, your waist size, and how much weight you gain after your early twenties—strongly influence your chances of having or dying from a heart attack, stroke, or other type of cardiovascular disease; of developing high blood pressure, high cholesterol, or diabetes; of being diagnosed with postmenopausal breast cancer or cancer of the endometrium, colon, or kidney; of having arthritis; of being infertile or having trouble getting an erection; of developing gallstones; of snoring or suffering from sleep apnea; or of developing adult-onset asthma. As shown in Figure 4, weight is directly linked with a variety of diseases in the Nurses' Health Study. With increasing body mass index—more about that later—the risks of heart disease, high blood pressure, gallstones, and type 2 diabetes all steadily increase, even among those in the healthy weight category. Above a body mass index of 30, which is the boundary between overweight and obesity, the risks continue to increase. Similar trends are seen among men in the Health Professionals Follow-up Study.

Given the importance of weight in staying healthy, no mention of weight in the USDA Food Guide Pyramid for a decade has been a serious omission.

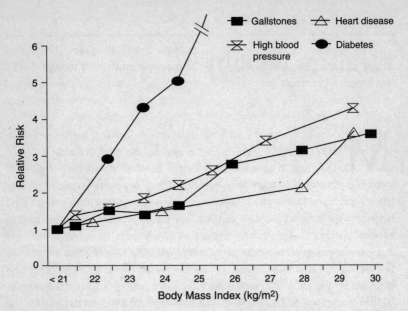

FIG. 4 Weight and Disease. Among women in the Nurses' Health Study, the chances of developing any of four common conditions increases with increasing body mass index.

What's more, weight recommendations in the current Dietary Guidelines for Americans are set too high for many people and may mislead some into thinking that substantial weight gains within the "healthy" weight categories are perfectly fine (see page 39).

THE OBESITY EPIDEMIC

Excess weight is a very personal problem. It shapes how you feel about yourself and how others treat you. It has a direct impact on your current and future health. It costs you (or at least your health insurance company) tens of thousands of dollars more in medical costs over the years. Excess weight is also a major public health problem. If current trends continue, we could call the first decade of the new millennium the obesity decade. Since the early 1960s, the proportion of Americans who are moderately overweight has stayed the same, hovering just over 30 percent. What has changed dramatically, though, is the number who are obese. About one-third of Americans now fall into this category, more than double the proportion from the early 1960s. Obesity among children is also on the rise, an alarming trend given that early obesity leads to diabetes and cardiovascular disease at a young age. As a nation, we spend more than $90 billion a year on medical care for obesity and its complications.

The situation isn't much better elsewhere around the globe. The World Health Organization calls obesity a worldwide epidemic. And though deadly famines and starvation make headlines, overweight, obesity, and their health consequences have begun replacing undernutrition and infection as the main causes of early death and disability in many developing countries.

WHAT IS A HEALTHY WEIGHT?

What seems to be a simple question turns out to be remarkably difficult to answer. Part of the problem is that a weight that may be perfectly fine for someone who is six feet one—say, 175 pounds—is way too much for someone who is five feet one. Another part is lingering confusion from the way healthy weights have been defined in the past.

A number called the body mass index, or Quetelet index, gets around the first problem. This measure of weight adjusted for height does a good job of accounting for the fact that taller people tend to weigh more than shorter people. If you like math, you can calculate your body mass index, or BMI, like this: Divide your weight in pounds by your height in inches; divide that number by your height in inches; and multiply that number by 703. You can also just look it up in the table on page 38 or have it calculated for you by any number of online BMI calculators, such as the one on the Harvard Health Publications Web site (www.health.harvard.edu/EDBH).

Setting guidelines for healthy BMIs has traditionally been done by examining death rates in large groups of people and then picking those BMIs with the lowest death rates as the "healthy range." This usually gives a U-shaped curve with increasing death rates on either side of some minimum. These curves imply that weighing too little is just as unhealthy as weighing too much.

There's certainly no argument about the too-much-weight side. Countless studies, one of which includes more than a million adults, have shown that BMIs above 25 increase the risk of dying early, mainly from heart disease and cancer. There is widespread agreement that BMIs from 25 up to 30 should be considered overweight and over 30 obese. It's the too-little-weight side of the curve, however, that has caused confusion.

CAN YOU BE TOO THIN?

Some experts have said the curves mean exactly what they show, that weighing too little also increases the risk of dying early. Others, including me, believe that

Body Mass Index Chart

Height (inches)	19	20	21	22	23	24	25	26	27	28	29	30	31	32	33	34	35
								Body Weight (pounds)									
58	91	96	100	105	110	115	119	124	129	134	138	143	148	153	158	162	167
59	94	99	104	109	114	119	124	128	133	138	143	148	153	158	163	168	173
60	97	102	107	112	118	123	128	133	138	143	148	153	158	163	168	174	179
61	100	106	111	116	122	127	132	137	143	148	153	158	164	169	174	180	185
62	104	109	115	120	126	131	136	142	147	153	158	164	169	175	180	186	191
63	107	113	118	124	130	135	141	146	152	158	163	169	175	180	186	191	197
64	110	116	122	128	134	140	145	151	157	163	169	174	180	186	192	197	204
65	114	120	126	132	138	144	150	156	162	168	174	180	186	192	198	204	210
66	118	124	130	136	142	148	155	161	167	173	179	186	192	198	204	210	216
67	121	127	134	140	146	153	159	166	172	178	185	191	198	204	211	217	223
68	125	131	138	144	151	158	164	171	177	184	190	197	203	210	216	223	230
69	128	135	142	149	155	162	169	176	182	189	196	203	209	216	223	230	236
70	132	139	146	153	160	167	174	181	188	195	202	209	216	222	229	236	243
71	136	143	150	157	165	172	179	186	193	200	208	215	222	229	236	243	250
72	140	147	154	162	169	177	184	191	199	206	213	221	228	235	242	250	258
73	144	151	159	166	174	182	189	197	204	212	219	227	235	242	250	257	265
74	148	155	163	171	179	186	194	202	210	218	225	233	241	249	256	264	272
75	152	160	168	176	184	192	200	208	216	224	232	240	248	256	264	272	279
76	156	164	172	180	189	197	205	213	221	230	238	246	254	263	271	279	287

Body Mass Index Chart

Height (inches)	36	37	38	39	40	41	42	43	44	45	46	47	48	49	50	51	52	53	54
									Body Weight (pounds)										
58	172	177	181	186	191	196	201	205	210	215	220	224	229	234	239	244	248	253	258
59	178	183	188	193	198	203	208	212	217	222	227	232	237	242	247	252	257	262	267
60	184	189	194	199	204	209	215	220	225	230	235	240	245	250	255	261	266	271	276
61	190	195	201	206	211	217	222	227	232	238	243	248	254	259	264	269	275	280	285
62	196	202	207	213	218	224	229	235	240	246	251	256	262	267	273	278	284	289	295
63	203	208	214	220	225	231	237	242	248	254	259	265	270	278	282	287	293	299	304
64	209	215	221	227	232	238	244	250	256	262	267	273	279	285	291	296	302	308	314
65	216	222	228	234	240	246	252	258	264	270	276	282	288	294	300	306	312	318	324
66	223	229	235	241	247	253	260	266	272	278	284	291	297	303	309	315	322	328	334
67	230	236	242	249	255	261	268	274	280	287	293	299	306	312	319	325	331	338	344
68	236	243	249	256	262	269	276	282	289	295	302	308	315	322	328	335	341	348	354
69	243	250	257	263	270	277	284	291	297	304	311	318	324	331	338	345	351	358	365
70	250	257	264	271	278	285	292	299	306	313	320	327	334	341	348	355	362	369	376
71	257	265	272	279	286	293	301	308	315	322	329	338	343	351	358	365	372	379	386
72	265	272	279	287	294	302	309	316	324	331	338	346	353	361	368	375	383	390	397
73	272	280	288	295	302	310	318	325	333	340	348	355	363	371	378	386	393	401	408
74	280	287	295	303	311	319	326	334	342	350	358	365	373	381	389	396	404	412	420
75	287	295	303	311	319	327	335	343	351	359	367	375	383	391	399	407	415	423	431
76	295	304	312	320	328	336	344	353	361	369	377	385	394	402	410	418	426	435	443

FIG. 5 BMI Tables. To use these tables, find your height in the left-hand column. Move across to a given weight. The number at the top of the column is your BMI.

such a simple cause-and-effect explanation is misleading. Here's why: Cigarette smokers tend to be leaner than nonsmokers, in part because smoking blunts the appetite. Because smoking is such a powerful risk factor for death, this will tend to make being lean look unhealthy. Also, in any large population, the leanest people are a mix of those with illnesses that are often accompanied by weight loss (such as cancer, heart disease, and emphysema) and a relatively small number of people who have managed to strike a long-term, low-weight balance between the number of calories they take in and the number they burn. In other words, low weights don't necessarily *cause* premature death but are instead often the *result* of diagnosed and undiagnosed illnesses that may be fatal.

One way of sidestepping these limitations involves looking only at nonsmokers and then ignoring in the data crunching any deaths that occur during the first few years of follow-up. A ten-year American Cancer Society study of more than three hundred thousand initially healthy men and women took this approach. The result was a straight-line connection between body mass index and death—death rates steadily declined with lower BMIs. A similar trend has been seen in the Nurses' Health Study—among nonsmokers, those with stable weights and BMIs as low as 17 (someone who is five feet five and weighs one hundred pounds) died at slightly lower rates than women with BMIs between 21 and 25. Using another approach, my colleagues and I looked at a large group of men by both BMI and level of physical activity. In the low BMI group, it was only those who were inactive, probably owing to a chronic illness, who had higher death rates. The physically active men with low BMIs had low death rates.

CURRENT WEIGHT GUIDELINES CAN BE TOO GENEROUS

In the Dietary Guidelines for Americans, healthy weights are those corresponding to BMIs between 18.5 and 25. BMIs above 25 are clearly labeled as unhealthy, but the guidelines dodge the issue of setting a lower healthy limit by not putting any label on BMIs below 18.5. (See Figure 6.)

In choosing these limits, the committee charged with setting the guidelines tried to balance scientific evidence with public policy and perception. That's a difficult job, because there is no simple breakpoint between healthy and unhealthy weights. Panel members agreed that the risk of heart disease, diabetes, and high blood pressure begins to climb at BMIs of 22 or so. But they didn't feel justified choosing such a low number as the cutoff between healthy and unhealthy weights, because doing so would have labeled a large majority of the U.S. population as overweight. Instead they chose a BMI of 25 as the upper bound of healthy weights, based on clear evidence that the risk of dying

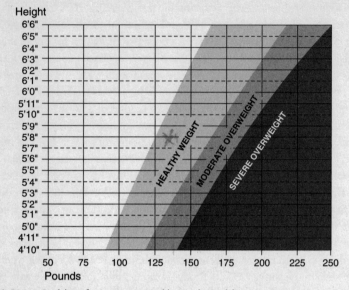

FIG. 6 Dietary Guidelines for Americans: Healthy Weight Guidelines

prematurely increases above that point. Thus almost everyone with a BMI over 25—except for extremely muscular body builders—would be healthier with a lower BMI, but many people with a BMI of 23–25 are not at their healthiest weight. Still, drawing the line at 25 means that two-thirds of adult Americans are overweight or obese.

Another problem with defining a range of BMIs from 18.5 to 25 as healthy is that this "allows" you to gain a fair amount of weight and still stay in the healthy range. For example, a woman who is five feet six and weighs 130 pounds (BMI of 21) could gain twenty-five pounds and still be in the healthy range (BMI of 25), whereas this much added weight poses clear health risks.

KEEP YOUR BMI LOW

The bottom line on healthy weight is this: If your weight corresponds with a BMI below 25, do everything you can to keep it there. More specifically, try to keep from gaining weight, even if you could add some pounds and still stay within the healthy BMI range. If your weight corresponds to a BMI above 25, you will do yourself a huge health favor by keeping it from getting larger and, if possible, by trying to bring it down. If you inhabit the low end of the BMI curve and your weight hasn't changed, great. But if you've been watching your weight slip downward and you aren't dieting or trying to lose weight, check with your physician to pin down why this is happening.

THE COLLEGE WEIGHT SCALE

If you could travel back in time and stand next to your twenty-year-old self, how would you measure up? Older and wiser, to be sure. But how about around the waist or on the bathroom scale? It's not an idle question—how much your weight and your waist have changed since your early twenties has a major bearing on your chances of staying healthy or developing a chronic disease.

Adding a few pounds here, a few there, during adulthood seems innocuous enough. It has its own catchy moniker—middle-age spread—and was once considered a sign of prosperity and success. It also seems to be an inevitable part of aging, affecting most Americans. In reality, adult weight gain is neither inevitable nor innocuous. In many cultures, gaining weight during adulthood just isn't the norm. In Japan, for example, men and women—especially women—tend to stay the same weight throughout their adult years. On a trip through Japan, I asked what would happen if a Japanese woman gained weight as she got older. The answer was a shocked "That would be one of the worst possible things for her." Even in the United States, we are beginning to see clear cultural differences in weight gain. The more education people have, the less likely they are to be overweight or obese.

Gaining more than a few pounds after your early twenties can nudge you down the path toward chronic disease. The more weight, the harder the push. In two long-term Harvard studies, the Nurses' Health Study and the Health Professionals Follow-up Study, middle-aged men and women who had gained between eleven and twenty-two pounds after age twenty were up to three times as likely to develop heart disease, high blood pressure, type 2 diabetes, and gallstones as their counterparts who gained five pounds or less. Larger weight gains meant even higher chances of developing these diseases.

These studies and others point to one of the big problems with the "healthy range" for weight and BMIs. Someone who was lean at age twenty—say, with a BMI of 19—can gain more than twenty-five pounds and still stay in the healthy range, even though this weight gain has serious health consequences.

WHY WE GAIN WEIGHT

Your weight depends on a simple but easily unbalanced equation: Weight change equals calories in minus calories out. Burn as many calories as you take in and your weight won't change. Take in more than you burn and your weight increases. Dieting explores the other end of the spectrum—consuming fewer calories than you burn.

Chalk up *why* you're the weight you are to a combination of what and how much you eat, your genes, your lifestyle, and your culture.

• *Your diet.* What and how much you eat affects your weight. I will talk about this in the rest of the book.

• *Genes.* Your parents are partly to thank, or to blame, for your weight and the shape of your body. Studies of twins raised apart show that genes have a strong influence on gaining weight or being overweight, meaning that some people are genetically predisposed to gaining weight. Heredity plays a role in the tendency to store fat around the chest and waist. It is also possible that some people are more sensitive to calories from fat or carbohydrates than others, though the evidence for this is still thin. I must stress the phrase *partly to blame,* though, because genetic influences can't explain the rapid increase in obesity seen in the United States over the last thirty years or the big differences in obesity rates among countries.

It's possible that our prehistoric ancestors shaped our physiological and behavioral responses to food. Early humans routinely coped with feast-or-famine conditions. Since it was impossible to predict when the next good meal might appear—like a ripe patch of berries or a catchable antelope—eating as much as possible whenever food was available may have been a key to surviving the lean times. This survival adaptation means that complex chemical interactions between body and mind that evolved aeons ago in response to routine periods of starvation may drive us to eat whenever possible. In this era of plenty, that means all the time.

• *Lifestyle.* If eating represents the pleasurable, sensuous side of the weight change equation, then metabolism and physical activity are its nose-to-the-grindstone counterparts. Your resting (basal) metabolism is the energy needed just to breathe, pump and circulate blood, send messages from brain to body, maintain your temperature, digest food, and keep the right amount of tension in your muscles. It typically accounts for 60 to 70 percent of your daily energy expenditure. Physical activity makes up most of the rest. If you work a desk job and do little more than walk from your car to your office and back again, you may burn ridiculously few calories a day.

• *Culture.* Ours is a culture of living large, of Texas-size appetites where quantity often edges out quality. Indulgence is tolerated, even revered. Love is food, and food is love—just imagine your grandmother urging you to have another helping or the pleasurable groans and belt loosening that end many holiday and regular meals. These are not universal tendencies. In France and throughout much of Asia, the cuisine emphasizes quality and presentation, not how much food can be crammed on a plate. People in many cultures also believe it is inappropriate or downright rude to eat until you are full, and teach their children to eat to 70 percent of capacity.

On top of that, we have what I call the overproduction problem. U.S. farmers produce 3,800 calories' worth of food a day for every man, woman, and child in America. That's nearly double what the average person needs. The almost inevitable consequence of this surfeit is a system that encourages full-tilt consumption: Producers and food manufacturers want us to eat more of their products, and they are competing with one another to exploit our weaknesses. The food industry spends tens of billions of dollars a year learning the best ways to entice us and then acting on that knowledge. The keen senses we have inherited for salt and sweetness that were once needed for survival (our taste for sweet things, for example, helped early humans sort through leaves to find the tender young ones with a ready supply of energy) are continually exploited. The sugar and salt content of products have been ratcheted up to increase our expectations for sweetness and saltiness and get us to eat, and buy, more. What's more, food is sold everywhere—gas stations sell doughnuts and sandwiches, bookstores and department stores offer coffee and sweets, and you can get full, belly-busting meals at baseball and other sporting events. Restaurants have also gotten into the act. The modest portions of nouvelle cuisine have been overshadowed by supersizing, and it isn't uncommon to be served a meal that contains 1,500 to 2,000 calories, about what you need for an entire day.

This incredible access to food and the nearly unlimited variety of food tests the willpower of even the most sensible eater. When combined with too little physical activity, it's a sure recipe for weight gain. And because weight control is the single most important factor in your good health (after not smoking), overeating can pose serious health risks.

APPLES AND PEARS

Some people store much of their fat around the waist and chest, others store it around the hips and thighs. These two different body shapes have been dubbed apple and pear. Magazine articles and Web sites make a big fuss out of these arbitrary categories, and several Web sites use your waist and hip measurements to calculate your waist-to-hip ratio, then use it as a key point in determining your health profile and risk of developing heart disease.

Fat that accumulates around the waist and chest (technically called abdominal adiposity) may pose more of a health problem than fat around the hips and thighs. Abdominal fat has been linked with high blood pressure, high cholesterol, high blood sugar, and heart disease. It is possible that this fat is metabolically more active than fat stored elsewhere. It is also possible that it isn't any worse than other kinds of fat but instead is a way of telling us about overall fatness that weight and height alone can't describe.

Where, exactly, is your waist? For clothing designers, it's the narrowest part of the torso. For scientists studying the health effects of body fat, it's the region near the navel, where fat is typically deposited. In large standardized health surveys, such as the ongoing National Health and Nutrition Examination Survey, researchers use a two-step process to measure a volunteer's waist: One, gently press the right hipbone to find its high point. Two, place the tape measure just above that point and extend the tape around the abdomen, *keeping it parallel to the floor.* (See Figure 7.) For most people, the top of the hipbone is generally in line with the navel. Others may need to pull the tape down a bit to the top of the hipbone.

The waist measure can be useful because many people—particularly men—find themselves converting their muscle to abdominal fat as they go through midlife. Even though weight may remain stable, an expanding waistline can be a warning sign of trouble on the horizon. So use your waist as a kind of low-tech biofeedback device—a waistwise expansion of two or three

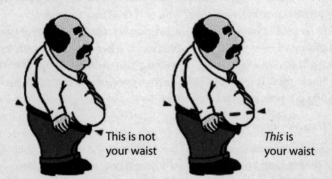

This is not
your waist

This is
your waist

FIG. 7 Measuring Your Waist. To measure your waist, wrap a flexible measuring tape around your midsection where the sides of your waist are narrowest. This is usually even with the navel. Make sure you keep the tape parallel to the floor.

inches over the years should trigger a warning that you need to reevaluate your diet and physical activity level.

Some researchers advocate calculating a waist-hip ratio (dividing the size of your waist by the size of your hips). Simply measuring your waist is probably just as useful. Many studies have shown that this single number is just as powerful at gauging the chances of developing chronic disease as the waist-to-hip ratio. It's also a lot easier to do.

A CALORIE IS A CALORIE IS A CALORIE

We eat food for two physiologic reasons, energy and chemical building blocks. The amount of energy a particular food can deliver to mitochondria—the tiny engines that power your cells—is measured in calories. Technically, a food calorie is the amount of heat needed to raise the temperature of a liter of water (just over a quart) from 14.5° C to 15.5° C. Practically, a food calorie is the amount of energy a 150-pound person burns each minute while sleeping.

If you read diet books or keep up with health and nutrition news, you've probably heard a lot about "fat calories" or "carbohydrate calories." The idea that fat calories are different from carbohydrate calories came from studies done under extreme conditions, such as consuming pure carbohydrate, protein, or fat. In these situations, the body converts dietary fat to body fat a bit more efficiently than it does carbohydrate or protein.

In a normal diet, though, your body converts all three to fat at the same rate. Like a kiss or a rose, a calorie is a calorie. So five hundred calories from ice cream, five hundred from red meat, and five hundred from pasta will have similar effects on your weight.

This calorie blindness is the result of a neat solution to a vexing problem faced by some of earth's early inhabitants—how to run a body on different fuels. Instead of having completely different intracellular systems for fats, carbohydrates, protein, and alcohol, the cells in your body use the same energy source. Much of what you eat is (or can be if needed) converted to the energy coin of the realm, a six-carbon sugar called glucose. When you eat, some of the glucose dumped into your bloodstream is used immediately by your cells. Some is linked into long chains, called glycogen, and stored in your muscles and liver. Any leftovers are converted to fat and squirreled away in special fat storage cells and padded in between muscles. If glucose is like cash in your pocket, ready to be spent when needed, glycogen is money in the bank, available with a bit of effort, and fat is money tied up in stocks or mutual funds.

Does Fiddling with the Form of Calories Help You Lose Weight?

Almost any kind of diet can lead to weight loss, at least for a few months. Some of the most absurd diets ever published have their champions who will testify, complete with eight-by-ten glossy color photographs, that the diet helped them lose weight. That's because even the oddest diet makes people pay attention to how much they are eating, rather than eating willy-nilly throughout the day. This mindfulness is often enough to limit daily calories, the single most important key to controlling weight. It is aided and abetted by the monotony imposed by many of these diets and their inability to please the palate. Most fad diets fail in the long run. For that matter, so do most middle-of-the-road, commonsense diets.

Diets usually vary in the way they deliver calories. Although a calorie is a calorie, how you get yours *may* make a difference in limiting your daily intake. The ultimate diet would be one that offers meals and snacks that rapidly lead to feeling pleasantly full (technically called satiety), delay the return of hunger pangs (technically called satiation), are pleasing and satisfying, meet the body's needs for energy and nutrients, and work to prevent chronic disease. That's a tall order. Countless books have been written claiming they'll give you all or part of this dietary nirvana. Most promise far more than they deliver.

Diets usually fiddle with the form of calories by focusing on one particular dietary villain or hero. The most common include low-fat, low-carbohydrate/high-protein, the glycemic index, and energy-density strategies.

LOW-FAT DIETS AREN'T THE ANSWER

A common, though incorrect, thread that runs through many diets is the idea that fat in food makes fat in the body. Limit "fat calories," so the thinking goes, and you'll be able to control your weight. Although there's a pleasant symmetry to the logic, and although many dietary guidelines focus on reducing dietary fat, there's no good evidence linking dietary fat with excess weight. In fact, there's plenty of evidence showing that the percentage of calories from fat has little to do with excess weight. That's why the Healthy Eating Pyramid doesn't ban fats across the board. Instead, it treats fats as one of the most important nutritional factors in your diet. What fats to choose and how much to eat are discussed in chapter 4.

To be sure, some countries with high fat intake have many overweight people. In the United States, for example, the average person gets about one-third of his or her daily calories from fat (a relatively high percentage), and almost two-thirds of the population is overweight. But in some parts of South Africa, where 60 percent of people are overweight, fat contributes barely one-quarter of calories.

I am not trying to absolve dietary fat or downplay its contributions to weight or weight gain. Dietary fat has an impact on energy, fat stores, and weight. But if you balance the number of calories you eat with the number of calories you burn, especially if part of the burn comes from exercise, then you won't gain weight on a diet that has 35 or even 40 percent of calories from fat. And if you are eating the right kinds of fat, you will help protect yourself from heart disease and other chronic conditions. (See chapter 4.)

LOW-CARBOHYDRATE DIETS MAY HELP

For almost thirty years, mainstream nutrition experts dismissed Dr. Robert Atkins's carbohydrate-shunning diets as an unhealthy fad. How in the world could a high-protein, high-fat, low-carbohydrate diet help with weight loss, the medical establishment reasoned, when everyone knew that *fat* was the dietary demon? Now that the Atkins diet is getting its day in court—the court of careful scientific testing—the good doctor appears to have been about half-right.

Limiting carbs and loading up on meat, cheese, and eggs gives the digestive system more work to do, and this may help you feel full longer. And by smoothing out the blood sugar/insulin roller coaster (see "Why Carbohydrates Matter" in chapter 5), it may stretch the time between hunger pangs. But eating unlimited amounts of beef, sausage, butter, and cheese—as promoted by the original Atkins diet—is a bad idea for overall optimal health. There are healthier ways to cut back on carbs. Following the Healthy Eating Pyramid and eating more fish, poultry, beans, nuts, fruits and vegetables, whole grains, and vegetable oils can work for weight control even as it reduces the risks of heart disease, diabetes, and several cancers. Even Atkins seems to have been heading in that direction before his untimely death in 2003, as his final book had shifted toward this version of a low-carbohydrate diet.

LOW-ENERGY-DENSITY DIETS MAY BE CONFUSING

When it comes to gaining or losing weight, is there any difference between eating a baked potato or a cookie that delivers the same number of calories? Several popular diet books say there is. They focus on energy density (sometimes called caloric density) as a key to controlling weight. The thinking here is that foods that deliver relatively few calories per bite, like soup or baked squash, fill you up faster than foods that pack more calories per bite, like meat or nuts. The faster you feel full with fewer calories, so the thinking goes, the less you will eat.

Calculating energy density is simple. You divide the number of calories in a particular food by its weight in ounces or grams. Apples, potatoes, cooked rice, and lettuce have low energy densities, largely because they are mostly water. Nuts, bagels, and cookies have high energy densities.

If people eat similar weights or volumes of food, no matter what the energy density, reducing the energy density decreases calorie intake. Pure fat has a relatively high energy density (nine calories per gram) compared with pure protein and carbohydrate (four calories per gram). Short-term successes with the energy density approach to weight loss have been used to champion the importance of low-fat diets. But we don't eat pure carbohydrates or pure fats—we eat mixtures of these. A salad with oil-and-vinegar dressing, or roasted vegetables sprinkled with olive oil, have low energy densities but high percentages of calories from fat. Likewise, many fat-free products have the same energy densities as their full-fat versions because the fat has been replaced with highly refined carbohydrates.

LOW-GLYCEMIC DIETS MAY BE PART OF THE ANSWER

When you eat carbohydrates, your blood sugar rises. How much it rises depends on what you eat, how much you eat, and how much insulin your body produces in response to sugar loads. White bread, cornflakes, and other highly processed carbohydrates trigger large, rapid increases in blood sugar (glucose), while whole grains, beans, and most fruits and vegetables generate smaller, slower increases. (See chapter 5.) Easily digested foods that cause sharp spikes in blood sugar also stimulate a matching production of insulin, leading to rapid removal of glucose from the blood. The sudden drop in glucose, along with other hormonal changes, generates new hunger signals.

In an elegant study involving a dozen overweight boys at Children's Hospital in Boston, those who ate specially prepared breakfasts enriched with easily digested carbohydrates snacked almost twice as much during the morning as those who ate breakfasts containing the same number of calories but fewer rapidly digested carbohydrates.

The glycemic index and glycemic load (see page 106) are measures of how different foods affect your blood sugar levels. People with diabetes have been using the glycemic index for years to plan meals and snacks that cause the smallest possible increases in blood sugar. Lately, though, these have become popular dieting tools. Both offer useful guides for choosing carbohydrates. Yet it isn't necessary to religiously follow the tables in planning meals or snacks. There are simpler rules of thumb: avoid highly processed sources of carbohydrates such as white rice and breads, pastries, and cereals made with white flour and include more whole-grain foods, fruits, vegetables, and beans.

THE HEALTHY EATING PYRAMID AIDS WEIGHT LOSS

Healthy eating (in moderation, of course) should be as good for losing and maintaining weight as it is for long-term health. Some solid research supports this idea.

One of the few studies to show a sustained weight loss was conducted by Kathy McManus and her colleagues at Harvard-affiliated Brigham and Women's Hospital. They randomly assigned 101 overweight volunteers to either a low-fat (20 percent fat) or a moderate-fat diet (35 percent), consistent with the Healthy Eating Pyramid. It included an abundance of vegetables, nuts, and whole grains flavored richly with herbs and olive oil. At six months, both groups had similar and impressive weight loss. After that, though, volunteers in the low-fat group began regaining weight, and most dropped out of the study. Those who stuck with the low-fat diet regained most of their weight by 18 months. In contrast, those following the moderate-fat diet based on the Healthy Eating Pyramid kept off the pounds they had shed. At 18 months, more than half were still sticking with the diet, and many maintained their weight loss even on to 30 months.

One reason this eating plan led to successful and long-term weight loss is that the participants reported being quite satisfied with the variety and flavors of their new way of eating and did not feel deprived.

THREE STEPS TO WEIGHT CONTROL

Given how easy it is to gain weight, and the food temptations that bombard us, how can you avoid gaining weight or lose it if you need to? I suggest a three-pronged strategy:

1. If you aren't physically active, get moving. If you are, try to increase the level of your activity.

2. Find an eating program that works for you. The strategies offered in this book are a place to start.

3. Become a defensive eater.

I wish I could give you a more precise set of instructions guaranteed to control weight. But I can't. Chalk that up to the wonderful diversity of the human race. People are as unique as snowflakes. They come in different sizes and shapes, have different metabolisms, like and dislike different tastes and textures. So no single formula can apply to everyone. You need to find what works for you and stick with it, using a scale and your waist size as guides.

What I *can* do is suggest different strategies that have worked for others and may work for you.

1. GET MOVING

• *Exercise counts most toward good health.* Although I have focused on the intake side of the energy balance equation so far, the expenditure side is critically important. After not smoking, exercise is the single best thing you can do to get healthy or stay healthy and keep chronic diseases at bay. Exercise is far more than merely a way to lose or control weight. A report by the U.S. Surgeon General, *Physical Activity and Health,* says that regular physical activity

- improves your chances of living longer and living healthier;
- helps protect you from developing heart disease or its handmaidens, high blood pressure and high cholesterol;
- helps protect you from developing certain cancers, including colon and breast cancer;
- helps prevent type 2 diabetes;
- helps prevent arthritis and may help relieve pain and stiffness in people with this condition;
- helps prevent the insidious bone loss known as osteoporosis;
- reduces the risk of falling among older adults;
- relieves symptoms of depression and anxiety and improves mood;
- helps prevent impotence; and
- controls weight.

• *Build muscle, burn fat.* Physical activity is essential to weight control for two main reasons: It burns calories that would otherwise end up stored in fat. And it builds muscle, or at least maintains muscle, an often ignored but absolutely essential ingredient in weight control.

Even when you are sleeping, your muscles are constantly using energy. When you walk, run, swim, lift weights, dance, play tennis, clean the house, or do anything active, they burn even more calories. Physical activity stimulates muscle cells to grow and divide, causing muscles to grow in strength and size. The more muscle you have, the more calories you burn, even at rest.

• *Without exercise, fat replaces muscle.* If you live a sedentary life, your muscles gradually waste away. It's the same kind of atrophy that occurs when you wear a cast on an arm or leg, only stretched out over years rather than weeks so it's impossible to feel or see. The less muscle you have, the less energy your body uses at rest and the easier it is to gain weight. To make matters worse, lost muscle is usually replaced by fat (see Figure 8). This starts a vicious and tough-to-break cycle. For a fifty-year-old person who isn't physically active, a ten-pound weight gain over the years may really mean a loss of five pounds of muscle and gain of fifteen pounds of fat. Unlike muscle, fat uses very little glucose and burns few calories. As the balance between muscle and fat shifts further and further in favor of fat, resting metabolism decelerates even more. And as the body needs less and less energy to take care of its basic needs, more and

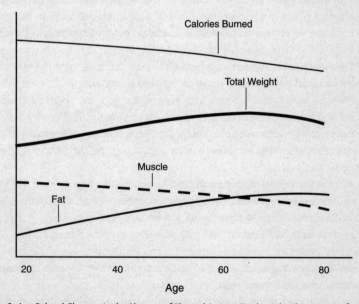

FIG. 8 Age-Related Changes in the Absence of Physical Activity. Total weight, the amount of muscle and fat, and the number of calories the body burns at rest tend to change with age (assuming no increase in physical activity). Muscle mass declines, owing to decreased production of sex and growth hormones. Less muscle mass means the body uses less energy at rest and accumulates more fat. An increase in physical activity can break this vicious cycle.

more food goes into fat stores. The extra weight may also act as a physical or mental impediment to activity, which further reduces resting metabolism. In other words, the shift from muscle to fat makes it easier to gain weight, makes it harder to maintain your weight, and increases your risk of heart disease and diabetes.

Not long ago, a colleague of mine saw her physician for one of those "big birthday" physical exams. Everything was fine, with one exception—her blood pressure was too high. When her doctor told her she needed to lose thirty pounds or so to get her pressure under control, she shot back, "Where were you when I was putting on those pounds?" It's a great question. The physical and physiological changes wrought by decreased muscle mass and increased weight are tough to reverse and in some cases may be irreversible.

• *Ounces of prevention are better than pounds of cure.* Over the last few decades, we've been learning that it is far easier to *prevent* weight gain than it is to lose excess weight. In fact, gaining weight makes your body more receptive to future weight gain and makes getting rid of extra pounds doubly difficult. To make matters worse, some of the effects of excess weight, such as diabetes, heart disease, or stroke, may not fully disappear even with successful weight loss.

The two big questions concerning exercise are these: What is the best kind of exercise? And how much exercise do we need each day?

• *Walk for health.* Not too long ago, experts thought that vigorous exercise was needed to keep the heart and circulatory system in shape. Recent research has tempered that idea. We are learning that brisk walking offers many of the same benefits as sweating it out in a noisy gym or jogging through your neighborhood.

Among women participating in the Nurses' Health Study, there is a very strong link between walking and protection against heart disease—women who walked an average of three hours a week at a brisk pace were 35 percent less likely to have had a heart attack over an eight-year period than women who walked infrequently. Vigorous exercise offered similar protection. Brisk walking also substantially cuts the risk of diabetes, while more vigorous exercise is associated with even lower risk.

What, exactly, is "brisk?" It means moving quickly enough so your heartbeat and breathing speed up, but not so fast that you can't carry on a normal conversation. It's moving as if you were late for an important meeting. If you are a counter or measurer, brisk walking is taking around one hundred steps a minute or walking at a clip of three to four miles per hour.

For many people, walking is an excellent alternative to other types of physical activity because it doesn't require any special equipment, can be done any time and any place, and is generally quite safe. More vigorous exercise such as running or bicycling lets you pack the same cardiovascular workout into a shorter period than you can with walking and also gives you a higher level of physical fitness. Although more vigorous activity than brisk walking may provide some added benefits, you can achieve much in the way of chronic disease prevention with a good daily walk.

• *Exercise at least thirty minutes a day.* According to the Surgeon General's report, you need to intentionally burn at least two thousand calories a week to begin reaping the benefits of physical activity. That's a difficult number to calculate. Most recommendations translate this into time—thirty minutes of physical activity on most, if not all, days of the week. There is no question that this much activity is far better than inactivity. But thirty minutes of activity a day isn't much when you think about how active our farmer or laborer forefathers and foremothers were. Even someone who runs five miles a day usually sits for most of his or her other waking hours. So consider thirty minutes of physical activity as a daily minimum for maintaining your health and weight. And keep in mind that most people will benefit from more.

A word of caution here: The *intensity* of your activity also matters. Sauntering through the mall for fifteen minutes beats sitting, and it may help your bones and mood. But it won't do much for your heart, lungs, and blood vessels. For an activity to help your cardiovascular system, it must speed up your heartbeat and your breathing.

• *Make your day more active.* There are many ways to inject more activity into your day. Some people choose to live close enough to their jobs so they can walk, run, or ride a bike to work. Not only does self-propelled commuting improve your health, but it makes a small contribution to others' health by cutting down on traffic congestion and air pollution. Restructuring your day can add small "activity bits" that add up. Possibilities include walking up the stairs at work instead of taking the elevator; parking in a far corner of the lot and walking; getting off your train or bus a stop or two early and walking the rest of the way; using a rake for leaves or a shovel for snow rather than a leaf- or snowblower.

• *It also helps to have fun.* Many people have turned walking into a social activity, a chance to touch base with a partner or friends several times a week. Others enjoy the challenge of learning new skills, like rowing or tennis, and pushing themselves to improve. If you make exercise a fun high priority, you'll find a way to fit in thirty minutes of activity a day, either in one long stretch or in several small bursts. It might help to consider this outlay of time as a solid investment that will offer an excellent return for your long-term health.

2. FIND A DIET THAT WORKS FOR YOU

If your weight has been holding steady in the healthy range, you are clearly doing many of the right things as far as the amount of food you are eating. Even so, you can probably fine-tune your diet so it's even healthier. The Healthy Eating Pyramid and information in the following chapters can help you choose the right foods to further improve your health.

However, if your weight has been creeping upward or if you are already overweight, a new direction is in order. Its compass points are eating fewer calories and burning more of them. Many people get lost. Some ignore exercise, a crucial part of losing weight and keeping it off. Others are overwhelmed by the legions of diets and diet books, have trouble following a particular diet, or try one and it doesn't work.

• *Diets low in refined carbohydrates work best.* For years we've been hearing that low-fat diets rich in carbohydrates are the best route to weight loss and improved cardiovascular fitness. For many people, just the opposite is true. As I describe in chapters 5 and 7, only people who are lean and active can tolerate a lot of carbohydrates. For others, too many carbohydrates don't promote weight loss or improve heart health.

The Atkins, South Beach, and other popular diets have you take drastic measures, at least at first, and stop eating virtually all carbohydrates. As long as you aren't gobbling no- or low-carb foods packed with saturated and trans fats, limiting or eliminating refined carbohydrates is a good step to take. Keep in mind, though, that these "crash" diets overemphasize short-term weight loss when the real goal should be finding a healthy eating pattern that can help you control your weight for years. The strategies described in this book are aimed at exactly that.

Giving up refined carbohydrates in favor of whole grains, vegetables, and some fruits such as apples will reduce the spikes of glucose and insulin that provoke hunger while also supplying important vitamins, minerals, fiber, and other phytonutrients. It can also reduce your chances of developing high blood pressure, type 2 diabetes, or heart disease. Avoiding saturated and trans fats and getting more monounsaturated and polyunsaturated fats can improve your cholesterol levels, help prevent blood clots, allow your arteries to work more effectively, and boost your muscles' response to insulin. Going easy on red and processed meats and eating in their place fish, nuts, beans, and poultry will reduce the risks for colon cancer, prostate cancer, diabetes, and heart disease, even if total fat remains high.

• *A healthy global diet.* An eating plan that borrows heavily from the Mediterranean and other traditional diets offers a healthy nutritional foundation (see chapter 11). Plenty of vegetables, moderate amounts of whole grains, and relatively little red meat offer reasonably low energy density. The abundance of vegetables and whole grains, as well as the relatively high percentage of fat (30 to 45 percent of calories, mainly from olive and other vegetable oils), makes for mild effects on blood sugar. Just as important, this kind of diet is open to creative interpretation. You can incorporate cuisines from around the world, as well as your own creations, into an eating pattern with enough variety and pleasure to last a lifetime.

• *It has to work for you.* One finding buried in the latest diet trials is that individual responses to weight loss strategies vary widely. In the *overall* results, low-carb participants lost an average of ten to fifteen pounds. That average hides what really happened. Some people in both the low-carb and low-fat groups lost more than twenty-five pounds each, some saw smaller changes in weight, and others didn't lose any weight at all. These differences, which are probably due to a combination of genetic, environmental, and psychological or social factors, are actually good news. Such individual differences are one reason why this book doesn't define healthy eating by a rigid breakdown of calories into percentages from protein, carbohydrate, and fat.

If you are one of the lucky folks who have successfully controlled weight with the first diet you try, thank your genes, your psyche, or your family. But if you try a diet and it doesn't work, don't give up! It may not have been right for your metabolism, eating habits, or social situation. Experiment with other weight control strategies, as long as they emphasize healthy sources of fat and protein and include regular physical activity. You should be able to find the one that's right for you.

3. PRACTICE DEFENSIVE EATING

Most people in our relatively sedentary society need to watch their calories as they age to avoid gaining weight. This involves more than just selecting certain types of foods or a particular kind of diet. It also means learning how to avoid overeating, which I call "defensive eating." Here are some suggestions that may be helpful:

- *Practice stopping before you are stuffed.* Recognize that we are victims of our culture, one that glorifies excess.
- *Be selective.* Don't eat things just because they are put in front of you.
- *Choose small portions.* In restaurants, realize that portions are often over-size and that a single meal can contain your daily caloric allowance. Consider sharing entrées, or order two appetizers instead of an entrée.
- *Beware of desserts.* A single slice of the Cheesecake Factory's Original Cheesecake packs almost eight hundred calories and an incredible 49 grams of fat (28 of them saturated, or 50 percent more than is recommended per day). And many people down that *after* eating an entire meal. If you want to order a rich dessert, skip the entrée altogether, or try sharing the dessert four ways. Better yet, have a healthy meal and finish it off with a piece of fruit or other lower-calorie option.
- *Slow down and pay attention to your food when you eat.* When you wolf down food, you effectively bypass the intricate set of "I'm full" signals that your digestive system is designed to generate. Eating at a moderate pace gives your stomach and intestines time to send these messages to your brain.
- *Be creative with low-calorie options to show you really care.* Don't love your family and friends to death with calories they don't need.
- *Keep track of the calories in the foods you eat.* I don't mean for you to for-mally count calories, just be aware of what you are eating and drinking. Sugary sodas and fruit drinks, for example, can be a big source of invisible calories that you can easily cut from your diet. A small glass of juice in the morning is per-fectly good for you, but drinking several glasses during the day can add hun-dreds of extra calories. Keep in mind that you would have to eat two oranges to get the same number of calories as you do from a glass of orange juice. Soda is worse because it gives you nothing but calories.
- *Spoil your appetite.* Have a snack or appetizer before eating a meal. Re-member the dreaded line *"It will spoil your dinner!"* that your mother used to ut-ter when you asked for a cookie or some popcorn late in the afternoon? She was right (of course). So use this principle to your advantage.
- *Minimize temptation.* Many of us find it hard to ignore chocolates, cook-ies, chips, or other goodies when they are sitting on a shelf or in the refrigera-tor. Out of sight doesn't necessarily mean out of mind. Out of the house or apartment, though, usually offers a great deterrent. In their place, keep a sup-

ply of low-calorie snacks such as apples, carrots, or whole-grain crackers on hand for when you really want to munch on something.

• *Be vigilant.* Don't forget that much of the food industry, because its goal is to sell more food, is out to exploit your weaknesses and destroy your defenses. You will need to be smart to avoid their traps.

• *Try keeping it simple.* Here's a truism from animal research: Rats fed "rat chow" or monkeys fed "monkey chow" don't weigh as much as animals that get to pick from a variety of foods. The same is probably true for humans. Think back to the last time you wandered through a cafeteria with great choices and you'll probably picture a tray piled with more food than you usually eat. There's no question that we need variety in our diets. Different foods offer different nutrients that are essential for good health. At each meal, though, simplicity may be a better strategy for some people. You may eat less if your entire meal is a chicken dish and vegetables than if you prepare several tempting dishes. Such simplification runs counter to trends in the marketplace, as the food industry offers an ever growing and ever beguiling variety of foods. But it may help reverse the ever expanding trend of your waistline.

Weight control isn't impossible, nor does it need to mean deprivation or a boring, repetitive diet. With conscious effort and creativity, most people can successfully control their weight long term with an enjoyable but reasonable diet and near daily exercise.

Why bother? There are several good reasons. You'll be in control of your body's machinery. That alone can give you a sense of accomplishment and determination that could pay off in other areas of your life. Watching your weight with a healthy diet and exercise can give you more energy. Finally, the trio of a healthy weight, healthy diet, and healthy exercise offers the safest, most effective way to prevent disease and live longer.

The Skinny on Popular Diets

Legend has it that King Arthur and his Knights of the Round Table searched fruitlessly for the Holy Grail. Today, millions of people are looking for its dietary equivalent—the one true combination of foods that will help them lose weight or stay healthy. Most search in vain, led astray by empty promises from dueling diet books and conflicting nutrition news. They try diets that work for a few weeks then stop working, or ones that don't work at all, and they end up frustrated and still overweight.

Disappointment with diets shouldn't come as a surprise. Part of the problem is the notion that there's a single diet that is right for everyone—an idea as mythical as the Grail. Genes, family, our environment, and many other factors influence how, why, what, and how much we eat. Another, bigger problem is that *anyone* can cook up a diet. You don't have to know anything about medicine, nutrition, or even physiology. All you need is an idea and the chutzpah to promote and sell it.

The graveyard of fad diets stands in silent testimony to the design flaws of most diets. Remember the cabbage soup diet, which claimed that the more cabbage soup you ate, the more weight you would lose? How about the rigid Scarsdale diet, which promised one-pound-per-day weight loss by limiting daily intake to about one thousand calories a day with the help of specified amounts of fruits, vegetables, and mostly lean sources of protein. The list goes on: the Hollywood 48 Hour Miracle Diet, the grapefruit diet, the caveman diet, the Subway diet, the Russian Air Force diet, the apple cider vinegar diet, a host of forgettable celebrity diets, and countless others.

The fact is, almost *any* diet will work—at least for a short time—if it helps you take in fewer calories. Diets do this in two basic ways:

- Defining "good" foods you should eat (like the grapefruit diet) or "bad" ones to avoid (think low fat or no carbs)
- Changing how you behave and the ways you think or feel about food

Most restrictive diets come with the seeds of failure planted and germinating. Hunger from eating less, not to mention cutting back on common or once-favorite foods or giving them up altogether, creates cravings that can lead to "cheating." This can trigger feelings of failure and hopelessness. These, in turn, undermine the effort and enthusiasm needed to stick with a diet.

Keep in mind that weight loss is only one spoke in the wheel of good health. You could put yourself on a hot dog diet and almost certainly lose weight. But it won't last or be good for you in the long run. What's really needed is a plan you can sustain for years. It should be as good for your heart, bones, brain, colon, and psyche as it is for your waistline. Its hallmarks should be plenty of choices, relatively few restrictions, and few "special" foods.

How do current diets measure up using this yardstick? Let's take a look at a few popular ones.

LOW-FAT DIETS

The average American gets about 33 percent of his or her calories from fat. Low-fat diets try to squeeze this down to 10 to 20 percent. There are two key ideas behind low-fat diets: fat makes you fat, and fat is bad for the heart. Neither one of these blanket statements is accurate. A moderate amount of healthy fats can promote weight loss as well as or better than a low-fat diet. On the heart disease front, some fats are good for the heart (see page 66), and eliminating them from the diet can cause problems.

One of the best-known low-fat diets is Dr. Dean Ornish's *Eat More, Weigh Less* plan. The "eat more" idea comes from the fact that fat contains 9 calories per gram while carbohydrates contain 4. By switching from fatty foods to carbohydrate-rich ones, especially fruits and vegetables, you can double your food intake without taking in more calories.

There is no question that following a low-fat diet can aid weight loss, at least for the short term. Some people manage to stick with such a diet for the long haul, but that takes real commitment. Why? Low-fat diets tend to be less flavorful than other eating strategies and more restrictive about food choices, especially when one is dining out. They can also leave you feeling hungry, one reason why low-fat diets usually call for high-fiber foods that increase the sensation of fullness as well as between-meal snacks.

Low-fat diets are touted as being excellent for the heart. That reputation is a holdover from a time when many experts believed that all fats were bad for the heart. This belief is fading in light of findings that unsaturated fats can improve cholesterol levels and snuff out potentially deadly heart-rhythm disturbances. The Ornish plan also got a boost from a small study Dr. Ornish conducted among thirty-five men and women with heart disease. It showed that a very-low-fat vegetarian, whole-grain diet, along with exercise, stress management, and group support, reduced blood-vessel narrowing better than less intensive changes. The improvement could have come from the low-fat diet. It could also have come from the other changes. Keep in mind that "doing Ornish" means forgoing refined grains in favor of whole grains, and exercising. Eating refined carbohydrates without exercising can increase triglycerides and decrease HDL (good) cholesterol, neither of which is good for the heart.

Bottom line: Some people lose weight and keep it off with a low-fat diet. Others lose weight then put it back on, or don't lose weight at all. Many people find it difficult to stick with a low-fat diet for a long time because it is so restrictive and because fats make food taste good. One of the hazards is replacing fat with easily digested carbohydrates. In some people, this interferes with weight loss. It can also cause problems with HDL cholesterol and triglycerides.

LOW-CARB DIETS

Over the past few years, carbohydrates have replaced fats as the great dietary demons. Thanks to Drs. Robert Atkins *(Dr. Atkins' Diet Revolution)* and Arthur Agatston *(The South Beach Diet)*, millions of Americans have given up bread, pasta, rice, and other carbohydrate unmentionables in their quest to lose weight.

The idea isn't new. In the mid-1800s, an obese British undertaker named William Banting happened on a low-carbohydrate diet. He tried it for a few months and watched with delight as the pounds slipped away without the gnawing hunger and cravings that other diets had caused him. Banting's "Letter on Corpulence, Addressed to the Public," written in 1863, became so popular that people began using the term "to bant" in place of "to diet."

Are bunless burgers the key to weight loss? Not necessarily. Some solid studies indicate that low-carb, high-protein diets are at least as good as low-fat diets—and in most cases better—at helping very overweight people shed pounds *for a short time.* How well they work over the long term is anyone's guess. Low-carb diets seem to be easier to stick with than low-fat diets and, contrary to experts' warnings, for most people they don't seem to cause harmful changes in blood cholesterol even when they contain fairly high amounts of fat.

Why do high-protein, low-carb diets seem to work more quickly than low-fat, high-carb diets? First, chicken, beef, fish, beans, and other high-protein foods slow the movement of food from the stomach to the intestine. Slower stomach emptying means you feel full longer and get hungrier later. Second, protein's gentle, steady effect on blood sugar avoids the quick, steep rise and the just as quick hunger-bell-ringing fall in blood sugar that occur after eating a rapidly digested carbohydrate like white bread or baked potato.

One big unknown is the long-term effects of eating a lot of protein. Bone loss is one potential complication. Too much protein could force the body to pull calcium from bone to neutralize the acid formed when protein is digested. The jury is still out on whether eating a lot of protein weakens bones, has no effect on them, or strengthens them. Protein also puts extra demands on the kidney. This probably isn't an issue for people with healthy kidneys, but it may pose problems for those with mild (and often undiscovered) kidney disease. People with high blood pressure are often in this category.

The other controversial element of the different high-protein, low-carb diets is what people choose to eat in place of refined carbohydrates. High-protein options such as fish, beans, and nuts are better than hamburgers, steak, and sausage, which deliver a lot of saturated fat. In addition, shying away from whole grains, fruits, and vegetables can lead to low intake of cereal fiber, fats, vitamins, and minerals—deficits that supplements can't possibly overcome.

The early Atkins diet banned carbohydrates in virtually every form and gloried in fat. The latest version of this diet allows some carbohydrates—mainly fruits, vegetables, and some whole grains—after an initial no-carb period. In this way it is much like the South Beach diet. One big difference between the two is their approach to fats: The Atkins diet allows almost unlimited fats, and doesn't adequately discriminate between good and bad fats, while the South Beach diet takes a harder line against bad fats.

Bottom line: A low-carb diet works for some people. It may make it easier to shed pounds quickly, but there isn't any evidence that it works any better in the long term than a low-fat diet. Low-carb diets can also be expensive: Following the portion sizes and ingredients in the Atkins and South Beach diets can nearly double your average grocery bill. Finally, some questions still need answers regarding these diets, such as:

- Do moderately or slightly overweight people see the same weight loss and blood fat improvements from low-carbohydrate diets as obese people?
- Could the abundant protein in an Atkins– or South Beach–style diet cause kidney damage or bone loss over time?
- What are the other broad long-term health effects of these diets?

RIGHT-CARB DIETS

Instead of banning carbohydrates, diets such as *Sugar Busters!* and *The Glycemic Revolution* embrace "correct" carbohydrates while shunning "harmful" ones. Briefly, this means eating plenty of fruits, vegetables, and whole grains and cutting way back on refined sugars (white sugar, high-fructose corn syrup, honey, molasses, etc.) and processed grains.

These and other right-carb diets rely heavily on the glycemic index and glycemic load (see pages 106–109). These scales measure how strongly a particular food boosts blood sugar and insulin levels. Foods with a high glycemic load make blood sugar and insulin levels rise quickly and then crash. This cycle can lead to the early onset of hunger pangs. In general, products made from refined grains, such as white bread, bagels, and crackers, along with white rice and baked potatoes, have high glycemic index and glycemic load values (above 70 for the glycemic index and above 20 for the glycemic load). Foods with a low glycemic index or glycemic load (under 55 for the glycemic index and under 10 for the glycemic load) have slow and steady effects on blood sugar and insulin. These foods include whole grains, beans, vegetables, and fruits. In theory, foods with a low glycemic load, which generate small but steady increases in blood sugar, help stave off hunger, while foods that cause large but fleeting increases quickly ring your internal hunger alarm.

Bottom line: In general, right-carb diets promote healthy eating by focusing on fruits, vegetables, and whole grains. Their reliance on the glycemic index, however, overly complicates choosing what to eat, especially when dining out. Plans that prohibit refined sugars also make dieting and healthy eating unnecessarily complex. Cutting back on foods with added sugars certainly makes sense. Losing weight on such a diet stems from the fact that restricting sugar helps to reduce calories, not that refined sugars are toxic. Traditional Mediterranean diets have a relatively low impact on blood sugar because they use plenty of fruits and vegetables, are higher in healthy fats, and are relatively low in easily digested carbohydrates. So does the Healthy Eating Pyramid.

PERFECT PROPORTIONS AND CORRECT COMBINATIONS

Several popular diets are based on the notion that specific proportions of nutrients or certain combinations of foods are essential to weight loss.

According to *The Zone*, achieving the right balance of carbohydrates, proteins, and fats at every snack and meal creates the hormonal balance that will lead to weight loss, improved energy, and other health benefits. You reach "the zone" by creating meals and snacks that contain 9 grams of carbohydrate for every 7 grams of protein and 1.5 grams of fat (40% carbohydrate, 30% fat, and 30% protein). There is little evidence that such a rigid approach to eating is necessary, or even helpful, for weight loss. This approach can be expensive, and makes it difficult to eat with your family or dine out. But if you like structure and rules, then the Zone might be right for you.

The *Eat Right 4 Your Type* diet takes an odd and even less scientific tack: that your blood type determines what you should eat (not to mention how you should exercise, what supplements you need, and what type of personality you have). According to this plan, people with type O blood need a high-protein, low-carb diet that's easy on the wheat and beans, while those with type A blood need a high-protein, low-carb diet that contains plenty of fish and beans but steers clear of red meat, dairy products, and wheat. Following this diet means remembering a lot of detailed information, including lists of good and bad foods. It isn't a balanced diet—something you can tell from the long list of recommended supplements. And it certainly isn't family friendly, since most families encompass more than one blood type.

Bottom line: Exact proportions or specific food combinations may help you lose weight. Any success is almost certainly because such diets force you to focus on what you are eating and to eat less each day, *not* because of any nutritional or physiologic secret the diet developers have uncovered. Their long-term health effects have not been studied.

DOES DENSITY MATTER?

Another approach to losing weight takes aim at "energy density"—the concentration of calories in each portion of food. The *Volumetrics Weight Control Plan* fiddles with satiety, the body's signals that it has gotten enough food. It does this by recommending foods that fill the belly without adding too many calories. These tend to be water-rich foods such as fruits, vegetables, low-fat milk, cooked grains, beans, lean meats, poultry, and fish. Soups, stews, casseroles, pasta with vegetables, and fruit-based desserts get the thumbs up, while high-fat foods like potato chips and dry, calorie-dense ones like pretzels, crackers, and fat-free cookies get the thumbs down.

Bottom line: The strategy of eating foods that fill you up without delivering many calories probably helps people lose weight the same way most other diets do: It narrows your choices so you take in fewer calories each day. Although the *Volumetrics* idea is appealing, it is much too simplistic. For example, a can of Coca-Cola has a low energy density. But it contributes plenty of calories that do little to fill you up or delay hunger. The energy-density concept doesn't take into account how rapidly a food is digested and absorbed, which can have a big impact on the return of hunger. Most important, its long-term effects on weight control haven't been evaluated.

BEHAVIOR CHANGE

Some weight-loss strategies focus as much on how, why, and when you eat as on what you eat. The attention isn't entirely misplaced. Some people use food for comfort. They overeat because they are sad, lonely, frustrated, nervous, bored, depressed, or any number of other triggers. Breaking an unhealthy relationship with food can help such individuals lose weight.

Dr. Phil McGraw's *Ultimate Weight Solution* offers "seven keys to permanent weight loss." These include right thinking, healing feelings, a no-fail environment, mastery over food and impulse eating, intentional exercise, a circle of support, and what Dr. Phil calls high-response cost, high-yield nutrition. The closest this plan comes to offering nutrition advice is promoting foods that take a long time to prepare and eat.

Another entry in this category is *The Automatic Diet,* which walks you through a form of self-analysis and then offers behavior modification techniques to reprogram the patterns that work against healthy eating. In theory, following this plan makes good eating habits as automatic as brushing your teeth or setting the alarm clock.

Bottom line: There is no question that your habits, behaviors, and relationships with other people and with food influence your ability to lose weight or maintain a steady weight. What and how much you eat, as well as whether you exercise, are also important. Not all overweight people have dysfunctional habits or relationships, and they need to focus on food and exercise.

THE EVIDENCE

The glut of diet plans hides an appalling scarcity of solid evidence on effective strategies for weight loss. As mentioned earlier, anyone can concoct and peddle a diet. No laws mandate that it be tested first. Some diet promoters try their plans on themselves, their family, and their friends. Those who lose weight become the success stories hyped in the books. But there's no hard-nosed evaluation of what percentage of people who start the diet stick with it or how many lose weight and keep it off.

An early glimmer of evidence on weight-loss strategies came from the National Weight Control Registry, a select "club" of almost 4,000 women and men who have lost more than 30 pounds and kept them off for at least a year. What was their secret?

- They switched to lower-fat diets, cut back on sugars and sweets, and ate more fruits and vegetables. (Keep in mind that most of those in the Registry enrolled during an era when low fat was the mantra for weight loss.)
- They ate fewer calories. On average, Registry volunteers consumed about 1,400 calories a day, significantly less than the average American's intake. This doesn't mean, however, that you should aim for 1,400 calories a day. What's right for you is based on your weight, height, and activity level.
- They exercised. Registry participants burned an average of 400 calories per day in physical activity. That's the equivalent of about an hour of brisk walking.

One of the main messages of this research is that successful weight loss is very much a "do it your way" endeavor.

A *Consumer Reports* survey of more than 32,000 dieters echoed these findings. Nearly one-quarter had lost at least 10 percent of their starting body weight and kept it off for at least a year. Most chalked up their success to eating less and exercising more. The vast majority did it on their own, without resorting to commercial weight loss programs or weight loss drugs. Interestingly, the successful dieters in the *Consumer Reports* survey tended to adopt low-carbohydrate/high-protein rather than low-fat diets.

What the Registry and *Consumer Reports* groups have in common is a focus on daily calories and exercise. In other words, successful dieters learn to manipulate energy in and energy out to lose or maintain weight.

A second thread of truly scientific evidence about dieting comes from a handful of randomized controlled trials, the gold standard of medical research. In these studies, researchers assign overweight people to one diet or another, using the equivalent of picking names out of a hat, and then follow their progress for a few weeks or a few months. Most of the trials to date have compared a standard low-fat diet to a low-carb/high-protein diet.

Overall, people who followed the low-carb/high-protein diet tended to lose weight faster than those who followed the low-fat diet. Interestingly, low-carb dieters didn't suffer harmful changes in blood cholesterol, even though they ate more fat than low-fat dieters. Instead, they actually had greater reductions in triglycerides (fat-carrying particles associated with heart disease) and greater increases in HDL (good) cholesterol, than low-fat dieters.

In the few studies that lasted for a year, though, weight loss was about the same *regardless of diet type.* Keep in mind that these studies focused primarily on weight, and were too short to track other important consequences of diet such as heart disease, diabetes, bone strength, and cancer.

Buried in the data from these trials is the finding that people respond differently to different diets. Low-carb diets work long term for some people, while low-fat diets work for others. There's an important lesson here: It's okay to experiment on yourself. If you give a particular diet your best shot and it doesn't work, it's possible that it isn't the right one for you, your metabolism, and/or your situation. At the same time, don't get too discouraged or beat yourself up because a diet that "worked for everybody" didn't pay off for you. Try another.

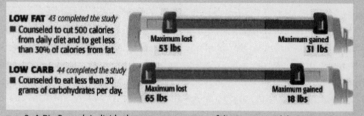

LOW FAT *43 completed the study*
■ Counseled to cut 500 calories from daily diet and to get less than 30% of calories from fat.
Maximum lost
53 lbs
Maximum gained
31 lbs

LOW CARB *44 completed the study*
■ Counseled to eat less than 30 grams of carbohydrates per day.
Maximum lost
65 lbs
Maximum gained
18 lbs

FIG. 9 A Big Spread. Individual responses to a year of dieting vary widely. In one controlled trial, people lost—and gained—weight on both low-carb and low-fat diets.

DO IT YOURSELF

Better yet, build your own plan. A reasonable one could be assembled from many of the diets discussed here, which include some valid and valuable strategies or philosophies even though the diets themselves are limited. The Ornish diet highlights the importance of lifestyle factors besides diet, which are important regardless of what you eat. Sugar Busters! offers help distinguishing good and bad carbs, while The Zone tackles good and bad fats. The Volumetrics approach emphasizes fruits and vegetables. Dr. Phil focuses on behavior, an often crucial component of eating, especially overeating.

A good diet should provide plenty of choices, relatively few restrictions, and no long grocery lists of sometimes expensive special foods. It should be as good for your heart, bones, brain, and colon as it is for your waistline. And it should be something you can sustain for years.

The principles of healthy eating presented in this book can give you the foundation for such a plan. They won't give you a quick fix. Instead they can offer you something better—a lifetime of savory, healthy choices that will be good for *you,* not just for parts of you.

CHAPTER FOUR

Surprising News About Fat

FEW PUBLIC HEALTH MESSAGES ARE as powerful and as persistent as this one: Fat is bad. Over the past four decades, fat has become a kind of dietary Public Enemy Number One, feared for its ability to cause disease and even kill. As a nation, we've taken that message to heart. The average American has substantially reduced the percentage of calories that she or he gets from fat over the past three decades. We spend billions of dollars a year on low-fat cookies, fake-fat chips, pills that block the absorption of fat from the digestive system, and all manner of fat-busting diets and cookbooks.

But we aren't any healthier for all of this effort. In fact, we're worse off for it. An astounding two-thirds of adult Americans are overweight. More than 30 percent of adults are so far overweight that they are classified as obese. Diabetes is on the rise. And the war on fat hasn't had any appreciable impact on rates of heart disease and cancer—the two main reasons for it in the first place.

SOME FATS ARE GOOD FOR YOU

One reason we aren't seeing a payoff is that we have lost sight of the critical fact that not all fats are the same. Or, to put it more bluntly, not all fats are bad. In spite of the scorn heaped upon dietary fat and the antifat recommendations from the country's leading health organizations, the truth is that **some fats are good for you, and it is important to include these good fats in your diet.** In fact, eating more good fats—and staying away from bad ones—is second only to weight control on the list of healthy nutritional strategies.

Eating the right kind of fat is a critical issue because dietary fat gets much of the blame for causing heart disease,* the number one killer in the United States and most developed countries and soon to be the leading cause of death around the world. In the United States, for example, more than a million

---

* Technically, the term *heart disease* encompasses a wide range of conditions ranging from chest pain to electrical problems and failure of the heart muscle to pump blood. In this book, the term *heart disease* refers to coronary heart disease, which stems from a blockage in one or more arteries that supply blood to the heart.

people have heart attacks each year, and heart disease and stroke account for about one-third of all deaths. The cost of heart disease and stroke tops $240 billion, not counting the costs of lost productivity. Diet, and specifically saturated fat, certainly isn't the *only* cause of heart disease—smoking is the single leading cause, while excess weight and inactivity also contribute a substantial share of deaths and disability. But after these, controlling the type of fat you eat is one of the most important ways to prevent heart disease.

Dietary Fat and Body Fat

You may be thinking, Hold on a second. Won't eating more fat make me fatter, something I know is definitely bad for my heart? Only if you merely add extra fat to your diet without cutting anything out of it. Remember, the goal here isn't getting more fat in your diet. Instead it is cutting back on bad fats (saturated and trans fats) while increasing good fats (monounsaturated and polyunsaturated fats) and keeping the number of daily calories constant. If you do that, you won't gain weight. If you are already following a low-fat diet, think about replacing some of the carbohydrates with unsaturated fat, especially if your HDL (good) cholesterol level is low or your triglyceride level is high.

There's a nice, intuitive feel to the notion that eating more fat makes you fatter. Given the evidence from different kinds of studies, though, it doesn't hold water.

- People on low-fat diets generally lose about two to four pounds after several weeks, but then gain that weight back *even while continuing with the diet.* Randomized trials of weight loss usually show little net weight change after a year.

- In country-to-country surveys across Europe, women with the lowest fat intake are the most likely to be obese, while those with the highest fat intake are the least likely; in European men, there is no relation between fat intake and obesity.

- In the United States, the gradual reduction in the fat content of the average diet, from 40 percent of calories to about 33 percent, has been accompanied by a gradual *increase* in the average weight and a dramatic increase in obesity.

In short, the fat in your diet doesn't necessarily make you fat. If you usually eat more calories than you burn off, you're going to gain weight regardless of whether your calories mostly come from fat, carbohydrates, or protein. Put into the context of this chapter, if you keep your calories constant, you won't gain weight if you cut back on saturated fat or carbohydrate and eat more unsaturated fat.

HOW DIETARY GUIDELINES HAVE DISTORTED THE FAT FACTS

The traditional link between diet and heart disease is a kind of scientific two-step that goes like this: 1) Too much fat in the diet increases cholesterol levels in the blood; and 2) Higher cholesterol levels increase the chances of having a heart attack or developing some other form of heart disease. If this is true, then eating less fat should decrease rates of heart disease.

This relatively simple diet-heart hypothesis leaves out a lot. An important omission is that different fats have different effects on cholesterol. What's more, there are many other ways that dietary fat can affect heart disease other than through the single channel of cholesterol. Dietary fats also influence how much high-density lipoprotein (HDL), the so-called good or protective cholesterol, is in your bloodstream, how your blood clots, how susceptible your heart is to erratic rhythms, how the inner lining of blood vessels responds to stress, and probably other pathways to heart disease we haven't yet discovered.

Tragically, the public policy that has been based on the simple diet-heart hypothesis doesn't cover these alternate pathways. For years we have been urged to use fats and oils "sparingly." We've been encouraged to choose diets that are low in saturated fat and cholesterol but haven't gotten any advice about the proven benefits of unsaturated fats.

None of this overly simplistic advice tells you that eating unsaturated fats instead of saturated fats can improve the levels of cholesterol and other fats in your bloodstream, fortify your heart against erratic heartbeats, or help counteract a number of processes that underlie atherosclerosis, the gradual clogging and narrowing of arteries.

SIMPLER DOESN'T ALWAYS MEAN BETTER

Back in 1957, with only a limited amount of hard data at hand, the American Heart Association (AHA) set out its first dietary guidelines. Though the AHA hedged its bets with liberal use of the word *may*, its first guidelines were remarkably on target. They said: 1) Diet may play an important role in the development of heart disease. 2) Both the fat content *and the total calories in the diet* (italics added) are probably important. 3) The ratio between saturated and unsaturated fats may be the basic determinant, and people should get more unsaturated fat and less saturated fat. 4) A wide variety of other factors besides fat, both dietary and nondietary, may be important.

Four years later the AHA was still suggesting that people increase their intake of unsaturated fat.

Over the years, though, as expert panels discussed (and sometimes fought over) the most effective public health message, the AHA, the National Cholesterol Education Program, and other influential groups decided that Americans just couldn't grasp a concept as nuanced as good fat/bad fat. Instead they settled on the simpler "all fat is bad" message.

There's no question that the public has heard and heeded this message. Today, fats and oils make up about 33 percent of the calories in the average diet, compared with 40 percent in the 1960s and 38 percent in the 1980s. If this reduction meant we were eating a lot less saturated fat, that would be great news and would show up as lower rates of heart disease. But we've thrown out the baby with the bathwater. Much of the reduction has been in beneficial unsaturated fats, one reason there has been little change in heart disease rates in recent years.

REPLACING FATS WITH CARBOHYDRATES CREATES A NEW PROBLEM

Reducing the amount of fat in your diet means adding something else. You do this unconsciously, even if you are planning to lose weight. If you follow the standard dietary guidelines, that something else is carbohydrates, usually simple or highly processed carbohydrates such as sugar, pasta, white rice, and potatoes. Replacing saturated fat with carbohydrates lowers total cholesterol levels, though only a little bit. But it also lowers levels of HDL (good) cholesterol.

The two trends encouraged by the standard dietary guidelines—increasing intake of carbohydrates and decreasing intake of all fats—have other troubling consequences beyond their harmful impact on HDL. Carbohydrates can, and do, increase weight every bit as effectively as fats if you consume more calories than you burn off. Equally bad, white bread, potatoes, pasta, and white rice cause large spikes in blood sugar (glucose) and insulin levels in the bloodstream, something that doesn't happen with fat, protein, and slowly absorbed carbohydrates like those from whole grains, fruits, and vegetables. A constant and heavy demand on the pancreas to make insulin appears to be a key ingredient for adult-onset diabetes, now called type 2 diabetes, especially when paired with lack of exercise. Finally, replacing fats with carbohydrates usually means forgoing foods such as nuts, avocados, salad dressings made with unsaturated oils, and other foods or products that contain beneficial monounsaturated and polyunsaturated fats, as well as vitamin E and other valuable nutrients.

THE BENEFITS OF EATING UNSATURATED FATS
IN PLACE OF SATURATED FATS

Eating less saturated fat and more unsaturated fat improves cholesterol levels across the board and helps prevent heart disease in other ways as well. It is this message I hope to hammer home against the "all fat is bad" drumbeat.

By steering clear of all fats, you eliminate a number of foods that can improve your long-term health. Don't get me wrong. I wholeheartedly agree with pruning out saturated and trans fats from your diet. But the same doesn't apply to unsaturated fats. Eating unsaturated fats instead of saturated fats or carbohydrates

- lowers levels of low-density lipoprotein (LDL), the so-called bad cholesterol, without also lowering levels of HDL (good) cholesterol;
- prevents the increase in triglycerides, another form of fat circulating in the bloodstream that has been linked with heart disease, that occurs with high-carbohydrate diets;
- reduces the development of erratic heartbeats, a main cause of sudden cardiac death; and
- reduces the tendency for blood-flow-blocking clots to form in arteries.

Unsaturated fats are so important to good health that they support the foundation of the Healthy Eating Pyramid. This acknowledges that fats and oils make up a substantial chunk of daily calories and can also have long-term health benefits.

TYPES OF FAT

Chemically speaking, the fat family is an extended clan. What the members of this group have in common is a chain of carbon atoms bonded to hydrogen atoms. Fats differ in the length and geometry of their carbon backbones, how the carbon atoms are connected to each other, and the total number of hydrogen atoms attached.

Almost all of the fats in our diet are triglycerides—three fatty acids bound together by a "glue" known as glycerol. There are four main categories of fatty acids—saturated, monounsaturated, polyunsaturated, and trans fatty acids. (See "Types of Dietary Fat" on page 71.) Throughout this book fatty acids will simply be referred to as fats.

Until the middle of the twentieth century, fats were thought to play one

Types of Dietary Fat

Type of Fat	Important Sources	State at Room Temperature	Effect on Cholesterol Compared with Carbohydrates
Monounsaturated	Olives and olive oil, canola oil, peanut oil; cashews, almonds, peanuts, and most other nuts; peanut butter; avocados	Liquid	Lowers LDL; raises HDL
Polyunsaturated	Corn, soybean, safflower, and cottonseed oils; fish	Liquid	Lowers LDL; raises HDL
Saturated	Whole milk, butter, cheese, and ice cream; red meat; chocolate; coconuts, coconut milk, and coconut oil	Solid	Raises both LDL and HDL
Trans	Most margarines; vegetable shortening; partially hydrogenated vegetable oil; deep-fried fast foods; most commercial baked goods	Solid or semi-solid	Raises LDL*

* Compared to monounsaturated or polyunsaturated fat, trans fat increases LDL, decreases HDL, and increases triglycerides.

main role in the body, that of providing fuel for cells. We now know that they have many other important jobs. Fats provide the raw materials for building cell membranes, the delicate yet sturdy skin that surrounds each cell and controls what gets in and what gets out. They make up the sheaths that surround and protect nerves. They are the raw materials from which some hormones are made, as well as other chemicals that control blood clotting and muscle contraction.

Fats in the Bloodstream

Your body depends on fats for a host of functions. Fats form a major energy source for cells. They make up adipose tissue, which stores energy, cushions and protects vital organs, and provides insulation. Cholesterol, which is technically not a fat, is needed to make cell membranes and the critically important sheaths around nerves and is a building block from which the body makes many hormones.

In order for all this to happen, fats must somehow get from your digestive system to your cells. This isn't as simple as it sounds. Like oil and water, fats and blood don't mix. If your intestines or liver simply dumped digested fats into your blood, they would congeal into unusable globs. Instead fat is packaged into protein-covered particles that mix easily with blood and flow with it. These tiny particles, called lipoproteins (lipid plus protein), contain some cholesterol to help stabilize the particles.

Like a highway at rush hour, your bloodstream carries many sizes and shapes of fat-transporting particles. Lipoproteins are generally classified by the balance of fat and protein they contain. Those with a little fat and a lot of protein are heavier and more dense than the lighter, fluffier, and less dense particles that are more fat than protein. The proteins do more than just shield fat from water. They also act like address labels that help the body route fat-filled particles to specific destinations.

With regard to heart disease, the most important lipoproteins are high-density lipoprotein (HDL), low-density lipoprotein (LDL), and very-low-density lipoprotein, which is composed of triglycerides.

LDL is often referred to as the bad cholesterol. When your bloodstream carries too many of these particles, they can end up inside cells that line blood vessels. Once there, LDL is attacked by highly reactive free radicals and transformed into oxidized LDL. Oxidized LDL can damage the artery lining and kick off a cascade of reactions that clog the artery and set the scene for artery-blocking blood clots.

In contrast, HDL particles sponge up excess cholesterol from the lining of blood vessels and elsewhere and carry it off to the liver for disposal. They also help the liver recycle other lipoprotein particles.

Triglycerides make up most of the fat that you eat and most of the fat that circulates in your bloodstream. Triglycerides are essential for good health, since your tissues rely on them for energy. But as is the case for cholesterol, too much triglycerides may be bad for the arteries and the heart.

When you have your cholesterol checked, the number you get back is usually your total cholesterol. This number tells you how much LDL and HDL are circulating in your blood. The ideal total cholesterol level is under 200 milligrams per deciliter (tenth of a liter) of blood. The National Cholesterol Education Program (NCEP) defines borderline high cholesterol as a total cholesterol level between 200 and 239 milligrams per deciliter and high cholesterol as 240 milligrams per deciliter or higher.

Because total cholesterol is a mix of bad and good, it doesn't tell the whole story. That's why many physicians also check HDL levels along with total cholesterol and then calculate the LDL level with a simple formula. The lower the LDL the better, with anything under 130 milligrams per deciliter considered healthy. For healthy people, levels between 130 and 159 milligrams per deciliter are borderline high, and 160 milligrams per deciliter or above are high. For people with heart disease or at high risk for it, the thresholds are lower. The opposite is true for HDL, with higher levels offering greater protection against heart disease. An HDL under 35 milligrams per deciliter is considered low, while a level over that is defined as healthy, though the risk of heart disease continues to fall with increasing HDL.

The role of triglycerides in heart disease has been controversial, but recent studies show that high levels increase the chances of developing heart disease. The NCEP defines normal triglycerides as a level below 150 milligrams per deciliter. Borderline high is between 150 and 199, and high is anything above 200 milligrams per deciliter.

The human body can build most of the different fats it needs from any other fat in the diet, or from carbohydrates, for that matter. A few, though, can't be made from scratch. These so-called essential fats, which are all polyunsaturated fats, must come directly from food.

• *Saturated fat.* The term *saturated* means that the carbon atoms in a chain hold as many hydrogen atoms as they can. This happens only when each carbon atom is connected to its carbon neighbors by single bonds. Saturated fats look like straight chains.

About two dozen different saturated fats exist in nature. They are abundant in meat and animal fat, dairy products, and in a few vegetable oils like palm and coconut oil. At room temperature, saturated fats are solid rather than liquid, something you see every time you let the drippings from cooked bacon or hamburger congeal in a pan.

When it comes to their effects on cholesterol and the artery-clogging process known as atherosclerosis, saturated fats come in gradations of bad. The saturated fats in butter and other dairy products most strongly increase LDL (bad) cholesterol. Those in beef fat aren't quite as powerful at boosting LDL, and those in chocolate and cocoa butter have an even smaller impact.

• *Monounsaturated fat.* The Greek prefix *mono,* meaning "one," hints at the structure of these fats. At one point along the carbon backbone, two carbons are connected by a double bond. This seemingly small change leads to several key differences. It reduces the number of hydrogen atoms the carbon chain can hold by two. It changes the shape of the molecule from a straight chain to a bent stick. And it makes the fat a liquid at room temperature. Basically, monounsaturated fats are oils. Olive oil, peanut oil, and canola oil are all high in monounsaturated fats. Avocados and most nuts (see page 122) are also excellent sources.

• *Polyunsaturated fat.* Two or more double bonds make a polyunsaturated fat. These hold even fewer hydrogen atoms than a monounsaturated fat with the same number of carbon atoms and look like a stick with a double bend. Polyunsaturated fats can be subdivided into the omega-3 or omega-6 groups, with the number referring to how far the first double bond is from the end of the carbon chain. Each type plays different roles in the body. Polyunsaturated fats are also liquid at room temperature. Our bodies don't make polyunsaturated fats, so we need to get these essential fats from plant oils like corn and soybean oil, seeds, whole grains, and fatty fish such as salmon and tuna.

• *Trans fats.* More than one hundred years ago, food chemists discovered that they could solidify a polyunsaturated vegetable oil by heating it in the presence of hydrogen gas and finely ground particles of nickel metal. During the process, called partial hydrogenation, hydrogen latches on to some—but not all—of the double-bonded carbons, changing them into single bonds. At the same time, some of the remaining double bonds twist into a new straightened shape, which gives the fat new chemical and physical properties.

Why did anyone bother figuring this out? It's easier to ship and store solidified vegetable oils than liquid oils, and partially hydrogenated vegetable oil can be used in place of butter or lard in baking. And a lesser degree of hydrogenation yields a still-liquid oil that doesn't become rancid as quickly as unprocessed vegetable oils. Without this process we wouldn't have had margarine or vegetable shortenings such as Crisco. We also would have less heart disease and at least thirty thousand fewer deaths from it each year (see "Trans Fats—A Special Concern" on page 81).

Not long ago, an FDA advisory panel said that trans fats are even more harmful than saturated fats. The Institute of Medicine went a step further, concluding that the safest amount of trans fats for humans is zero.

TRACING THE DANGERS OF SATURATED FATS

Until the middle of the last century, when infectious diseases like tuberculosis and influenza were leading causes of death, calorie-rich diets laden with fat

Eggs

Not long ago, eggs were considered a perfect food, the centerpiece of solid breakfasts, the hearty garnishes atop salads and side dishes. The discovery of cholesterol and its link with heart disease sullied that reputation. With more than 200 milligrams of cholesterol in each egg yolk—two-thirds of the daily recommended intake—eggs were branded as unhealthy, to be eaten sparingly. Per capita egg consumption tumbled from more than 400 per year to 250 per year (see Figure 10), and many people today eat them with a side order of guilt.

In many ways, the dangers of eggs aren't all they're cracked up to be. Controlled feeding studies have shown that adding an *extra* 200 milligrams of cholesterol a day to the diet increases blood cholesterol levels only slightly and therefore might theoretically boost the risk of heart disease by about 10 percent. However, the focus on cholesterol has ignored the fact that eggs aren't just packets of cholesterol. They are very low in saturated fat and contain many other nutrients that are good for you—protein, some polyunsaturated fats, folic acid and other B vitamins, and vitamin D. So their effect on heart disease risk can't be predicted by considering only their cholesterol content. Also, people

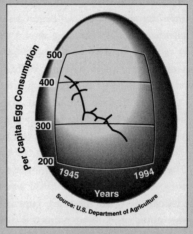

FIG. 10 Per Capita Egg Consumption

respond in different ways to cholesterol in their food. For some people, let's call them responders, the amount of cholesterol in the diet has a direct effect on the amount of cholesterol in the bloodstream. Nonresponders, though, can eat and digest cholesterol with only small or immeasurable changes in the amount of cholesterol in the bloodstream. It also appears that eating eggs has relatively little effect on small, dense LDL, the class of bad cholesterol that poses the greatest risk to cardiovascular health.

No research has ever shown that people who eat more eggs have more heart attacks than people who eat few eggs. And recent research suggests you needn't feel so guilty about eating them. The most comprehensive study to date looked at the egg-eating habits of almost 120,000 men and women. Healthy men and women who ate up to an egg a day were no more likely to have developed heart disease or to have had a stroke over many years of follow-up than those who ate less than one egg a week. For those with diabetes, though, there did seem to be some connection between eating an egg a day and the development of heart disease.

While this study, and others like it, don't give the green light for daily three-egg omelets, they should be reassuring to people who enjoy eggs. If your breakfast choices are an egg, a doughnut fried in trans fat–rich oil, or a bagel made from refined flour, the egg is the better choice, especially if it is fried in healthy vegetable oil.

were thought to provide some protection against disease and aid in recovery. As late as the 1950s, a healthy diet meant eggs, bacon, and butter-slathered toast for breakfast, roast beef and mashed potatoes with gravy for dinner.

Our comfortable, almost thoughtless relationship with food was forever changed by separate threads of research that came together after World War II. Large studies in the late 1940s and early 1950s began to focus on diet as a cause of the skyrocketing rates of heart disease. In 1956, a midwestern scientist named Ancel Keys began an international survey called the Seven Countries Study. It showed a strong connection between saturated fat and heart disease—in general, the higher the amount of saturated fat in a country's diet, the higher the rate of heart disease. Curiously, Keys and his colleagues didn't find any connection between the *total* amount of fat in the diet and heart disease. In fact, the area with the lowest rate of heart disease in the study, Crete, had the highest average total fat intake (about 40 percent of calories), mostly due to liberal use of olive oil. At around the same time, the Framingham Heart Study started tracking the health and habits of more than five thousand men and women living in the town of Framingham, Massachusetts. One of its early findings was that high levels of cholesterol in the bloodstream were often an early signal of impending heart disease. These important studies and others pointed to diet as a key element in the path to heart disease.

Without turning this into a textbook of nutritional epidemiology, I'll briefly describe the consistent evidence from several kinds of studies showing the harmful effects of saturated and trans fats and the benefits that can come from replacing these harmful fats with unsaturated fats.

CROSS-CULTURAL SURVEYS:
THE MORE SATURATED FAT, THE MORE HEART DISEASE

The country-by-country surveys of Ancel Keys and others showed that heart disease rates varied more than tenfold between Crete and Finland, the country with the highest rates. And the more saturated fat in a country's average diet, the more heart disease. Although the Seven Countries and Framingham studies pointed to something about diet and lifestyle as being a major cause of heart disease, other factors linked with saturated fat could have been responsible. Because the highest heart disease rates were seen in the richer Western countries, cigarette smoking, lack of activity, or other aspects of diet could have contributed to the large difference in rates.

METABOLIC STUDIES:
GOOD FATS CAN IMPROVE YOUR CHOLESTEROL PROFILE

In the 1950s and 1960s, dozens of carefully controlled feeding studies among small groups of volunteers showed conclusively that when saturated fat replaced carbohydrate in the diet, total cholesterol levels in the blood rose; and when polyunsaturated fat replaced carbohydrate, total cholesterol levels fell. Thus, for decades we have known that all fats should not be considered equal. Unfortunately, at that time the importance of other blood lipids—HDL in particular—was not appreciated. So those studies gave an incomplete picture

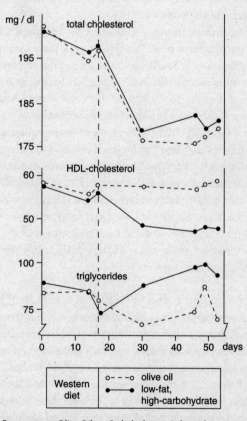

FIG. 11 Blood Fat Responses to Olive Oil vs. Carbohydrates. A diet rich in unsaturated fat (olive oil) improved HDL cholesterol and triglyceride levels compared with a diet rich in carbohydrates.

at best. One of the most compelling pieces of evidence to challenge the emphasis on cutting back on all fat and eating more carbohydrates comes from an experiment by two Dutch scientists. They recruited forty-eight volunteers for an eight-week study. For the first seventeen days, all of the volunteers ate a typical Western diet with about 40 percent of calories from fat. For the next thirty-six days, half of the volunteers were assigned to a diet rich in olive oil and lower in saturated fat, while the other half got a low-fat, high-carbohydrate diet. In both groups, total cholesterol levels plummeted. (See Figure 11.) But in the high-carbohydrate group, levels of HDL (good) cholesterol also fell, while triglycerides rose—both changes that increase the chances of having a heart attack or developing some other form of heart disease. In the olive oil group, the same healthy trend was seen for total cholesterol without the unhealthy changes in HDL and triglycerides.

A later, longer study from the University of Washington took a different approach but got similar results. In this one, 444 men with high cholesterol were asked to follow one of four diets, containing either 30 percent, 28 percent, 22 percent, or 18 percent of fat. After a year, all four diets had lowered LDL (bad) cholesterol. But the two lowest-fat diets also dropped the level of HDL (good) cholesterol and raised the level of triglycerides.

The more we learn about cholesterol, the more we realize that even though total cholesterol is a decent red flag for heart disease risk, what really count are the different cholesterol subtypes. The best cholesterol profile is one with a low level of LDL cholesterol and a high level of HDL. This relationship is neatly captured as a ratio of LDL (or total cholesterol) to HDL. The ratio should be less than 4.5, and the lower the better. The Dutch study, and the many others that have repeated this test, leave no doubt that replacing saturated fats with carbohydrates has little effect on the ratio of LDL to HDL, while replacing saturated fats with unsaturated fats improves it.

COHORT STUDIES: THE MORE GOOD FATS, THE LESS HEART DISEASE

I have had the privilege of being involved in several long-term studies of specific groups (cohorts) of volunteers. Two of these are the Nurses' Health Study and the Health Professionals Follow-up Study (see page 32). Both have yielded valuable information on diet and health. In 1997, we looked at the kinds and amounts of different fats eaten by more than 80,000 nurses who, in 1980, had never been diagnosed with cancer, stroke, or heart disease. Between 1980 and 1994, 684 of these women survived heart attacks, and 281 died from heart disease. The amount of *total* fat in the diet wasn't linked with heart attacks or heart disease deaths because the benefits of the good fats balanced out the hazards of the bad ones. But the amounts of specific types of fats did make a difference. Women who ate more unsaturated fat instead of saturated fat had fewer heart problems. We calculated that replacing 5 percent of total calories as saturated fat with unsaturated fat would reduce the risk of heart attack or death from heart disease by about 40 percent. That would be like eating an ounce of mixed nuts instead of a half cup of ice cream. In contrast, replacing saturated fat with carbohydrates showed much smaller reductions in risk. This study also demonstrated the dangers of trans fats—replacing just 2 percent of total calories from trans fats with the same number of calories from unsaturated fats would cut the risk by 50 percent. That's akin to eating six trans-free Triscuits instead of a larger serving of French fries.

CLINICAL TRIALS:
REPLACING SATURATED FATS WITH UNSATURATED FATS SAVES LIVES

The results of clinical trials looking at overall fat reduction (most of which have been done in people who already have heart disease) are less than impressive. When viewed as a group, they show that eating less total fat—usually by increasing carbohydrate intake—does little for the heart and blood vessels. Total cholesterol levels, an important gauge of heart disease risk, drop only slightly, as does the development of heart disease itself. In stark contrast, clinical trials in which volunteers were randomly assigned to either a standard diet or a diet in which some saturated fat was replaced with unsaturated fat have yielded positive results, including lower total and LDL cholesterol levels and, most important, reductions in heart disease of one-third or more with five years of treatment.

One example of such a trial is the Lyon Diet Heart Study. (See Figure 12.) Begun in 1988, this French trial set out to test whether a so-called Mediterranean diet could reduce second heart attacks or heart-related deaths among 605 men and women who had survived a first heart attack. Half were asked to follow an American Heart Association diet for five years, while the other half were asked to follow a Mediterranean diet that included more whole-grain bread, more root vegetables and green vegetables, more fish and poultry, less red meat, fruit every day, olive oil, no cream, and a special margarine supplied by the study in place of butter. This margarine was made so it contained a similar amount of monounsaturated fat as olive oil. It was low in saturated and trans

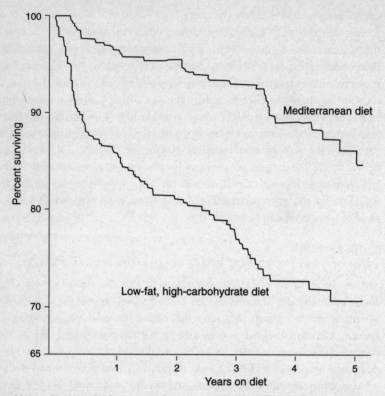

FIG. 12 Lyon Diet Heart Study. Heart attack survivors eating a Mediterranean-type diet had fewer second heart attacks and deaths from heart disease than those on a low-fat, high-carbohydrate diet.

fats and rich in unsaturated fats, especially the essential n-3 polyunsaturated fat known as alpha-linolenic acid. Just two and a half years into the trial, the study's ethics and safety committee ordered it stopped early because the benefits of the Mediterranean diet were so compelling—a 70 percent reduction in deaths from all causes. When the investigators checked in on the study participants several years later, the benefits—including a reduced risk of cancer— seen after two and a half years were still in evidence. Interestingly, most members of the experimental group were still following the study's Mediterranean diet even though the trial was long over.

PLENTY OF PROOF FOR THE BENEFITS OF UNSATURATED FATS

The popular view of science is that if you assemble the facts, they will give you clear, definite answers. The reality of science isn't anything like that, especially when it comes to human nutrition and its connection with disease. We have an ocean of existing facts and a steady deluge of new data, but only a few solid answers. That's because studies are always open to criticism, and their results to interpretation. It is standard operating procedure to conclude that "more research is needed," a phrase I have often used in reporting the results of a study or writing an editorial or review on specific aspects of diet and disease.

I don't feel that way at all about what people should be doing with dietary fat. **Cutting back on all types of fat and eating extra carbohydrates does little to protect against heart disease and will ultimately harm some people. Instead, replacing saturated fats with unsaturated fats is a safe, proven, and delicious way to cut the rates of heart disease.**

TRANS FATS—A SPECIAL CONCERN

In addition to saturated fats, there's another family of fats to stay away from—the trans fats. These are mostly man-made fats that have almost invisibly become a substantial part of the American diet. A century ago, the average American ate a negligible amount of trans fats, getting tiny amounts of naturally occurring ones in meat and milk. Today, they contribute 4 to 7 percent of calories from fat. They're abundant in many margarines, vegetable shortenings, fast-food French fries, doughnuts, commercial baked goods such as packaged pastries and cookies, and countless other foods.

You can think of these as stealth fats because food makers have never had to list trans fats content on food labels. The only way you would know they are in a particular food is to scrutinize the ingredients list and recognize "partially hydrogenated vegetable oil" or "vegetable shortening" as the giveaways for trans fats.

That's changing. After a long, drawn-out review, the Food and Drug Administration (FDA) is finally requiring that food labels list trans fats along with total and saturated fats. (See Fig. 13.) That's certainly a step in the right direction. The new labels will let consumers know what kinds of fats are in the foods they buy and help them avoid those that contain trans fats (see "Cutting Back" on page 92).

The FDA should go even further and remove man-made trans fats from

Nutrition Facts

Serving Size 1 cup (228g)
Servings Per Container 2

Amount Per Serving

Calories 260　　Calories from Fat 120

	% Daily Value*
Total Fat 13g	**20%**
Saturated Fat 5g	**25%**
Trans Fat 2g	
Cholesterol 30mg	**10%**
Sodium 660mg	**28%**
Total Carbohydrate 31g	**10%**
Dietary Fiber 0g	**0%**
Sugars 5g	
Protein 5g	

Vitamin A 4%	•	Vitamin C 2%
Calcium 15%	•	Iron 4%

*Percent Daily Values are based on a 2,000 calorie diet. Your Daily Values may be higher or lower depending on your calorie needs:

		Calories:	2,000	2,500
Total Fat	Less than		65g	80g
Sat Fat	Less than		20g	25g
Cholesterol	Less than		300mg	300mg
Sodium	Less than		2,400mg	2,400mg
Total Carbohydrate			300g	375g
Dietary Fiber			25g	30g

Calories per gram:
Fat 9　•　Carbohydrate 4　•　Protein 4

FIG. 13　New Label for Trans Fats. Instead of hunting for the term "partially hydrogenated" in ingredient lists as a marker of trans fats, you'll be able to see trans fats at a glance on food labels beginning in 2006.

the list of foods and food additives that are generally recognized as safe. They were added to this list in the 1970s, before studies began indicating they were harmful.

How bad are trans fats? Like saturated fats, trans fats raise levels of LDL (bad) cholesterol. They are particularly good at boosting levels of small, dense LDL particles, the kind that are most damaging to arteries. They also elevate levels of triglycerides and lipoprotein (a), which aren't healthy trends since higher levels of each have been linked with heart disease. At the same time, trans fats lower levels of HDL, the protective form of cholesterol, something that saturated fats don't do.

To make matters worse, trans fats make platelets (blood cell fragments that are important in clotting) stickier than usual and so more likely to form clots inside blood vessels in the heart, brain, and elsewhere. The latest research indicates that trans fats also fire inflammation, an overactivity of the immune system that plays key roles in the development of heart disease, diabetes, and probably other leading causes of death and disability.

This double, triple, or even quadruple whammy from trans fats should translate into higher rates of heart disease. It does. The rise in the amount of trans fats made and eaten in the United States suspiciously parallels the rise in heart disease throughout much of this century. Even stronger evidence comes from the Nurses' Health Study. Women who ate the most trans fats (about 7 grams of trans fats, or about 3 percent of daily energy) were 50 percent more likely to have developed heart disease over a fourteen-year period than those who ate the least (slightly over 1 percent of daily energy). Women with the lowest intake of trans fats and the highest intake of polyunsaturated fats were 70 percent *less likely* to have developed heart disease when compared with women who ate the most trans fats and the least polyunsaturated fats.

Trans Fats in Typical Processed Foods

FOOD	SERVING	WEIGHT GRAMS	TRANS FAT GRAMS*
Red Lobster Admiral's Feast	one	—	22
Long John Silver's Fish & More	one	—	14
KFC Chicken Pot Pie	one	370	8
Burger King French Fries**	large	160	5
Dunkin' Donuts			
Old Fashioned Cake Donut	one	71	6
Cinnabon	one	170	6
Van de Kamp's Breaded Fish Sticks	6 pieces	105	5
McDonald's French Fries**	large	170	3
Little Debbie Swiss Cake Rolls	2 rolls	60	4
KFC Biscuit	one	56	4
Pillsbury Grands! Buttermilk Biscuit	one	60	4
Burger King BK Big Fish Sandwich	one	255	3
McDonald's Chicken McNuggets	9 pieces	160	3
Ore-Ida Tater Tots	9 pieces	85	2
Burger King Chicken Sandwich	one	230	2
Nabisco Oreos	3 cookies	33	2
Nabisco Chips Ahoy!	3 cookies	32	2
Nabisco Triscuits	7 crackers	30	2
Nabisco Wheat Thins	16 crackers	28	2
Orville Redenbacher's			
Natural Popcorn	4 cups	30	2
Nabisco Nilla Wafers	8 cookies	30	1
Nabisco Ritz Crackers	5 crackers	16	1
Doritos Corn Chips**	1 ounce	28	0.1

* Note: Federal rules requiring that trans fat be listed on food labels beginning in 2006 have prompted many companies to reduce or eliminate trans fats from many products.

** Analyzed at Harvard School of Public Health, July 2003.

Source: Wootan, M., Liebman, B., Rosofsky, W. "Trans: The Phantom Fat." *Nutrition Action Health-letter* (September 1996).

The Great Butter Battle

Many people accepted the demise of butter in stride, ruing the loss of its savory flavor but agreeing that the effects of its saturated fat on the heart might be too high a price to pay. They dutifully switched to margarine, as researchers and nutritionists suggested. When later reports highlighted the hazards of margarine, though, many people felt betrayed or duped.

There never was any good evidence that switching from butter to margarine cut the chances of having a heart attack or developing heart disease. Making the switch was a well-intentioned guess, given that margarine had less saturated fat than butter, but it overlooked the large amounts of trans fats in margarine.

Today the butter-versus-margarine issue is really a false one. From the standpoint of heart disease, butter is on the list of foods to use sparingly mostly because it contains so much of the kind of saturated fat that aggressively raises levels of LDL (bad) cholesterol. Margarines, though, aren't so easy to classify. Those that are high in trans fats—the older stick margarines that are still widely sold—are worse for you than butter. Some of the newer margarines that are low in saturated fat, high in unsaturated fat, and free of trans fats are fine as long as you don't use too much (they are still rich in calories). Before you reach for either butter or margarine, though, think about whether you could use olive oil or another liquid vegetable oil instead.

Using the Food and Drug Administration's own data, the Center for Science in the Public Interest estimates that removing trans fats from the food supply will prevent between eleven thousand and thirty thousand premature deaths and save $50 billion in medical costs a year. These are almost certainly underestimates, since they were based only on the negative effects of trans fats on LDL (bad) cholesterol and HDL (good) cholesterol and don't take into consideration newer evidence showing other potentially harmful effects and an increased risk of diabetes with higher trans fats consumption.

In Europe, the food industry responded rapidly to concerns over trans fats with commitments to reduce the trans fat content of food. By 1995, margarines in Europe were mostly free of trans fats, and other improvements are ongoing. Denmark, for example, has banned trans fats. In the United States, trans fats in margarines decreased a bit in the 1980s and 1990s as companies began making some margarines and spreads that were higher in polyunsaturated fats and, incidentally, lower in trans fats. These gains have been offset, though, by the fast-food industry's decision to switch the fat they use for deep-frying from beef fat to heavily hydrogenated vegetable oils high in trans fats.

Some U.S. companies have responded to the special hazard from trans fats by removing them from their products. Snack food giant Frito-Lay has removed partially hydrogenated oil from many of its products. Kraft is removing trans fats from Triscuits and other foods. Pepperidge Farms now makes trans-free Goldfish crackers. Even Crisco sells a vegetable shortening free of trans fats.

On the restaurant front, Legal Seafoods, Ruby Tuesday, and a few other farsighted chains use liquid vegetable oil, which is free of trans fats, for deep-frying. Most major chains, though, including McDonald's, Burger King, Dunkin' Donuts, Red Lobster, and others, continue to use trans-rich partially hydrogenated shortening for deep-frying. Interestingly, in countries such as Denmark, which restrict the use of trans fats, McDonald's and Burger King use trans-free cooking oils.

OMEGA-3 FATS—A SPECIAL BENEFIT

One class of polyunsaturated fat deserves individual attention even though it makes up only a minority of the fats in our diet. These are the omega-3 fatty acids (also called the n-3 fats). They are *essential* fats. That means your body needs them for normal functions, and it can't make them from scratch. There are three main types of omega-3 fats in our diets. Since their names are a bit tricky, I'll use their abbreviations: ALA (alpha-linolenic acid), EPA (eicosapentaenoic acid), and DHA (docosahexaenoic acid).

All three are unsaturated fats, meaning they have one or more extra-strong double bonds joining neighboring carbon atoms. The first double bond is on the third carbon from the end (*omega* is Greek for "end," thus the name). Omega-3 fatty acids have the first double bond three carbons from the end. ALA, with eighteen carbons, is sometimes called a medium-chain omega-3; EPA and DHA are sometimes called long-chain omega-3 fats because EPA contains twenty carbons and DHA contains twenty-two.

ALA is the main omega-3 fatty acid in most Western diets. It's found in a variety of vegetable oils and nuts, leafy vegetables, and some animal fat, especially in grass-fed animals (see the table on page 86). EPA and DHA come mainly from fish and so are sometimes referred to as the marine omega-3s. Your body uses ALA mainly for energy, but it can also transform this omega-3 fat into EPA and DHA. The reverse doesn't happen.

What makes omega-3 fatty acids so special? For one thing, they help make up cell membranes throughout the body, especially in the eye, the brain, and sperm cells. For another, they provide the starting point from which some hor-

Alpha-Linolenic Acid in Various Foods

Food	Serving	Weight Grams	Alpha-Linolenic Acid Grams
Flaxseed oil	1 tbsp.	13.6	6.91
English walnuts	1 ounce	28	1.90
Canola oil	1 tbsp.	14	1.30
Soy oil	1 tbsp.	13.6	0.95
Mayonnaise	1 tbsp.	14	0.85
I Can't Believe It's Not Butter!	1 tbsp.	14	0.76
Generic soy margarine	1 tbsp.	14	0.49
Italian salad dressing	1 tbsp.	14	0.45
Shedd's Spread Country Crock	1 tbsp.	14	0.44
Olivio Spread	1 tbsp.	14	0.43
Beef	6 ounces	170	0.38
Benecol Light	1 tbsp.	14	0.38
Brussels sprouts, raw	1 cup	88	0.18
Corn oil	1 tbsp.	13.6	0.14
Promise Soft Margarine	1 tbsp.	14	0.11
Almonds	1 ounce	28	0.11
Kale, raw	1 cup	67	0.09
Olive oil	1 tbsp.	13.5	0.08
Hazelnuts	1 ounce	28	0.06
Cashews	1 ounce	28	0.06
Safflower oil	1 tbsp.	13.6	0.05
Whole milk	1 cup	244	0.05
Cheddar cheese	1 ounce	28	0.05
Chocolate	1 bar	44	0.04
Spinach, raw	1 cup	30	0.04
Peanuts	1 ounce	28	trace

Source: Connor, W. "Alpha-Linolenic Acid in Health and Disease." *American Journal of Clinical Nutrition* (May 1999): 827–28; and analyses performed at Harvard School of Public Health.

mones are made. Omega-3-derived hormones include ones that regulate blood clotting, contraction and relaxation of artery walls, and inflammation. Equally important, these fats have been shown to help prevent or treat heart disease and stroke. They may also help control lupus, eczema, and rheumatoid arthritis and may play protective roles in cancer and other conditions.

The evidence for a protective effect on heart disease is the strongest. Omega-3 fatty acids play a critical role in keeping the heart beating at a steady clip and not lapsing into dangerous, sometimes fatal erratic rhythms. These arrhythmias, as they are called, cause many of the two hundred thousand–plus sudden cardiac deaths that occur each year in the United States—half of which happen to people with no history of heart disease. The story of this discovery begins with a British physiologist's trip to the Arctic to visit Eskimos, a group once remarkable for their low rates of heart disease despite their high-fat diet. Since then, dozens of studies have shown that omega-3 fatty acids prevent heart attacks and sudden cardiac deaths by several mechanisms: preventing erratic rhythms, making blood less likely to form clots inside arteries (the ultimate cause of most heart attacks), improving the balance of cholesterol and other fat particles in the bloodstream, and limiting inflammation (which plays a role in the development of atherosclerosis).

A large randomized trial from Italy bolstered the benefits of omega-3 fatty acids. In the Gruppo Italiano per lo Studio della Sopravvivenza nell'Infarto Miocardio (known as the GISSI Prevention Trial), more than eleven thousand men and women who had survived a heart attack took a 1-gram capsule of omega-3 fatty acids or a placebo capsule every day for more than three years. At the end of this period, the omega-3 group had 10 percent less deaths (especially sudden deaths, which were cut by half), second heart attacks, and strokes.

One popular book, *The Omega Diet* by Artemis Simopoulos and Jo Robinson, is based on the idea (but not on direct evidence in people) that a balance of unsaturated fatty acids is the key to good health. These authors worry that eating too much omega-6 fats and not enough omega-3s can pose problems. The most abundant omega-6 fat in the average American diet is linoleic acid, which is found mainly in vegetable oils. There's no doubt that many Americans could benefit from getting more omega-3 fatty acids. But there is also strong evidence that omega-6 fatty acids, which make up the majority of the polyunsaturated fats in our diet, help shape healthy cholesterol levels and reduce heart disease. In the Nurses' Health Study, the ratio of omega-3 to omega-6 fatty acids wasn't linked with risk of heart disease because both of these were beneficial.

Of course, too much of a good thing can pose problems, and we really don't know the upper limit of healthy omega-6 (or omega-3) fatty acid intake for optimal health. We do know, though, that reducing omega-6 fatty acids from the current amounts in the average American diet is likely to wipe out many of the gains we have made in preventing deaths from heart disease over the last thirty years.

Research on prostate cancer raises questions about a different kind of balance. Results from the Health Professionals Follow-up Study and others have shown that men whose diets are rich in EPA and DHA—the marine omega-3s—are less likely to develop prostate cancer. The story for ALA, though, is a bit worrisome. Some studies show an increase in prostate cancer and advanced prostate cancer among men with high intakes of ALA. Before you pour out your canola oil or trash your walnuts, though, keep in mind that several other studies show no link with ALA, and one large Dutch study showed that ALA helped protect against prostate cancer. Clearly, more research is urgently needed to determine if the heart-protective benefits of ALA are partly offset in men by an increase in prostate cancer.

Given the wide-ranging importance and benefits of omega-3 fatty acids, try to eat at least one good source of them a day. Daily doses of omega-3 fatty acids are especially important for women who are pregnant or hoping to become pregnant. From conception onward, a developing child needs a steady supply of omega-3 fatty acids to form the brain and other parts of the nervous system.

Unfortunately, omega-3 fatty acids aren't as plentiful in the average diet as they once were. Food companies purposely destroy them in vegetable oils to make foods last longer on the shelf without turning rancid. (The process by which this is done, partial hydrogenation, creates trans fats [see page 74]). Meat from cows and chickens now contains fewer omega-3 fatty acids. Where most animals used for food once foraged on wild plants and seeds, which are rich in omega-3 fatty acids, today they are fed grains that are low in them.

The best source of omega-3s is fish, especially fatty fish such as salmon, mackerel, herring, and sardines. Yet the relatively high price now puts fish beyond the budget of many households. Contamination with mercury and other pollutants is also a concern for some. So what's a body to do?

Eating fish twice a week is a good target for almost everyone. Eating more than that adds little extra protection against heart disease. Young children and women in their childbearing years need to pay extra attention to the types of fish they eat and focus on types low in mercury (see "Fish, Mercury, and Fish Oil," page 89). As research in this area continues to unfold, including in your

Fish, Mercury, and Fish Oil

If you like to eat seafood, or think you should eat more of it, you may feel you're caught between the devil and the deep blue sea these days. Fish is a great choice for many reasons—it tastes good, it's a healthier source of protein than red meat, and the omega-3 fats in many types of seafood help the heart. Yet some species contain mercury, polychlorinated biphenyls (PCBs), and other contaminants. Should you stop eating fish? Cut back? Hold the line? The answer depends on who you are.

Mercury and PCBs are definitely dangerous at the high doses you'd see in an industrial accident. In the small amounts found in fish, their effects aren't as clear-cut.

Young children and women who are pregnant, might become pregnant, or who are nursing need to be the most careful about mercury. This metal, which comes from natural sources, industrial emissions, and burning coal, can harm the developing brain and nervous system. Yet getting enough omega-3 fats is especially important during pregnancy and when nursing because they are needed to build a developing child's nervous system.

What about PCBs, which were banned in the 1970s but are still present in the environment? High doses kill fish and cause cancer in laboratory rats. Low doses may cause subtle developmental problems in babies. Studies in adults haven't linked PCBs to cancer or other diseases.

To be on the safe side, it makes sense for children and women of child-bearing age to stay away from shark, swordfish, king mackerel, or tilefish (sometimes called golden snapper or golden bass) because they contain high levels of mercury. But that doesn't mean avoiding seafood altogether. The Food and Drug Administration and Environmental Protection Agency suggest eating up to twelve ounces (two average meals) a week of a variety of fish and shellfish that are lower in mercury, such as salmon, pollock, catfish, and shrimp. Canned tuna warrants special attention because it is easy and inexpensive—making it something that people tend to eat often—and contains intermediate amounts of mercury. Canned albacore (white) tuna has more mercury than light tuna. To be prudent, eat it no more than once a week. (For more information, visit the Food and Drug Administration's Web site on mercury in fish, www.cfsan.fda.gov/~dms/admehg3.html.)

What about men and older women? If you're old enough to worry about heart disease, the definite benefits from eating seafood greatly outweigh the possible (and possibly minuscule) risks from mercury and PCBs. It's prudent to limit seafood species known to carry high levels of mercury to once a month, and you might not want to eat fish every single day.

Fish oil supplements are an alternative if you don't like to eat fish or are worried about contamination. They deliver plenty of EPA and DHA, without the mercury—several chemical analyses of fish oil supplements show negligible amounts of the metal. However, they don't deliver the same benefit that fish can as a replacement for a less healthy source of protein such as steak. You might consider talking with your doctor about taking a fish oil supplement that contains 600–800 milligrams of EPA plus DHA if you:

- have angina (chest pain), have had a heart attack, or are at high risk for one. (You can calculate your risk of having a heart attack using an online calculator provided by the National Heart, Lung, and Blood Institute, hin.nhlbi.nih .gov/atpiii/calculator.asp.) Results from the GISSI trial indicate that fish oil supplements are good for people with heart disease.

- engage in high-intensity sports or activities. Even though the overall risk of heart disease is generally low among people who exercise hard, fatal heart rhythms can appear during and shortly after intense activity. Formal studies haven't yet been done on the effect of fish oil supplements in this group. Even so, it's prudent to have plenty of omega-3 fats aboard in these situations.

diet a good source of ALA on most days of the week ensures an adequate intake of omega-3 fats. Common ways to do this include eating walnuts, flaxseeds, or foods made with or cooked in canola or soybean oil.

DIETARY FAT AND CANCER: A WEAK CONNECTION

The same kind of international comparisons that sparked the dietary fat–heart disease hypothesis have also generated strongly held beliefs about a connection between dietary fat and cancer. Countries with lower average fat intakes (mostly developing or less affluent nations) tend to have lower rates of breast, colon, or prostate cancer than countries with higher average fat intakes. But better, more direct evidence linking diet and cancer has weakened support for this connection.

Throughout the 1960s and 1970s, international comparisons pointed to a link between dietary fat and breast cancer. Keep in mind that many other lifestyle differences between women in traditional cultures and those in Western countries could be responsible, such as age of first menstruation, physical activity, smoking, and other dietary factors like fruit and vegetable or fiber consumption. Case-control studies—those in which women who developed breast cancer were compared with women who did not—also tended to find a connection, although weaker ones than those found in the international comparisons.

Based on a limited number of studies, the U.S. National Research Council concluded back in 1982 that reducing the fat content of the diet from 40 to 30 percent of calories would reduce the number of women diagnosed with breast cancer. Two years later, the National Cancer Institute made this the focus of a major health-promotion campaign. These efforts have borne little fruit in lowering breast cancer, perhaps because they were based on inadequate data.

Later, larger studies of cancer have not supported the dietary fat–breast cancer connection. In the Nurses' Health Study, more than five thousand of the participants have developed breast cancer since 1980. So far we have not seen an increase in breast cancer with higher dietary fat. In fact, the rate of breast cancer among women who ate the most dietary fat was slightly *lower* than the rate among women who ate the least. An analysis of all the large cohort studies from around the world also found no connection between dietary fat and breast cancer, except for an unexpected increase among the small numbers of women with the lowest fat intake.

Most studies into the connection between dietary fat and breast cancer involved postmenopausal women. That makes sense, because breast cancer is more common in older women. But it also can strike younger women, who may be susceptible to different dietary influences. So my colleagues and I examined information collected as part of the Nurses' Health Study II, which includes women between twenty-six and forty-four years old. Over an eight-year period, 714 of the more than 90,000 women developed breast cancer. High intake of animal fat, especially fat from red meat and dairy products, increased the chances of having breast cancer. High intake of vegetable fat did not. I'll talk more about unsettling findings about dairy products in chapter 9.

The clearest and most consistent finding from both animal and human studies is that too many calories, *regardless of food source,* are far more important to the development of breast cancer than dietary fat.

Some early studies suggested a link between dietary fat and colon cancer, the third leading cause of cancer deaths in the United States. But this, too, hasn't been bolstered by more detailed work. There are some strong hints that eating a lot of red meat increases the risk of colon cancer. This could stem from the types of fats in red meat or the cancer-causing chemicals generated by cooking red meat at high temperatures. So far, too many calories in relation to exercise levels is the strongest dietary link with colon cancer—people who are overweight are more likely to develop this cancer than people who aren't. On the flip side, regular physical activity decreases your chances of getting colon cancer. So does not smoking and getting plenty of folic acid, one of the B vitamins (see chapter 10).

The situation for prostate cancer is murkier, partly because there have been relatively few studies in this area. International comparisons show that Asian men, who eat relatively low-fat diets, have substantially lower rates of prostate cancer than their Western counterparts. Although Asian men do experience some increases in prostate cancer when they move to the United States, rates in this group always stay lower than among Caucasians, suggesting that some genetic factors play an important role. If there is a connection between dietary fat and prostate cancer, it seems to be mainly related to animal fat or some other component of red meat. That's good news, because it means that olive oil and other unsaturated fats that decrease the risk of heart disease would not increase the risk of prostate cancer.

It is impossible to prove that there's absolutely no connection between dietary fat and cancer. If fat does influence the development of cancer, though, evidence from large cohort studies with many years of follow-up show that the effect is small. Given the strong and consistent association that has been observed between type of fat and heart disease, I think it makes sense to focus on dietary fats for their proven impact on heart disease, not for their hypothetical connections with cancers that so far have not been supported by good evidence.

SELECTING HEALTHY FATS

The phrase *heart-healthy diet* often conjures up images of steamed rice and vegetables, a platter of baked fish, lots of pasta—easy on the sauce, please—and only dreams of fried onion rings.

If you believe, as I do, that a low-fat diet isn't the way to a healthier heart, there's another option. This one requires a bit of cutting back, just as traditional low-fat diets do, but it also means consciously adding some fats to your diet. This takes some practice at first, but the effort will be well worth it, both in taste and health.

• *Cutting back.* Avoid trans fats whenever and wherever you can, and limit your intake of saturated fats.

Trans fats are everywhere. Until recently, all vegetable shortenings were packed with trans fats. So were most brands of stick margarine. Some companies now offer brands that are low in saturated fat and are virtually trans fat–free. Unfortunately, the bulk of trans fats that we eat—somewhere around 70 percent—is hidden in commercially baked goods like crackers, muffins, and cookies, in other prepared foods, and in fried foods prepared in restaurants. Until now, the only way you could have found these stealth trans fats was by searching the ingredient list of food labels for the words *partially hydrogenated vegetable oils* or *vegetable shortening* or by grilling waiters or cooks while eating out. Now that the FDA is requiring food makers to specifically list trans fats on food labels, you will be able to see what foods contain them. (See Figure 13.) One source of confusion can be that a product is allowed to proclaim itself as "trans fatty acid–free" if it contains less than one-half gram of trans fat per serving—in this case the label will still say "partially hydrogenated vegetable oil." Don't be fooled by labels that proclaim a product as cholesterol-free—it can be high in trans fats and contain no cholesterol. In restaurants, foods "cooked in vegetable oil" aren't necessarily free of trans fats, because these oils may still be heavily hydrogenated.

Now that fast-food restaurants use heavily hydrogenated vegetable fats for deep frying, they are one of our country's largest sources of dietary trans fats. Slipping into the double-digit range doesn't take much effort at all. Eating a doughnut at breakfast (3.2 grams of trans fats) and a large order of French fries for lunch or dinner (6.8 grams of trans fats) represents just under 5 percent of total calories for someone whose usual diet contains two thousand calories.

Limiting saturated fats in your diet basically means going easy on, or avoiding, red meat and whole-fat dairy products. It isn't worth making yourself crazy to eliminate all traces of saturated fat from your diet. For one thing, that's almost impossible to do, since the sources of monounsaturated and polyunsaturated fats also contain some saturated fat. For another, as the Lyon Diet Heart Study and others have shown, eating saturated fats in the right proportion with unsaturated fats is perfectly fine. Try to keep your saturated fat intake below 8 percent of calories, or around 17 grams a day. That's the amount in seven pats of butter, one Pizza Hut Personal Pan Pizza, or three glasses of regular milk.

It isn't necessary to count fat grams or whip out a calculator to compute percentage of calories from fat. You have better things to do with your time, the payoff is very small, and so far there's no solid evidence for adopting exact numerical goals for total fat intake. It does make sense to know what is in the foods you eat, or plan to eat, so you can make healthy choices. But I don't recommend keeping precise tallies all day long.

• *Adding in.* Once you have a handle on the saturated and trans fats in your diet, you'll find there are plenty of easy and delicious ways to replace them with unsaturated fats. The healthiest mix of monounsaturated and polyunsaturated fats hasn't yet been determined. For now, a combination of these

Percentage of Specific Types of Fat in Common Oils and Fats*

OILS	SATURATED	MONO-UNSATURATED	POLY-UNSATURATED	TRANS	ALPHA-LINOLENIC ACID**
Canola	7%	58%	29%	0%	12%
Safflower	9	12	74	0	0
Sunflower	10	20	66	0	2
Corn	13	24	60	0	1
Olive	13	72	8	0	1
Soybean	16	44	37	0	7
Peanut	17	49	32	0	1
Palm	50	37	10	0	0
Coconut	87	6	2	0	0
COOKING FAT					
Original Crisco	25	36	30	11	2
Lard	39	44	11	1	0
Beef fat	39	49	3	8	3
Chicken fat	27	41	31	0	0
Butter	64	29	6	3	1
MARGARINES/ SPREADS					
Imperial Stick	18	2	29	23	4
Fleischmann Tub	19	31	46	6	1
Shedd's Country Crock Tub	21	27	49	5	6
Promise 60% Tub	21	26	51	3	1

* Values expressed as percent of total fat; data are from analyses performed at Harvard School of Public Health Lipid Laboratory and USDA publications.

** Alpha-linolenic acid is also included in polyunsaturated fat.

is a good strategy and gives you plenty of flexibility in your diet. (See the table above.)

One of the best sources of monounsaturated fats is olive oil, which is every bit as versatile as butter. You can sauté vegetables in it, use it for stir-frying chicken or fish, add it as the base for salad dressings, even dip bread in it at the table instead of using butter, as is done in Spain, Italy, and Greece. Different olive oils have different flavors, so it also gives you a wider range of tastes. Other good sources of monounsaturated fats include canola oil, peanut oil, avocados, walnuts, peanuts, and most other nuts.

The main sources of polyunsaturated fats include vegetable oils such as corn and soybean oil, legumes such as soybeans and soy products, and seeds. One easy way to replace saturated fats with unsaturated fats is to use fish, poultry, nuts, and seeds in place of red meat wherever possible. Also, chicken fat is much higher in polyunsaturated fat than beef fat, probably the main reason why substituting chicken for red meat is related to a lower risk of heart disease. (See recipes.)

PUTTING IT INTO PRACTICE

- Remember that some fats are good for you—unsaturated fats protect against heart disease and other chronic conditions.
- Make decisions about dietary fats based on their proven impact on heart disease, not by their weak—if any—connection with cancer.
- Limit the amount of saturated fat in your diet, as the American Heart Association, National Cholesterol Education Program, and others recommend. But there is no good evidence that replacing saturated fat with carbohydrates will protect you against heart disease, while there is solid proof that replacing saturated fat with unsaturated fats will help.
- Reduce saturated fats by limiting the amount of full-fat dairy products you eat and by replacing red meat with nuts, legumes, poultry, and fish whenever possible.
- Use liquid vegetable oils in cooking and at the table.
- Eat one or more good sources of omega-3 fatty acids every day—fish, walnuts, canola or soybean oil, ground flaxseeds or flaxseed oil.

FAT SUBSTITUTES

The pinnacle of the all-fat-is-bad movement may have been the widely hyped introduction of the fake fat known as olestra. From a scientific standpoint, olestra is a marvel of food engineering. From a public health standpoint, olestra—sold under the misleading trade name Olean—could have been a disaster had it ever caught on.

The basic idea behind fat substitutes—that fats are intrinsically unhealthy—is fundamentally wrong. Some fats, the saturated and trans fats, are indeed unhealthy. But unsaturated fats, which make up the majority of fats we eat, actually

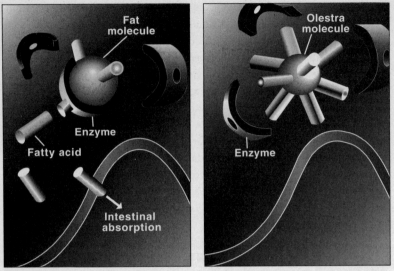

FIG. 14 Natural Fat vs. Olestra. Digestive enzymes break apart natural fats by snipping off fatty acids from the fat molecule's central core. Olestra's shape makes it impossible for these enzymes to surround and remove the fatty acids.

reduce cholesterol levels and protect against heart disease and stroke. America's fat phobia has been further fueled by the misguided notion that only dietary fat makes us fat. What really counts is total calories, regardless of food type.

An ordinary fat molecule consists of a three-carbon core (glycerol) attached to three fatty acid arms. Olestra is completely different. Its starts out as an ordinary 12-carbon molecule of table sugar (sucrose). The sucrose is then chemically processed so it is attached to six to eight fatty acids. These fatty acids surround and protect the sucrose center. (See Figure 14.)

In your mouth, olestra acts much like the fats made by plants and animals—its fatty acid arms trigger the same sensations on your taste buds. In your digestive system, though, olestra is a completely different beast. The enzymes that break down fats are designed for the natural models. They snip off the fatty acid arms where they join the glycerol core. These small fats then pass through the intestinal wall and into the bloodstream. Olestra, though, is a foreign invader that your digestive system can't recognize. Like a football team's defensive line, the fatty acids in olestra crowd together and prevent the enzymes from zipping in and clipping the connection between the sucrose core and the fatty acid arms.

And because the intact olestra molecule is much too large to pass through the intestinal wall, it slides unchanged through the digestive system.

This certainly sounds innocent enough. A bag of potato chips fried in olestra delivers to your bloodstream none of the fat found in a similar-size bag of chips fried in corn oil. (Keep in mind that olestra doesn't interfere a bit with your ability to digest and store away the carbohydrates.) According to studies done by olestra's maker, Procter & Gamble, the use of fake-fat snacks could lower the proportion of fat calories in the diet by 1 percent to 3 percent. That certainly won't translate into long-term weight loss for several reasons. People eating chips or other snacks made with olestra might be inclined to eat more than usual—because they are *fat-free!* That's often what happens to people who eat fat-free cookies. They forget that the carbohydrates in these snacks are easily turned into fat. Also, people unconsciously tend to keep their caloric intake at the same level, olestra or no olestra.

The real problem with olestra is its effect on fat-soluble vitamins and other phytochemicals. Vitamins A, D, E, and K, as well as beta-carotene, lycopene, and a host of other plant pigments and phytochemicals, can't get into the bloodstream unless they are ferried through the intestinal wall aboard fat molecules. Olestra soaks up these fat-loving substances in the digestive system and whisks them out into the stool. This robs the body of a host of substances that play roles in preventing heart disease, cancer, dementia, and other chronic diseases. Procter & Gamble is adding vitamins A, E, and K to make up for these losses, but this won't do anything for the other carotenoids and as-yet-unnamed substances that are important for long-term health.

Olestra's nutrient-robbing effect isn't just theory. Eating a small one-ounce bag of chips made with olestra every day dramatically lowers carotenoid levels in the bloodstream. If this fake fat is ever used in fast-food restaurants, something for which Procter & Gamble once petitioned the FDA, or as a replacement for Crisco or other vegetable shortenings at home, it could have a major negative effect on public health. Although olestra managed to slide through our FDA (with the help of intensive lobbying), it is officially banned in Canada.

Several other fake fats are also on the market. Simplesse, made by Monsanto, is protein from milk whey that's been heated and whipped until the particles are microscopic. These tiny particles roll over the taste buds just like fat and trick them into thinking they are tasting fat. Because this airy mixture deflates and loses its creamy qualities when heated, it is used mostly in ice cream, sour cream, and other cool foods. It is usually listed on the food label as whey protein. A gram of Simplesse yields just over a calorie, compared with nine calories per gram of fat. Simplesse could be a nutritional plus if used in place of animal or trans fats, but its limited applications mean it probably won't have a major impact on health.

Oatrim, a fat substitute devised by George Inglett, a chemist with the USDA's Agriculture Research Service, is made by cooking oats, separating the soluble fiber, then drying the sticky slurry and grinding it into a powder. When mixed with water and whipped, it turns into a heavy, creamlike liquid that can be used in baked goods, salad dressings, sauces, and ice cream. Oatrim is rich in beta-glucans, a group of soluble fibers that contribute to the cholesterol-lowering properties of oats and barley.

Fat substitutes like olestra offer health hazards rather than improvements. Those such as Oatrim, however, could be beneficial if they are used in place of saturated or trans fats. Oatrim's soluble fiber could further reduce cholesterol levels. An equally healthy solution is to use liquid vegetable oils in place of saturated or trans fats. The bottom line is that we don't need new gimmicks or fake foods in order to have healthy diets. We can do this today in a way that makes eating a pleasure.

CHAPTER FIVE

Carbohydrates for Better and Worse

LIKE AN EASY MIDDLE CHILD, carbohydrates were once overlooked. Fats got most of the attention and fruits and vegetables the praise. That changed with the emergence and incredible popularity of the Atkins, South Beach, and other low-carb diets. Almost overnight, carbohydrates plummeted from being the "go to" foods for healthy eating and weight loss to culinary creeps.

As is the case with so many popular fads, the case against carbs began with a kernel of good science that has since been lost in hype and in the tragic generalization that all carbohydrates are the same.

In most parts of the world, carbohydrates provide the lion's share of calories. They contribute more toward weight maintenance or weight gain than any other nutrient. By wielding control over blood sugar, they have a critical influence on the development of diabetes, one of the fastest-growing chronic diseases in the United States and around the world. Last, but certainly not least, the type of carbohydrate in your diet may be as important as the type of fat in the development of heart disease, or protection against it, something largely ignored in the popular media.

In fact, eating the right type of carbohydrate—meaning grains that are as intact and unprocessed as possible—stands right next to maintaining your weight and choosing the right kind of fat in the foundation of a healthy diet.

Until the low-carb diet returned from oblivion a few years ago, the prevailing attitude was that all so-called complex carbohydrates are good, or at least benign, compared with fats. This idea came from rather simplistic looks at diet and disease in China and other developing countries. In general, the Chinese eat mostly carbohydrates, with a sprinkling of protein and fat. They also have very low rates of heart disease. Putting one and one together, some dietary experts concluded that the low rates of heart disease in China were the result of the high-carbohydrate, low-fat diet and transplanted that idea to the West. The "carbohydrates are good" message has been a key part of the recommendations from the American Heart Association, American Cancer Society, and World Health Organization. It has also traditionally formed the base of the USDA's dietary recommendation.

Like many transplants, though, this one isn't doing so well on foreign soil. Even as we tried to cut back on fat and ate more carbohydrates, we got fatter as a nation. The steady decline in rates of death due to heart disease that occurred during the 1970s and early 1980s has slowed. And the percentage of adult Americans with diabetes has almost tripled over the last 20 years. This tough-to-manage disease now affects an estimated 18 million Americans. Around the world, the number of adults with diabetes is expected to jump from 135 million in 1995 to 300 million by 2025.

THE WRONG TYPES OF CARBOHYDRATES
DO MORE HARM THAN GOOD

Why isn't a higher-carbohydrate diet paying off for us the same way it appears to for the Chinese? On average, the Chinese weigh less and are much more physically active than we are. Weight and exercise matter—high-carbohydrate diets have different effects on lean, active people than they do on overweight, sedentary people. So simply eating a high-carbohydrate diet doesn't offer blanket protection against heart disease, cancer, and diabetes, something the Chinese are also learning. In Beijing, for example, there has been a 400 percent increase in diabetes over the last few years as desk jobs replace manual labor and carbohydrate intake remains high.

The other big problem is that little attention has been paid to the *types* of carbohydrates we eat. A diet high in refined carbohydrates that are quickly digested and absorbed can have damaging consequences. These include higher levels of blood sugar, insulin, and triglycerides, and lower levels of HDL (good) cholesterol. In other words, more cardiovascular disease and diabetes. In the Healthy Eating Pyramid, refined carbohydrates are in the "Use Sparingly" category, meaning you will do yourself a favor by expanding your diet to include intact, whole-grain carbohydrates at most meals.

Carbohydrates from grains, fruits, and vegetables can give you a good share of your daily calories. For optimal health, though, it is important to rely on carbohydrates from whole grains, things like whole-wheat bread, brown rice, whole-grain pasta, and other possibly unfamiliar grains like kasha, quinoa, whole oats, and bulgur. Not only will these foods help protect you against a range of chronic diseases, they can also expand the palette of tastes, textures, and colors you can use to please your palate.

NOT JUST SIMPLE VS. COMPLEX

Carbohydrates have traditionally been divided into two categories: simple and complex. Simple carbohydrates have been portrayed as the bad boys of nutrition, while complex carbohydrates are regarded as the golden children. This is a gross oversimplification. Not all simple carbohydrates are bad, and not all complex carbohydrates are good. Later in this chapter I will describe two far more useful ways of categorizing carbohydrates: by their effect on blood sugar (the glycemic index) and by whether they come from refined or whole grains.

Simple carbohydrates are sugars. The simplest simple carbohydrates are glucose (sometimes called dextrose), fructose (also called fruit sugar), and galactose (a part of milk sugar). Table sugar is sucrose, which is made by joining a molecule of glucose with one of fructose. Milk contains lactose, which is made by joining a molecule of glucose with one of galactose. Simple carbohydrates provide us with energy and little else.

Complex carbohydrates are more . . . well, complex. In essence, they are long chains of linked sugars. Although there are many types of complex carbohydrates in our food, the main one is starch, a long chain of glucose molecules. The human digestive system can break down complex carbohydrates like starch into their component sugars. Others are quite indigestible and pass largely unchanged through the stomach and the intestines. These indigestible carbohydrates, called fiber, are an important part of our diet.

WHY CARBOHYDRATES MATTER

In the average American diet, carbohydrates contribute about half of all calories. And a staggering half of these "carbohydrate calories" come from just eight sources:

- soft drinks, sodas, and fruit-flavored drinks;
- cake, sweet rolls, doughnuts, and pastries;
- pizza;
- potato chips, corn chips, and popcorn;
- rice;
- bread, rolls, buns, English muffins, and bagels;
- beer and;
- French fries and frozen potatoes.

Corn Syrup Isn't to Blame

One of the many dramatic changes in the American diet over the past forty years has been in how we satisfy our craving for sugar. Until the 1970s, we relied almost exclusively on sucrose (table sugar) from sugar cane and sugar beets, with a bit of honey, maple sugar, and molasses thrown in for variety. Today, more than half comes from corn, most of it in the form of high-fructose corn syrup. It's found in everything from sugared sodas to ketchup and baby food.

Why the change? High-fructose corn syrup tastes sweeter than sucrose. It's easier to blend into beverages. And it costs a few pennies less per pound than sucrose.

Some people see a downside to high-fructose corn syrup. It's been cast as one of the villains behind the obesity epidemic for two main reasons: The jump in its use closely parallels the trajectory of obesity rates. And the body metabolizes fructose differently from glucose.

There's just one problem. Table sugar contains glucose and fructose in equal proportions, since sucrose is made of one glucose molecule joined to one fructose molecule. High-fructose corn syrup is pure glucose mixed with pure fructose in almost equal proportions. So it's likely that table sugar and corn sweeteners have much the same physiological impact on blood sugar, insulin, and metabolism.

Some people claim that they've lost weight by cutting high-fructose corn syrup from their diets. That may be so, but it probably isn't because they eliminated corn sweeteners, but because by doing so they took in fewer added sugars and thus fewer calories.

So far, high-fructose corn sweetener doesn't seem to be a greater dietary disaster than any other kind of added sugar. What's important is limiting your intake of *all* added sugars. Keeping these well under 10 percent of daily calories (roughly ten teaspoons), the World Health Organization recommendation, is a good goal.

In other words, many of our calories come from sugars or highly refined and easily digested grains.

When you eat a slice of bread, a potato, or a candy bar, the digestible carbohydrates it contains are broken down to their sugar components. Glucose molecules are rapidly absorbed into the bloodstream and swiftly shuttled to the farthest reaches of the circulation. Because these simple sugar molecules are the primary fuel for most of the body's tissues, complex mechanisms are in place to make sure that the level of glucose in the bloodstream doesn't shoot too high or drift too low.

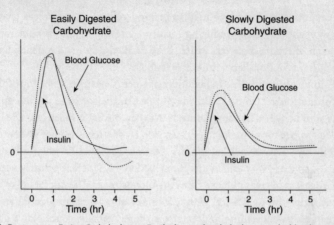

FIG. 15 Response to Eating Carbohydrates. Easily digested carbohydrates make blood sugar and insulin rise faster and higher—and fall further—than slowly digested carbohydrates.

The rise in blood sugar (glucose) is followed quickly by a parallel rise in insulin. (See Figure 15.) This hormone, produced by special cells in the pancreas, ushers glucose inside of muscle and other cells. As cells sponge up glucose, blood sugar levels fall first, followed closely by insulin levels. Once your blood sugar hits its baseline, the liver begins releasing stored glucose to maintain a constant supply.

Several hours after a snack or meal brimming with easily digested carbohydrates, the resulting flood of insulin can drive glucose levels too low. If there isn't any more digestible carbohydrate in the stomach or intestines, your gut and brain start sending out hunger signals to make you grab for more food even as the liver starts releasing stored glucose. A meal of slowly digested whole-grain carbohydrates and protein smooths out this glucose-insulin roller coaster. Because it takes longer for the digestive system to break these carbohydrates into sugar molecules, blood sugar and insulin levels rise more slowly and peak at lower levels. A more drawn-out process also means it may take longer to get hungry again.

THE PROBLEM OF INSULIN RESISTANCE

In a growing number of people, the body's tissues don't respond to insulin as they should and resist its "open up for sugar" signal. This resistance to insulin keeps blood sugar at high levels for longer periods and forces the pancreas to produce extra insulin in order to jam glucose into cells. Like an overworked, undermaintained pump, the insulin-making cells in the pancreas may wear out and eventually stop producing insulin. Faltering insulin production is an early sign of type 2 diabetes, which is also called non-insulin-dependent diabetes and was once called adult-onset diabetes.

Four things contribute to insulin resistance. Obesity is at the top of the list. The further you get from a healthy body mass index (see page 38), the more difficulty your body has handling glucose. Next on the list is inactivity. The less active you are, the lower the ratio of muscle to fat you have, even if your weight is perfectly fine. Muscle cells, especially if they are exercised regularly, handle insulin and glucose very efficiently. Fat cells don't. So the less muscle you have, the harder it is to clear glucose from the bloodstream. Dietary fats play a modest role in insulin resistance, with low intake of polyunsaturated fat and high intake of trans fats leading to greater resistance. Finally, genes play a part. Insulin resistance is more common among Native Americans, Pacific Islanders, and other people of Asian heritage than it is among those of European descent. But people with a genetic predisposition to insulin resistance can beat the condition by staying lean, being physically active, and eating the right diet.

Insulin resistance isn't just a blood sugar problem. It has also been linked with a variety of other problems, including high blood pressure, high levels of triglycerides, low HDL (good) cholesterol, heart disease, and possibly some cancers.

HIGH-CARBOHYDRATE DIETS ARE ESPECIALLY BAD
FOR PEOPLE WHO ARE OVERWEIGHT

People who are overweight appear to fare worse on a diet high in carbohydrates than do lean people. In the Nurses' Health Study, for example, eating a lot of easily digested carbohydrates is most strongly connected to increased odds of having a heart attack among women who are overweight. What's more, experiments in which volunteers were asked to follow high-carbohydrate, low-fat diets ended up with heart-unhealthy changes in levels of HDL and triglycerides, not to mention higher levels of blood sugar and insulin, and these changes were the most pronounced in overweight people.

Put more plainly, a low-fat, high-carbohydrate diet may be among the worst eating strategies for someone who is overweight and not physically active. The Healthy Eating Pyramid recommends a diet that includes fewer refined carbohydrates, more good fats, and more carbohydrates from intact grains. Whether or not you are overweight, the switch from refined to whole grains will be healthy because of the increased intake of micronutrients.

THE GLYCEMIC INDEX:
HOW DO CARBOHYDRATES AFFECT YOUR BODY SUGAR?

Some foods containing carbohydrates make blood sugar spike in a flash. Others yield their sugars more slowly, acting like those sustained-release cold capsules you may have seen advertised on television.

Not long ago, the rule of thumb was that sugars triggered rapid rises in blood sugar and insulin, while complex carbohydrates caused more delayed responses. But nutrition researcher David Jenkins and his colleagues at the University of Toronto turned this conventional wisdom on its head by systematically testing the impact of different carbohydrates on blood sugar levels compared with white bread. (See "Measuring the Glycemic Index and Glycemic Load.") The carbohydrate ranking they developed, called the glycemic index (GI), counters the notion that all complex carbohydrates are good and all simple ones are bad. The higher a food's glycemic index, the faster and stronger it affects blood sugar and insulin levels. As a reference point, pure glucose—the rapidly digested essence of blood sugar—is assigned a score of 100. On this scale, anything below 55 or so is considered a low-glycemic-index food. A low glycemic load is considered to be anything below 10.

Some of the glycemic index rankings are exactly what you might expect. An apple has a glycemic index of 38. A serving of old-fashioned (not instant) oatmeal has a glycemic index of 58. Ten jelly beans have a glycemic index of 78. Other rankings come as a surprise. Cornflakes, surely a complex carbohydrate, are in the 80s, while ice cream and a Snickers bar—which most people would assign to the simple carbohydrate camp—have lower glycemic index rankings than white bread, a classic complex carbohydrate. Perhaps surprisingly, dark bread can have just as high a glycemic index value as white bread if the flour is finely ground. However, its higher content of fiber and other nutrients sets it apart as a healthier choice.

Foods with a high glycemic index can offer a fast energy boost by quickly increasing blood sugar levels. (That's one reason some people who use insulin to treat diabetes are urged to carry glucose tablets when they travel or exercise.) But such foods also promote equally swift drops in blood sugar that may trigger the early return of hunger. In contrast, the steadier, more sustained release of glucose associated with low–glycemic index foods may stave off hunger for longer periods. They may also help keep diabetes at bay.

Glycemic Index and Glycemic Load Values for Commonly Eaten Foods (Relative to Glucose)

The glycemic index and glycemic load offer information about how a food affects blood sugar and insulin. The lower the glycemic index or glycemic load, the less the food affects blood sugar and insulin levels. A glycemic index below 55 and a glycemic load below 10 are considered low.

Foods	Serving Size	Glycemic Index (%)	Carbohydrate (grams)	Glycemic Load*
Pancake	2 six-inch	83	56	46
Cornflakes	1 cup	81	48	38
Total	1 cup	76	40	31
Grape-Nuts	1/2 cup	71	41	29
Coca-Cola	12 ounces	63	39	25
Cranberry juice	1 cup	68	36	24
White rice	5 ounces	64	36	23
Jelly beans	1 ounce	78	28	22
Snickers bar	1 bar (2 ounces)	68	32	22
Raisin Bran	1 cup	61	35	21
Pasta	1 cup	42	47	20
Shredded Wheat	2 biscuits	75	20	15
Potatoes, mashed	1 cup	74	20	15
Cheerios	1 cup	74	20	15
Oatmeal (rolled oats)	1 cup	58	22	13
Banana (ripe)	1 medium	51	25	13
Orange juice	1 cup	52	23	12
White bread	1 slice	70	14	10
Strawberry jam	1 tbsp	51	20	10
Pizza Hut Super Supreme Pizza	2 slices	36	24	9
Whole-wheat bread	1 slice	71	13	9
English muffin	1 muffin	77	11	8
Ice cream	1/2 cup	61	13	8
All-Bran	1/2 cup	42	21	8

Foods	Serving Size	Glycemic Index (%)	Carbohydrate (grams)	Glycemic Load*
Sugar, table	1 tsp	68	10	7
Baked beans	1 cup	48	15	7
Apple	1 medium	38	15	6
Pumpernickel (dark rye bread)	1 slice	41	12	5
Milk, skim	1 cup	32	13	4
Carrots	½ cup	47	6	3

* The glycemic load is calculated by multiplying the grams of carbohydrate by the glycemic index.

Source: Foster-Powell K., Holt, S. H., and Brand-Miller, J. C. "International Tables of Glycemic Index and Glycemic-Load-Values." *American Journal of Clinical Nutrition* 62 (2002): 5–56. The entire list is available for free at www.ajcn.org/cgi/content/full/76/1/5. The University of Sydney (Australia) maintains a free searchable database of glycemic index and glycemic load values at www.glycemicindex.com.

GLYCEMIC LOAD: THE *AMOUNT* OF CARBOHYDRATE MATTERS, TOO

Although the glycemic index of a food is helpful information, it is only part of the story. The full effect of a food on blood glucose and insulin levels depends on both the amount of carbohydrate and the glycemic index of that carbohydrate (protein and fat have small effects on blood glucose). For this reason, my colleagues and I developed the concept of "glycemic load." This is the amount of carbohydrate in a food multiplied by the glycemic index of that carbohydrate. Glycemic load better reflects a food's effect on your body's biochemistry than either the amount of carbohydrate or the glycemic index alone. This is important—some popular diet books warn against eating carrots because they were initially thought to have a high glycemic index. Even if they do, carrots are mostly water, with only a small amount of carbohydrate. Finally, it's important to consider the other nutrients in a food. For example, the glycemic load of most commercial whole-wheat bread is only slightly lower than for white bread because the starch is pulverized into fine particles in both products. But the whole-wheat bread is a better choice because the fiber and other nutrients are removed from the white bread. Best of all would be a coarsely ground whole-grain bread.

While the glycemic load is a useful tool for deciding what to eat, don't build your whole diet around it. Some carbohydrate-rich foods deliver far more than just blood sugar. Fruits and vegetables offer fiber, vitamins, minerals, and plenty of active phytochemicals. The same is true for intact or slightly processed grains. The biggest value of the glycemic load may be for deciding among various options. When picking a snack or meal, choosing foods with a low glycemic load is excellent for your heart and your insulin-making cells.

WHAT DETERMINES A FOOD'S GLYCEMIC INDEX AND GLYCEMIC LOAD?

One general trend you can see in the glycemic index table is that products made from refined grains, things like white bread, bagels, and crackers, have a rapid and strong influence on blood sugar. Those that are less refined, such as

Measuring the Glycemic Index and Glycemic Load

Building the library of glycemic index values for foods has been a relatively slow, painstaking effort. That's because each food must be tested on a number of volunteers, and each volunteer must be tested several times. The basic steps are the same. A healthy volunteer fasts overnight. The next morning he or she drinks a glass of water in which 50 grams of glucose have been dissolved (or, alternately, eats 50 grams of white bread). Over the next two hours, blood samples are taken at regular intervals to measure the rise and fall of glucose and insulin. On another day, the same volunteer eats enough of the test food— cooked potato, whole-grain bread, kiwi fruit, ice cream, and so on—to consume 50 grams of carbohydrates and sits through another two hours of blood sampling. The glycemic index for that food for that individual is calculated by dividing his or her blood sugar response to the test food by the response to pure glucose or white bread. The numbers in the tables, then, represent percentages. For example, black beans have a glycemic index of 30. This means that they boost blood sugar only 30 percent as much as pure glucose.

Because everyone processes food and responds to glucose a little differently, the glycemic index published in tables is usually the average of eight to ten volunteers.

Once a food's glycemic index is in hand, calculating the glycemic load is easy. It involves multiplying the glycemic index by the amount of carbohydrate actually consumed. One-quarter of a cantaloupe, then, with a glycemic index value of 65 and 5.6 grams of carbohydrate, would have a glycemic load of about 3.7 (65 percent times 5.6). A mashed potato, with a glycemic index of 74 and 20 grams of carbohydrate, would have a glycemic load of 15.

whole-grain breads and cereals, have relatively lower glycemic indices, as do beans, vegetables, and fruits.

Several things determine how rapidly the carbohydrates in a particular food are broken down and the resulting glucose absorbed into the bloodstream:

• *How swollen (gelatinized) the starch grains are.* Starch grains swollen to the bursting point with water or heat, such as those in a boiled or baked potato, are more easily digested than the relatively unswollen starch grains found in brown rice.

• *How much the food has been processed.* Grinding wheat into superfine flour dramatically increases the attack rate of digestive enzymes. Not only does flour have greater surface area than coarsely ground wheat grains, but it has been stripped of the protective, hard-to-digest, fibrous outer coat that temporarily fends off enzymes from digesting the starch inside. Regular oatmeal, which is made of smashed oat grains, has a higher glycemic index than oats that are intact or sliced, usually sold as steel-cut oats.

• *How much fiber it contains.* As indigestible fiber passes through the intestine, it carries along partly digested food, shielding it from immediate digestion. This spreads out the release of glucose into the blood.

• *How much fat the snack or meal contains.* Fats tend to increase the time it takes for food to leave the stomach and enter the intestine. So a food that contains fat may temper the rise in blood sugar.

GLYCEMIC INDEX AND GLYCEMIC LOAD: BEYOND HEART DISEASE AND DIABETES

As people with diabetes come to know, chronically high levels of blood sugar and insulin aren't good for the body. They contribute to many of the complications of diabetes, such as nerve damage, loss of vision, kidney disease, sexual dysfunction, and wounds that won't heal. Recent research suggests that the excess blood sugar and insulin that come from eating a high-glycemic diet contribute to other chronic conditions besides heart disease and diabetes. These include breast cancer, colon cancer, and polycystic ovary syndrome.

For now, though, the main benefits for managing your glycemic load are preventing heart disease and diabetes and controlling weight.

REFINED GRAINS VS. INTACT GRAINS

Webster's defines the word *refined* as "free from impurities." That certainly applies to grains. Unfortunately, the "impurities" removed by refining include fiber, vitamins, minerals, and a variety of other micronutrients and phyto-chemicals.

Let's look at wheat as an example. Wheat is a gigantic relative of the grass that grows in yards and parks all across America. The hollow stem supports a seed head that's tightly packed with many individual wheat grains. Our ancestors often used these grains as they came from the plant, and many people still use these "wheat berries" with meals or in breakfast porridges. Today, though, most wheat is processed and refined. The milling process first cracks the wheat grains, then pulverizes them with a series of rollers. In this way the starchy, carbohydrate-rich center, called the endosperm, is separated from both the dark, fibrous bran and the wheat embryo, called the wheat germ.

At each stage of milling, something is lost. Removing the wheat germ pulls out vitamins and unsaturated fats. Whacking away the branny outer layer removes fiber, magnesium, and more vitamins. By the time whole-wheat grains have been turned into white flour, the final product is a pale shadow of the original, literally and nutritionally. (See Figure 16.)

If intact grains are so healthy, why did we stop eating them and shift to highly refined grains? It's partly a function of perception. Once it became possible to refine wheat, it was marketed as being purer than whole-grain flour. At first, white flour was a novelty for the upper classes. The bread and pastries it made were lighter and airier than their whole-grain cousins. In time, buying white flour became a symbol of moving up in the world. The shift was also driven by the reality of storage—white flour, with almost none of the healthy oils found in whole-grain flour, keeps longer. Whole-grain flours must be used more quickly and/or refrigerated.

For the past decade my colleagues and I have been studying the health effects of refined and intact grain foods with the dedicated help of the men and women participating in the Nurses' Health Study and Health Professionals Follow-up Study. The result of this work is compelling—compared with a diet high in refined carbohydrates, eating intact grain foods is clearly better for sustained good health and offers protection against a variety of chronic diseases. Other research around the world points to the same conclusion.

WHOLE GRAINS PROTECT AGAINST DIABETES

Eating whole grain products helps keep the body's sugar control system on track. In both the Nurses' Health Study and the Health Professionals Follow-up Study, participants who ate the most cereal fiber from grains (about 7.5

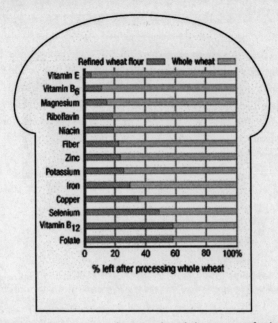

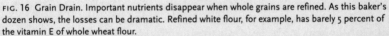

FIG. 16 Grain Drain. Important nutrients disappear when whole grains are refined. As this baker's dozen shows, the losses can be dramatic. Refined white flour, for example, has barely 5 percent of the vitamin E of whole wheat flour.

grams per day, the equivalent of a bowl of oatmeal and two pieces of whole-wheat bread) were 30 percent less likely to develop type 2 diabetes than those who ate the least grain fiber (less than 2.5 grams per day). The combination of low cereal fiber and high glycemic load more than doubled the risk of developing diabetes. (See Figure 17.) In these studies, eating high-fiber cold breakfast cereal seemed to have a protective effect on the development of diabetes, while soft drinks, white bread, white rice, French fries, and cooked potatoes were all associated with increased risk of diabetes.

INTACT GRAINS MEAN LESS HEART DISEASE

Other research from the Nurses' Health Study looked at the link between intact grains and heart disease. Women who reported eating the most intact grain foods, an average of 2.5 servings a day, were 30 percent less likely to develop heart disease than women eating the fewest, about 1 serving a week. Most of

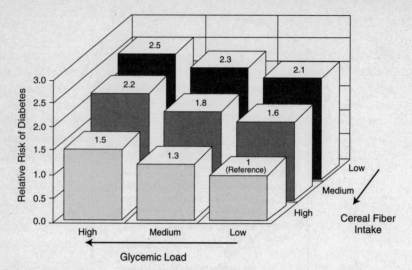

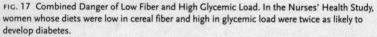

FIG. 17 Combined Danger of Low Fiber and High Glycemic Load. In the Nurses' Health Study, women whose diets were low in cereal fiber and high in glycemic load were twice as likely to develop diabetes.

the whole grain came from whole-grain breakfast cereals, brown rice, and whole-grain bread. We estimated that eating a bowl of cold breakfast cereal that supplies about 5 grams of fiber cuts the chances of heart disease by about one-third. The protective effect was larger in overweight women than it was in lean women. These benefits have also been seen consistently in other long-term studies of heart disease.

THEY IMPROVE GI HEALTH, TOO

Constipation is the number one gastrointestinal complaint in the United States. It accounts for more than two million physician visits a year, and we spend close to $1 billion a year on over-the-counter laxatives. By keeping the stool soft and bulky, the fiber in intact grains helps prevent this troubling problem. Two other common GI problems are diverticulosis, the development of tiny, easily irritated pouches inside the colon, and diverticulitis, the often painful inflammation of these pouches. Fiber from cereals, as well as from fruits and vegetables, adds bulk to the stool and softens it. Together, these actions decrease pressure inside the intestinal tract and help prevent diverticular disease.

UNCERTAIN EFFECTS ON CANCER

Although a number of early studies suggested that whole-grain consumption reduces the chances of developing mouth, stomach, colon, gallbladder, and ovarian cancer, later and larger ones haven't borne this out. If whole grains ultimately turn out to provide some protection against colon cancer, fiber probably isn't the reason. Recent analyses from the Nurses' Health Study, the Health Professionals Follow-up Study, and a compilation of large cohort studies from around the world showed that men and women with the highest fiber intake did not have lower risks of colon cancer.

Even if whole-grain, high-fiber foods have no effect on cancer, their impact on heart disease and diabetes is reason enough to eat grains in this form instead of their stripped-down counterparts.

HOW DO WHOLE GRAINS DO THIS?

It may be almost impossible to isolate the ingredient or ingredients in whole grains that reduce the risks of heart disease and diabetes. A few contenders, though, have been identified. The fiber in whole grains delays absorption of glucose and eases the workload for the insulin-making cells in the pancreas. Fiber helps lower cholesterol levels in the blood. It may also rev up some of the body's natural anticoagulants and help prevent the formation of small blood clots that trigger heart attacks or strokes. Antioxidants like vitamin E in whole grains prevent cholesterol-containing low-density lipids from reacting with oxygen, a key early step toward the formation of cholesterol-clogged arteries. Phytoestrogens, or plant estrogens, may protect against some cancers. The bran layer of many grains contains essential minerals such as magnesium, selenium, copper, and manganese that may be important in reducing the risk of heart disease and diabetes.

SEPARATING THE WHEAT FROM THE CHAFF

Exactly what is a whole-grain food? This shouldn't be a trick question, but it is. Part of the problem is our lack of knowledge about the foods we eat. The other is that food makers, eager to promote any health benefits that might sell their products, jumped on the fiber/whole-grain bandwagon several years ago and haven't gotten off. Stroll the aisles of your favorite grocery store and you'll see what we mean. General Mills Total is a whole-grain breakfast cereal, Quaker Puffed Wheat isn't. Nabisco Triscuits and Wheat Thins are whole-grain crack-

Don't Be Fooled by the Low-Carb Frenzy

Will the low-carb fad truly help people lose weight and keep it off? Will it lead to long-term health? I can't really say. But one thing is for certain: It has thinned the wallets of those caught up by it and fattened the bank accounts of those seeking to cash in on it.

Food companies and entrepreneurs are rushing to introduce new products before the fad fizzles. You can buy low-carb bread, bagels, cereal, pasta, ice cream, chocolate bars, and beer. There are more than one hundred books and two monthly magazines to teach you how to follow the low-carb lifestyle. Some restaurants list the carbohydrate content of their menu items (though hardly any list what you really need to know—calories). You can even take a low-carb cruise! By one estimate, Americans buy more than one billion dollars worth of branded, low-carb products per year.

And that's without the blessing of the FDA, which hasn't been keen on allowing food companies to use the term "low carb" on food labels because it hasn't been precisely defined. This hasn't stopped savvy marketers, who bypass this roadblock with terms like "carb smart," "carb friendly," and "net carbs."

Some so-called low-carb products are ones we have been eating for years that are naturally low in carbohydrates, such as salad dressings and peanut butter, dressed up with new labels. Others have been engineered or reformulated to carry fewer digestible carbohydrates. Companies do this in several ways. They can replace refined wheat flour with fiber, soy protein, or lower-carbohydrate, higher-protein soy flour; replace sugar with less digestible sugar alcohols, such as sorbitol; or add more fat.

These changes aren't necessarily bad, although there's some question about the long-term effects of eating large amounts of sugar alcohols, which are sometimes used as laxatives. But they can be misleading. Many consumers erroneously equate low carb with low calorie. In fact, many low-carb products deliver just as many calories as their normal-carb counterparts, and sometimes more. Add in their higher cost—following a low-carb diet can nearly double what you pay for food—and it's questionable whether you are getting the best nutritional bang for your buck.

ers, while Nabisco Wheatsworth crackers are mostly refined wheat. (While you are checking ingredients, be on the lookout for trans fats. These can affect the benefits of whole grains.)

Some choices are easy. Brown rice is whole grain, white rice isn't. Most of the time, though, it takes a savvy shopper to separate the whole grain from the refined. You have to read food labels with the discriminating eye of a food critic, alert for subtle nuances that spell the difference between whole grain and refined grain. If the label says "made with wheat flour," it may be a whole-grain product or it may just be an advertising gimmick—the silkiest, most refined white cake flour is made with wheat flour. True whole-grain products should list as the main ingredient whole wheat, whole oats, whole rye, or some other whole-grain cereal.

Bran cereals and wheat germ aren't technically whole-grain foods. Bran cereals lack the vitamin- and oil-rich germ, while wheat germ lacks the fiber-rich bran. Both are missing the starchy endosperm. If your diet is high in refined grains, adding bran and wheat germ makes sense. But this strategy doesn't give you the full benefits of eating intact grains, such as a protective shield that slows down the absorption of the starch inside the grain.

As you can see from the Healthy Eating Pyramid, it's important to include generous amounts of these healthy foodstuffs in your daily diet.

PUTTING IT INTO PRACTICE

Given the myriad health benefits of eating whole grains, and the fact that they are the third most important thing you can do for a healthier diet, why do 80 percent of Americans eat less than one serving a day?

For one, we aren't used to eating whole grains. For another, they haven't been that easy to buy. Until relatively recently, you could find products such as whole-grain pasta, whole-grain couscous, or bulgur only in health food stores, co-ops, or organic-type grocery stores. Finding them in restaurants or cafeterias was even harder. A third barrier has traditionally been time—many intact grains take longer to cook than their refined counterparts. Brown rice, for example, takes twice as long to cook as white rice.

The food industry, always on the lookout for new markets and marketing ideas, is helping break down the last two barriers. More and more mainstream grocery stores now carry a fair selection of whole-grain products. And you can now get quick-cooking brown rice, or brown basmati rice, that's ready in the same twenty minutes as white rice. (You can also make the old-fashioned, slow-cooking kind a day or more in advance.)

Here are a few suggestions for adding more intact grains to your diet. (See page 227 for more ideas and details.) Start slowly and add new grains or products as your appetite grows for these tasty foods:

• *Eat whole grains for breakfast.* Make a habit of starting the day with a bowl of whole-grain cereal. If you're partial to hot cereals, try old-fashioned or steel-cut oats. Quick and instant oatmeals are better than many choices, but they have a higher glycemic index than less-processed oats. If you'd rather have cold cereal, look for one that lists something whole—wheat, oats, barley, or other grain—first on the ingredient list. A few possibilities are Wheaties, Great Grains, Wheat Chex, Grape-Nuts, Shredded Wheat, and Kashi.

• *Discover whole-grain breads.* Choose breads made from whole grains instead of from refined grains. Again, check the label to make sure the first ingredient has the word *whole.* You can now buy whole-grain pita bread and sandwich rolls.

• *Forget the French fries.* Instead of potatoes or white rice, cook up some brown rice to accompany a meal. Or get really adventurous and try some "newer" grains like kasha, bulgur, oat groats, wheat berries or cracked wheat, millet, quinoa, or hulled barley.

• *Whole-wheat pasta can be a delicious alternative.* Look for whole-wheat pasta in your grocery store. If it's a bit too chewy for you, Eden, Prince, and other companies make pasta that is half whole-wheat flour and half white flour.

• *Bake with whole-wheat flour.* If you bake, try substituting whole-wheat flour for white flour. Start with a mixture that's one part whole wheat to three parts white flour. If you like the results, try increasing the ratio of whole wheat to white flour. Some companies sell a "white wheat" whole grain flour that has a milder taste and texture than traditional whole wheat flour. Precooked whole-wheat pizza shells are also showing up in grocery stores.

• *Pester your grocery store's manager or the chefs of your favorite restaurants.* If you have a hard time finding whole-grain products at the store, or ordering them in restaurants, ask the owner, manager, or chef to add some to their inventory or menu. You may be the first person to make such a request. You certainly won't be the last. The more they hear patrons ask for whole-grain products or dishes, the more likely those foods will start appearing.

CHAPTER SIX

Choose Healthier Sources of Protein

W E KNOW FAR LESS ABOUT protein in healthy diets and the role it plays in the onset of disease than we do about fats and carbohydrates. Not because protein is unimportant—quite the contrary, it's very important—but because it has been studied far less intensively than the other main components of food in relation to long-term health and disease. Much of the focus to date has been on the minimum amount of protein that children need for healthy development and that adults need to keep from slowly breaking down their own tissues. Far less attention has been paid to other important questions, like how much protein is best or if it matters whether your protein comes from animal or vegetable sources or whether a high-protein diet is better for losing or controlling weight than a low-fat, high-carbohydrate diet. Intriguing research on soy and weight loss strategies has kindled new interest in protein that is yielding better information.

As we wait for the full answer, eating more protein from fish, chicken, and vegetable sources like beans and nuts and getting less from red meat and dairy products is fourth on the list of healthy eating strategies.

WHAT IS PROTEIN?

Your hair and skin are mostly protein. Ditto your muscles, the oxygen-carrying hemoglobin in your blood, and the multitude of enzymes that keep you alive and active. In fact, your body is home to at least ten thousand different proteins.

On the molecular level, proteins are long, intricate chains fashioned from just twenty or so basic building blocks called amino acids. Because our bodies are constantly making new proteins and because we don't store amino acids as we do fats, we need a near daily supply of protein.

Some dietary proteins are complete, meaning they contain all the amino acids needed to make new protein. Others are incomplete, lacking one or more essential amino acids—ones we can't make from scratch or convert from other amino acids. Meat, poultry, fish, eggs, and dairy products tend to be good sources of complete proteins, while vegetable protein is often incomplete. That's why vegetarians need to eat combinations that complement each other, such as rice and beans, peanut butter and bread, tofu and brown rice.

HOW MUCH PROTEIN DO YOU NEED?

The latest dietary guidelines from the Institute of Medicine set the recommended daily allowance (RDA) for protein at 0.8 grams per kilogram of body weight, or just over 7 grams per 20 pounds. Translated to real body weights, that would mean 50 grams of protein a day for a 140-pound person and almost 65 grams for a 180-pound person. You can hit this goal almost without thinking, given the abundance of protein-containing foods. (See the table below.) For

Dietary Sources of Protein

Food	Serving Size	Weight (grams)	Protein (grams)	% Daily Value*	Calories	% Calories from Protein
Tuna, water-packed	3 ounces	84	22	43	99	88
Chicken, roasted	3 ounces	84	26	52	139	75
Cottage cheese, low fat	4 ounces	113	14	28	81	69
Beef, top sirloin, broiled	3 ounces	84	26	52	166	62
Salmon, fillet	3 ounces	85	22	43	155	56
Egg	1 large	50	9	18	74	49
Hamburger patty, 90% lean	3 ounces	82	21	42	178	47
Tofu, firm	1/2 cup	126	10	20	97	42
Milk, skim	1 cup	245	8	17	83	40
Yogurt, low-fat	1 cup	245	13	26	154	34
Lentils, cooked	1/2 cup	99	9	18	115	31
Soy milk	1 cup	245	9	18	120	31

Food	Serving Size	Weight (grams)	Protein (grams)	% Daily Value*	Calories	% Calories from Protein
Broccoli, cooked	5-inch stalk	140	3	7	49	27
Black beans	½ cup	86	8	15	114	27
Cheddar cheese	1 ounce	28	7	14	114	25
Cheese pizza	2 slices	126	15	31	281	22
Whole milk	1 cup	244	8	16	146	22
Peanuts	1 ounce	28	7	15	161	18
Whole-wheat bread	2 slices	56	5	11	138	16
Macaroni, cooked	1 cup	140	7	13	197	14
Corn, cooked	1 ear	77	3	5	83	13
Baked potato	1 medium	173	4	9	161	11
Almonds	1.5 ounces	42	6	12	246	10
Walnuts	1.5 ounces	42	7	13	278	9
Brown rice, cooked	1 cup	195	5	9	218	8

* Based on daily value of 50 grams in 2,000-calorie diet

Source: U.S. Department of Agriculture, Agriculture Research Service, National Nutrient Database for Standard Reference, Release 17, 2004 (www.nal.usda.gov/fnic/foodcomp)

example, a cup of yogurt at lunch and a serving of chicken plus rice and beans for dinner adds up to about 60 grams of protein. Because it is so easy for us to get protein, it's uncommon for healthy adults in this country to have a protein deficiency.

Aside from the minimum amount of protein needed to keep the body running, there's little guidance on the *ideal* amount of dietary protein or the healthiest proportion of calories contributed by protein. Country-to-country comparisons of protein intake and health aren't much help because diets around the world tend to have similar amounts of protein. In the average American diet, which we tend to think of as meat-centered, about 15 percent of calories come from protein. In the largely vegetarian, rice-based diets that are common throughout Asia, about 12 percent of calories come from protein. (Rice, which we think of as a carbohydrate, is about 8 percent protein.) Other types of human studies haven't paid that much attention to protein. And diet fads further confuse the issue, with competing claims for high-protein, low-carbohydrate diets and low-protein, high-carbohydrate diets.

Until there's a good reason to change, getting 7–8 grams of protein per twenty pounds of body weight is a good guide for most people.

PROTEIN AND CHRONIC DISEASES

Protein in general has been linked at one time or another with a variety of chronic diseases. Protein intake probably isn't intimately related to the development of cancer, though it may influence the role of heart disease, diabetes in children, obesity, and gastrointestinal disorders. Specific proteins in food, the air, and elsewhere are responsible for a variety of allergies, though we don't discuss that topic in detail here.

• *Protein and cancer.* There's no good evidence that eating a little or a lot of protein influences the risk of cancer in humans. You may have heard about low cancer rates in Japan, where the average diet contains a bit less protein, and certainly less animal protein, than the average American diet. In reality, total cancer rates in traditional Japan are about the same as they are here, though the *types* of cancers that are the most common in each country are different. Several prospective studies have suggested that diets higher in methionine, one of the building blocks of protein, may help reduce risks of colon and possibly breast cancer. Just how much methionine provides maximal benefit remains to be determined. A report from the Nurses' Health Study suggests that among women who have been diagnosed with breast cancer, those who eat more protein (and thus less carbohydrates) may live longer than those with lower-protein, higher-carbohydrate diets. But this work clearly needs to be confirmed by other research.

• *Protein and heart disease.* Cutting back on carbohydrates and replacing those calories with protein lowers the levels of triglycerides, which would be good for heart disease and also boosts HDL, the protective form of cholesterol. (The same things happen when you replace carbohydrates with monounsaturated or polyunsaturated fat, so it may well be that levels of blood fats are actually responding to less carbohydrate rather than to more protein or more fat.)

So far, the Nurses' Health Study is the only large prospective study to have examined the link between dietary protein and cardiovascular disease. Over the course of fourteen years, we asked more than eighty thousand initially healthy women about what they ate. The group of women who ate the most protein, accounting for about a quarter of daily calories, were 25 percent less likely to have had a heart attack or to have died of heart disease than the women who ate the least protein, about 15 percent of calories. It didn't seem to matter if the protein came from animals or vegetables, and the apparent protective effect applied equally to women on low-fat and high-fat diets. While this needs to be confirmed, it offers strong reassurance that even eating a lot of protein doesn't harm the heart.

• *Protein and diabetes.* The amount of protein in the diet doesn't seem to have an effect on the development of type 2 (adult-onset) diabetes. One or more specific proteins found in cow's milk may—and I stress the *may*—play a role in the development of type 1 diabetes in children, one reason cow's milk isn't recommended for infants.

• *Protein and other chronic diseases.* The medical literature is full of reports linking allergic responses to specific protein sources with conditions ranging from arthritis and breathing problems to chronic digestive disorders. Eggs, fish, milk, peanuts, tree nuts, and soybeans are known to cause allergic reactions in some people. A startling and well-documented report published in the *New England Journal of Medicine,* for example, showed that something in cow's milk causes an allergic response leading to severe chronic constipation in some young children. In a group of sixty-five toddlers with chronic constipation, two weeks' worth of soy milk in place of cow's milk cleared up the problem in two-thirds of the children. A return to cow's milk led to the return of constipation. What's more, the "responders" were also more likely to have had constant runny noses, bronchospasm, and skin inflammation when drinking cow's milk. This may be a sentinel report pointing the way to other links between specific proteins and chronic disease.

EMPHASIZE VEGETABLE SOURCES OF PROTEIN
INSTEAD OF ANIMAL SOURCES

The debate over which type of protein is better rumbles on two levels: personal health and environmental health.

• *Personal health:* In terms of your health, there isn't enough evidence to argue that one type of protein is better for you than another. Worldwide surveys of protein consumption and heart disease death rates hint that the more animal protein in the diet, the more heart disease, and the more vegetable protein, the less heart disease. But different dietary and lifestyle habits from country to country—things like consumption of saturated fat or smoking rates or amount

Go Nuts

The next time you're racking your brain over what to have for a snack or make for dinner, think nuts. Your taste buds and your heart will thank you.

Contrary to popular opinion, nuts aren't junk food. They're actually a great source of protein and other nutritional goodies. An ounce of almonds, walnuts, peanuts, or pistachios gives you about 8 grams of protein, the same as a glass of milk. True, nuts have quite a bit of fat, but these are mostly unsaturated fats that reduce LDL cholesterol and keep HDL cholesterol high.

One of the more surprising findings from nutrition research over the past decade is that people who regularly eat nuts are less likely to have heart attacks or die from heart disease than those who rarely eat them. That's not just an interesting but oddball result. Several of the largest cohort studies, including the Adventist Study, the Iowa Women's Health Study, and the Nurses' Health Study, have shown a consistent 30 to 50 percent lower risk of heart attacks or heart disease associated with eating nuts several times a week. Regularly including nuts in the diet also seems to help prevent type 2 diabetes and gallstones.

The evidence is strong enough for the FDA to let food companies claim on food labels that "eating 1.5 ounces per day of most nuts as part of a diet low in saturated fat and cholesterol may reduce the risk of heart disease." The FDA limited this claim to six types of nuts—almonds, hazelnuts, peanuts, pecans, pistachios, and walnuts. (See table, page 124) Other nuts, including Brazil nuts, cashews, macadamias, and pine nuts, didn't make the FDA's grade because they contain more than 4 grams of saturated fat. I think this is a trivial and misleading distinction. The amount of healthy unsaturated fat in these nuts far outweighs the saturated fat and so makes them healthy choices, too.

How do nuts help the heart? There are plenty of possibilities. Their unsaturated fats help improve levels of LDL (bad) and HDL (good) cholesterol. One particular unsaturated fat found in walnuts, an omega-3 fatty acid known as alpha-linolenic acid, seems to prevent clots and reduce potentially deadly erratic heartbeats. (See page 85, "Omega-3 Fats—A Special Benefit".) Nuts are also rich in arginine, an amino acid needed to make a tiny but important molecule called nitric oxide. Nitric oxide helps relax constricted blood vessels and ease blood flow. It also makes blood platelets (tiny, blood particles that are involved in clotting) less sticky and less likely to form clots in the bloodstream. Vitamin E, folic acid, potassium, fiber, and other phytonutrients found in nuts may also contribute to the benefit of including them in your diet.

However it happens, the message is the same—nuts are good for you. *If you eat them the right way.*

Here's the wrong way—gobbling nuts on top of your usual snacks and meals. At 160 calories an ounce, eating a handful of almonds a day without cutting back on anything could translate into a ten-to-twenty-pound weight gain over the course of a year. This weight would cancel out any benefit from nuts and tip the scales toward, not away from, heart disease.

Here's the right way—eat nuts instead of chips or chocolate as a snack. They'll take the edge off hunger every bit as well as junk food, they taste as good as or better than junk food, and they give you healthy nutrients to boot. Better yet, use nuts instead of meat in main dishes. Mediterranean and other traditional cuisines use nuts this way in all sorts of delicious dishes and sauces.

of physical activity—make these surveys difficult to interpret. The only large prospective study of protein and heart disease showed that eating more animal or vegetable protein was linked with a lower risk of heart disease.

Given what we know today, the bottom line is that animal and vegetable protein all by themselves have roughly equivalent effects on health. What matters is the protein *package*. Beef is a good source of complete animal protein. It's also an excellent source of saturated fat. The same is true for whole milk or dairy products made from whole milk. If you like beef, choose the leanest cuts you can find. Chicken, turkey, and fish are better options. Beans, nuts, whole grains, and other vegetable sources of protein are better yet, because they are generally low in saturated fat and high in fiber. If you intend to get most of your protein from nuts, legumes, vegetables, and grains, choose a variety of these foods to be sure that no essential components of protein are missing. If you enjoy milk and other dairy products, low- or no-fat versions are healthier choices than full-fat products.

There's more to the protein package than fats. Preliminary studies hint that people who regularly eat hot dogs, bologna, bacon, and other processed meats are more likely to develop type 2 diabetes than those who don't. Men whose diets include a lot of red meat—upward of four ounces a day—and dairy products seem to be more likely to develop prostate cancer, especially quickly spreading (metastatic) prostate cancer, than men who eat less meat and dairy products. In contrast, men who eat fish more than three times a week (and so who eat less red meat) have almost half the risk of developing prostate cancer as men who rarely eat fish.

Finally, frying and grilling meat, poultry, and fish to a well-done degree may increase cancer risk by generating a group of known carcinogens called heterocyclic amines. Whether this risk is large enough to worry about hasn't been clearly determined.

Fats in 1¹/₂ Ounces of Various Nuts and Seeds

TYPES (#PIECES/ 1¹/₂ OUNCES)	CALORIES	TOTAL FAT GRAMS	SATURATED FAT GRAMS	MONO-UNSATURATED FAT GRAMS	POLY-UNSATURATED FAT GRAMS	RATIO OF UN-SATURATED TO SATU-RATED FATS
Almonds (30–36)	246	21.5	1.6	13.7	5.2	11.8
Brazil nuts (9–12)	279	28.2	6.4	10.4	8.8	3.0
Cashews (24–28)	241	20.0	3.5	10.8	3.6	4.1
Flaxseed	89	6.1	0.6	1.2	4.0	8.7
Hazelnuts (27–30)	267	25.8	1.9	19.4	3.4	12.0
Macadamia nuts (15–18)	305	32.2	5.1	25.0	0.6	5.0
Mixed nuts (30–36)	253	21.9	2.9	13.3	4.6	6.2
Peanuts (42–45)	241	20.9	2.9	10.4	6.4	5.8
Peanut butter (smooth, 2 tbsp.)	192	167	3.2	7.9	4.8	4.0
Pecans (27–30 halves)	294	30.6	2.6	17.3	9.2	10.2
Pine nuts (~240)	286	29.1	2.1	8.0	14.5	10.7
Pistachios (73–77)	237	18.9	2.3	9.9	5.7	6.8
Sesame butter (tahini, 2 tbsp.)	190	16.2	2.2	6.1	7.2	6.0
Sesame seeds	240	20.8	2.2	4.0	13.7	8.0
Walnuts (12–16)	278	27.7	2.6	3.8	20.1	9.2

Source: U.S. Department of Agriculture, Agriculture Research Service, National Nutrient Database for Standard Reference, Release 17, 2004 (www.nal.usda.gov/fnic/foodcomp)

• *Global health:* Eating vegetable protein is a lot more efficient, not to mention kinder to the earth, than eating meat. Feeding grain to cattle to make steaks and hamburgers is terribly inefficient. That inefficiency doesn't much matter when cattle graze on plants growing all by themselves on land that isn't usable for much else. More and more, though, we eat beef, pork, and chicken that have been grown for us. They've been fed grains sowed and reaped specifically for this purpose, which requires increasingly large amounts of petroleum, fertilizers, herbicides, and pesticides. They are given hormones and antibiotics, which show up in milk and meat. The concentrated wastes from feedlots pose substantial pollution problems.

If you want to consider the total cost of protein, *The Consumer's Guide to Effective Environmental Choices* (Three Rivers Press, 1999), a book from the Union of Concerned Scientists, is an eye-opener. According to this report, the second most environmentally costly consumer activity—behind how we transport ourselves from place to place—is our consumption of meat. It takes 20 pounds of feed, usually corn, to make 1 pound of edible beef. Pork and chicken require 7 and 4 pounds, respectively. The Union of Concerned Scientists calculates that, compared with its caloric equivalent in pasta (made from flour), 1 pound of beef creates 17 times more water pollution and 20 times more habitat alteration.

Fish is a healthy alternative to meat and poultry, but our burgeoning appetite for this protein source is severely depleting many fish stocks and destroying once abundant fishing grounds. Fish farming may be able to expand our supply of this food, but the environmental implications of this practice on a large scale aren't yet clear.

Eating a diet that is largely plant based won't solve all of these problems, especially with the world population headed to seven billion in the not too distant future. But it could help sustain food production in both developing and developed countries as we search for new and better ways to make food.

PROTEIN AND WEIGHT CONTROL

As I described in chapter 3, a high-protein, low-carbohydrate diet tends to work better than a low-fat, high-carbohydrate diet for helping people shed pounds quickly. There are two reasons for this: First, chicken, beef, fish, beans, or other high-protein foods slow the movement of food from the stomach to the intestine. Slower stomach emptying means you feel full for longer. Second, protein's rather gentle, steady effect on blood sugar avoids the quick, steep rise in blood sugar and just as quick hunger-bell-ringing fall that occurs after eating a rapidly digested carbohydrate like white bread or baked potato.

There's no need to go overboard on protein and eat it to the exclusion of everything else, as the early Atkins diet used to recommend. By avoiding fruits, vegetables, and whole grains, you would miss out on fiber, vitamins, minerals, and other phytonutrients you can't always get from protein. Pills can add some of the big ones back in, but they leave out hundreds of others that may be equally important for long-term health. You also need to pay attention to what's coming along with your protein. A serving of salmon gives you 19 grams of protein plus 2 grams of unhealthy saturated fat and 7.4 grams of healthy unsaturated fats. A standard hamburger delivers the same amount of protein but with more than double the saturated fat (4.5 grams) and only 5 grams of unsaturated fat. Choosing high-protein foods low in saturated fat will help your heart even as it helps your waistline.

PROTEIN IN MODERATION

The latest high-protein diet craze, and its precursor twenty years ago, ignore a potential problem—the more protein you eat, the more calcium you excrete. The connection is complicated. At normal levels of protein intake, calcium and other agents in the blood neutralize acids formed by the digestion of protein. At higher levels, though, extra calcium is needed to neutralize these protein-related acids. This calcium is pulled mostly from bone, the body's calcium storehouse. The amount of calcium you lose by following a high-protein diet for a short time—say, a few weeks—probably won't have any disastrous consequences on the strength and density of your bones. But eating lots of protein for a long time may. In the Nurses' Health Study, for example, women who ate more than 95 grams of protein a day (more than 25 percent of daily calories) had more broken wrists than those eating an average amount of protein, less than 68 grams a day (less than 15 percent of daily calories).

The final answer on high-protein diets isn't in, but these results should at least flash a yellow light.

THE SCOOP ON SOY

Ten years ago you probably wouldn't have touched tofu with a ten-foot fork, let alone chugged a cold glass of soy milk. Odds are, though, that you've recently tried a soy product or at least have been tempted to. It's hard to resist the siren song of soy, given the press it's been getting. Here's a sampling of the headlines:

- HEY, HEALTHY BOY, LET'S HEAR IT FOR THE SOY (*Omaha* (Neb.) *World Herald,* May 10, 2004)
- SOY VEY: VEGGIE PUSH FOR SCHOOLS (New York *Daily News,* May 4, 2004)
- NOT MILK? SOY IS BECOMING THE MILKY WAY FOR SOME (*Milwaukee Journal Sentinel* July 18, 2001)

- SOY PROTEIN MAY STOP BREAST CANCER (*Los Angeles Times,* January 21, 2000)
- SOY COMPOUNDS MAY HELP IN FIGHTING PROSTATE CANCER (*Columbus Dispatch,* November 8, 1999)
- ENJOY SOY TO CUT RISK OF HEART DISEASE (*Detroit News,* November 4, 1999)
- THE MENOPAUSE MENU: CHANGE OF DIET CAN EASE CHANGE OF LIFE (*Rocky Mountain News,* May 25, 1999)
- SOY TO THE WORLD—GO BEYOND TOFU: HEALTHY DIET MOVES INTO LAND OF FAKIN' BACON AND NOT DOGS (*Boston Herald,* March 4, 1998)
- TOUTING THE JOYS OF SOY: STUDIES OF THE PROTEIN-RICH BEAN'S POSITIVE EFFECTS ON CHOLESTEROL MAY BE ONLY THE BEGINNING (*The Washington Post,* August 15, 1995)

Once grown mainly for animal food, soybeans in one form or another are being eaten by more and more Americans. The draw of these products is the many health benefits pegged to soy. These include lower cholesterol, less heart disease, easing hot flashes and other menopause-related problems, preservation of memory, and protection against breast, prostate, and other cancers.

There isn't particularly terrific evidence for any of these. The soy-cholesterol connection was bolstered a decade ago by an article in the *New England Journal of Medicine.* It looked at almost forty studies in which people ate soy protein in place of animal protein. Some—but not all—of the studies showed that soy protein reduced cholesterol levels. Overall, eating about 50 grams of soy protein a day instead of that much animal protein reduced total cholesterol levels by 9.3 percent, LDL cholesterol by 12.9 percent, and triglycerides by 10.5 percent. Soy's cholesterol-lowering ability was even greater for people with cholesterol levels up near 300 mg/dL. If sustained over time, this could translate into a 20 percent reduction in the risk of having a heart attack or developing other forms of heart disease.

The FDA relied heavily on this report to approve a "health claim" for soy. Foods that contain at least 6.25 grams of soy per serving can carry a claim on the label stating "Diets low in saturated fat and cholesterol that include 25 grams of soy protein a day may reduce the risk of heart disease."

IT TAKES A LOT OF SOY

There are three key things to keep in mind about these results: First, to meet the FDA's target for soy—which is half that described in the *New England Journal of*

Medicine report—you would need to drink four 8-ounce glasses of soy milk a day (along with a whopping six hundred calories) or eat almost a pound of tofu. Second, soy protein can't atone for the sins of a diet that's high in calories and saturated fat or for lack of exercise. It will work only if it is part of an otherwise healthy diet. Third, later studies don't fully back this health claim, with some trials showing that soy protein has little or no effect on cholesterol levels.

IS SOY A WOMAN'S DEFENSE AGAINST BREAST CANCER?

The bigger buzz about soy has to do with breast and other cancers. Early international studies showed that Japanese women, who eat lots of soy, have low rates of breast cancer. Later laboratory studies showing that substances in soy protein can inhibit the growth of breast cancer cells further heightened interest in soy.

Biologically speaking, there's a sound reason why soybeans and soy products might act against cancer. Soybeans are rich in compounds called phytoestrogens, literally plant estrogens. There are two main types of phytoestrogen, isoflavones and lignans. In soybeans and the other plants that make them—flax, some other grains, and fruits and vegetables—phytoestrogens act as growth-regulating hormones. In the human body, phytoestrogens act like weak estrogens. Exactly what they do depends on the amount of phytoestrogens and where they are. In some tissues, phytoestrogens mimic the action of estrogen, while in other tissues they block it. Estrogen stimulates the growth and multiplication of breast and breast cancer cells. So the estrogen-blocking effects of soy estrogens could protect against breast cancer.

But the simplistic explanation that plenty of soy in the diet accounts for the low rates of breast cancer in Japan is almost certainly wrong. Breast cancer rates have been low throughout Asia (at least until recently), and soy isn't a staple in many Asian countries. This suggests that other things, such as differences in childbirth patterns, amount of physical activity, or other components of lifestyle or nutrition, are the real protective agents.

When it comes to soy and breast cancer, the ever accumulating studies haven't provided a clear picture. Some show a benefit, and these tend to be trumpeted in the media. Those that show no benefit at all—and there are quite a few of these negative studies—get very little press. One informative negative study comes from the Shanghai Cancer Institute in China. An international team of researchers interviewed more than eight hundred women with breast cancer, along with an equal number of similar-age women without breast cancer, asking about their diets. The women with breast cancer, it turned out, ate the same amount of soy as the women without it. Two large prospective studies in Japan offer conflicting results. In one, women who ate more tofu—another soy product—did not have a lower risk of breast cancer during more than ten years of follow-up, while a more recent one suggested that soy offers some protection against breast cancer.

In the United States, women who are Seventh-Day Adventists develop breast cancer at the same rates as other women, despite eating more soy protein and avoiding alcohol. In fact, among Seventh-Day Adventists who are vegetarian (and who therefore eat even more soy protein), the risk of breast cancer tends to rise with increasing years as a vegetarian. We hope that other large prospective studies now under way will serve up solid information about soy and breast cancer.

CHILLING HOT FLASHES

Menopause is a time of dwindling estrogen production. If the same phyto-estrogens thought to block the effects of estrogen in breast tissue could mimic the effects of estrogen elsewhere in the body, they could provide a natural way to cool the hot flashes and ease other problems that plague many women during menopause. A few studies show that phytoestrogens from soy relieve hot flashes. Even more show they don't work any better than sugar pills. In these kinds of studies, comparison with a placebo is essential because hot flashes often improve with time, whether or not soy is part of the picture.

THE BRAIN AND BEYOND

Can soy keep your memory sharp as you get older? It's an interesting idea. Estrogen-related factors have been implicated in thinking and memory. Naturally falling estrogen levels in women and men, then, could be one of the causes of aging-related memory loss and cognitive problems. A few studies, mostly using isoflavone supplements, suggest that getting more soy could preserve memory and thinking skills. Others say that more soy won't make any difference.

Similar contradictory evidence exists for prostate cancer, with some research showing that something in soy prevents this common cancer and other research showing that eating plenty of soy does nothing for the prostate.

SOY MAY HAVE A DARK SIDE

The flip-flopping research on soy and breast cancer wouldn't be a huge concern if eating soy protein was completely and totally safe and free of side effects.

That may not be the case. Two disconcerting reports suggest that in some situations, overdoing soy protein could do more harm than good. In one randomized trial, forty-eight women with a suspicious breast lump were randomly assigned to either their normal diet or their normal diet plus a soy supplement containing 45 milligrams of isoflavones a day for the fourteen days until a scheduled breast biopsy. Breast tissue removed from women taking the soy supplement showed substantially more cell growth and division than the tissue removed from women not taking soy. There is some evidence that genistein, the most abundant isoflavone in soy, can stimulate the type of breast cancer known as estrogen-receptor positive (ER+) to grow. It may also interfere with the cancer-killing effects of tamoxifen, an important drug used against breast cancer.

Another troubling study, this one among older persons of Japanese ancestry living in Hawaii, showed that those who continued to eat the traditional soy-based diet were more likely to have memory loss and other cognitive problems than those who had made the switch to a more Western diet. This finding cannot be readily dismissed because estrogens play a role in maintaining normal mental functions, and it is possible that too much antiestrogen in the wrong place at the wrong time could be harmful.

Clearly both of these studies must be confirmed. But they point out the absolutely critical need to learn more about how soy protein affects different tissues at different life stages. The estrogen-blocking activity of phytoestrogens may be beneficial for young women, whose breast, ovarian, and other tissues are bombarded by more powerful human estrogens. Yet it would be a shame to make blanket recommendations for soy as a way to prevent breast cancer if phytoestrogens also stimulate the growth of breast cancer cells later in life, when the natural output of estrogen is dwindling.

SOY, TOO, IN MODERATION

I'm cautious about soy, specifically about eating a lot of it. As a food, soy can be a good alternative to meat. Just don't overdo it. Aim for a few servings a week, not a few a day. For women in the midst of menopause or beyond who are plagued by hot flashes or other problems related to estrogen loss, boosting soy intake for a while may help a bit. For now, though, this should not become a long-term habit. And the current evidence suggests that women diagnosed with breast cancer probably shouldn't be eating lots of soy.

One thing we know for certain about soy is that the phytoestrogens it contains are potent biological agents. Whether they trigger, suppress, or have no effect on breast cancer, prostate cancer, or memory is unfortunately an open question. That's why you should treat concentrated soy supplements or isoflavone pills with the same caution as you would a totally untested new drug.

PUTTING IT INTO PRACTICE

• *Mix up your proteins.* You need a minimum amount of protein every day, but almost any reasonable diet will provide this. If most of your protein comes from plants, make sure you eat a good mix of beans, nuts, whole grains, and vegetables.

• *Balance carbohydrates and protein.* Cutting back on carbohydrates and increasing protein improves levels of blood triglycerides and HDL and so may reduce your chances of having a heart attack, stroke, or other form of cardiovascular disease. Too much protein, like the amounts in high-protein, low-carb diets, though, can draw calcium out of the skeleton and possibly lead to osteoporosis and broken bones.

• *Eat soy in moderation.* Soy protein is a good replacement for animal protein. But given how little we know about its effect on breast cancer and memory loss, it's wise not to go overboard eating soy products. Two to four servings a week of a soy-based food such as tofu or soy milk is a good target. Don't take pills that deliver concentrated soy protein or pure isoflavones. Use of larger amounts of soy for a few months to soothe hot flashes and other menopause-associated problems probably won't do any harm. At the same time, it probably isn't much more effective than the tincture of time.

CHAPTER SEVEN

Eat Plenty of Fruits and Vegetables

A S A CHILD, YOU HATED to hear it. As a teenager, you promised yourself you'd never say it to your own children. Yet as a parent, it—*Eat your vegetables, they're good for you*—springs out of the mouth unbidden, like wisdom that must be passed from generation to generation.

That's actually a good description. "Eat plenty of fruits and vegetables" is timeless advice that science is only now catching up to. It is a simple, easy-to-remember, and tasty morsel of superb dietary advice that ranks high on the list of smart and healthy nutritional habits.

With apologies to Elizabeth Barrett Browning, how do fruits and vegetables help thee? Let me count the ways. A diet rich in fruits and vegetables can

- decrease the chances of having a heart attack or stroke;
- lower blood pressure;
- help you avoid constipation and the painful intestinal ailment called diverticulitis;
- guard against two common aging-related eye diseases—cataract, the gradual clouding of the eye's lens, and macular degeneration, the major causes of vision loss among people over age sixty-five;
- delay or prevent memory loss and a decline in thinking skills;
- help you feel full with fewer calories and so control your weight and waistline; and
- add variety to your diet and enliven your palate.

Notice that I keep saying "fruits and vegetables." Pills that contain one or two or ten substances made by plants just won't do. Why not? Plants make a seemingly endless cornucopia of compounds that have biological activity in the human body. So far, only a tiny minority have been flagged as agents that may be responsible for the health benefits of fruits and vegetables, sometimes on the basis of surprisingly little solid evidence. The vast majority of these phyto-chemicals (literally, chemicals made by plants) have yet to be discovered, named, chemically characterized, and biologically evaluated. The odds are high that the benefits just listed emanate from many different substances found in plants and quite possibly from the interactions among them.

BUT FIRST, EXACTLY WHAT ARE FRUITS AND VEGETABLES?

To a botanist, a fruit is any plant part that contains seeds. By the process of elimination, a vegetable is everything else: leaves, stems, flowers, roots, and bulbs. Things get hazy in the kitchen, though, because many of what are com-monly called vegetables are technically fruits—think of the seeds in avocados,

Why Supplements Are Not a Substitute for Fruits and Vegetables

So far, no one has found a magic bullet that works as well as fruits and vegeta-bles against heart disease, cancer, and a host of other chronic diseases. In theory, one could cram all of the good things that plants make—essential ele-ments, fiber, vitamins, antioxidants, plant hormones, and so on—into a pill. But it would have to be a very large pill, and no one can honestly say it is known exactly what should go into such a pill. Or in what proportions.

The benefits of eating fruits and vegetables probably come from combina-tions of compounds that work together. Take the antioxidant pigments known as carotenoids, for example. When you eat a tomato or carrot, the different carotenoids it contains eventually work their way into different types of cells and different parts of each cell. This offers antioxidant protection throughout the cell and to a wide variety of cell types. When eaten in the proportions usu-ally found in foods, carotenoids and other phytochemicals probably work to-gether and protect cells at different levels. But when delivered in unnatural proportions—say, via a poorly designed supplement pill—an oversupply of one carotenoid or phytochemical could block the activity of others. This isn't to say that vitamin and mineral supplements are worthless. As described in chapter 10, vitamin supplements are excellent insurance. But they aren't a substitute for a healthy diet.

Health issues aside, the biggest drawback is that a pill would always taste like a pill. It can't give you the earthy smell and taste of a fresh ear of corn, the sweetness of a juicy tomato still warm from the afternoon sun, the crunch of an apple, the festive green of a snap pea or broccoli floret, or the smooth, nutty taste of an avocado. Stick with real fruits and vegetables—they taste better and contain a bounty of phytochemicals that do not come in capsules.

Fruit or Vegetable?

The "is it a fruit or a vegetable" controversy has been around for years. Back in 1893, the U.S. Supreme Court ruled that tomatoes were a vegetable, and they've remained so ever since. Why was the highest court in the land asked to make a legal and somewhat unscientific rule like this? Fruit importers John, George, and Frank Nix sued New York's collector of customs taxes, Edward Hedden, to recover taxes he had levied on a shipment of tomatoes the Nixes had imported from the West Indies. Back then, imported fruits weren't taxed, while vegetables were. In its decision, the Court acknowledged that tomatoes were technically fruits. But "in the common language of the people," the Court determined that tomatoes, as well as cucumbers, squashes, beans, and peas, "are vegetables which are grown in kitchen gardens" and are usually served at dinner with the main part of the meal and not as dessert.

cucumbers, eggplants, squashes, and tomatoes, to name just a few. In this book I will stick with the culinary concept of fruits as sweet, dessert- or snack-like foods, and vegetables as savory, salad- or dinner-type foods.

I am not including potatoes in the vegetable category, even though they are the most popular vegetable in America. I'm sticking with that position even though the potato is one of the few vegetables mentioned by name in the Dietary Guidelines for Americans, and even though the USDA considers batter-coated frozen potatoes—the ones used to make French fries—to be a fresh vegetable. Like rice and pasta, potatoes are mostly easily digested starch. Studies show that eating potatoes isn't linked with the same health benefits as is eating other fruits and vegetables.

FAMILY NUTRITION

When studying the connection between fruits, vegetables, and health, it helps to talk about groups of plants. One of the most common classification schemes is by "family." Those plant families you usually find in the market or on the table include the following:

- The crucifer family (Cruciferae), which gets its name from the tiny cross you can see if you look at a recently sprouted seed. It includes a number of those vegetables that children (and some adults) instinctively but unwisely avoid—broccoli, Brussels sprouts, cabbage, cauliflower, collard greens, kale, kohlrabi, mustard greens, radishes, rutabaga, turnips, and watercress. Members of the crucifer family are excellent sources of isothiocyanates, indoles, thiocyanates, and nitriles, chemicals that may protect against some cancers.

- The melon/squash family (Cucurbitaceae) includes cucumbers, summer squashes such as zucchini and pumpkin, winter squashes such as acorn and butternut, and cantaloupes and honeydew melons.
- The legume family (Leguminoseae) includes alfalfa sprouts, beans, peas, and soybeans. Legumes have plenty of fiber, folate, and substances called protease inhibitors, all of which may offer some protection against heart disease and cancer.
- The lily family (Liliaceae) includes asparagus, chives, garlic, leeks, onions, and shallots. These vegetables contain a number of sulfur-containing compounds, especially allicin and diallyl sulfate, that may fight cancer.
- The citrus family (Rutaceae) encompasses grapefruits, lemons, limes, oranges, and tangerines. Citrus fruits are high in vitamin C and also contain the compounds limonene and coumarin, which have been shown to have anticancer properties in laboratory animals.
- Members of the solanum family (Solanaceae) include eggplant, peppers, potatoes, and tomatoes. As you can see from the list, this is a very diverse group. Tomatoes contain high amounts of lycopene, a type of antioxidant (see page 176) that may play a key role in preventing prostate and other cancers.
- The umbels (Umbelliferae) include carrots, celeriac, celery, parsley, and parsnips. Carrots are an excellent source of beta-carotene, which the body uses to make vitamin A. Several studies have also raised the possibility that beta-carotene and other related compounds called carotenoids help prevent some cancers or heart disease and maintain memory into old age.

While any one fruit or vegetable contains dozens, maybe hundreds, of different compounds that your body uses for something besides energy, no single fruit or vegetable contains all of the substances you need. That's why it's a good idea to get a few servings a week from each of these major groups.

It's also a good idea to eat for color variety as well. Painting your diet with the bold colors of ripe red tomatoes, crisp orange carrots, creamy yellow squash, emerald-green spinach, juicy blueberries, indigo plums, violet egg-plants, and all shades in between not only makes meals more appealing but also ensures that you get a variety of beneficial phytonutrients.

USDA AND OTHER GUIDELINES GIVE LITTLE REAL GUIDANCE

Back in 1991, the National Cancer Institute launched its 5-a-Day public health campaign. Through grocery store banners, labels on fruits and vegetables, public service announcements in the media, and educational materials for school-children, it urges us to eat five servings of fruits/vegetables a day. This campaign, which is still going strong, has been incorporated into the Dietary Guidelines for Americans, as well as into guidelines from the American Heart Association, American Cancer Society, World Health Organization, and others.

Five a day is a good start. But it gives no real guidance on what qualifies for five a day. Two glasses of orange juice, an apple, an order of French fries at lunch, and a potato with dinner meets the 5-a-Day target. While that's better than no fruits and vegetables at all, it doesn't offer the full dose of health benefits described here.

Instead, use five a day as a minimum, not a goal. Don't include potatoes in your daily tally. And try to vary the fruits and vegetables in your diet. (See "Putting It into Practice.")

NOT MEASURING UP

Few of us take advantage of the incredible bounty of fruits and vegetables grown in this country and elsewhere. The average American relies on roughly a dozen different fruits and vegetables. Daily consumption is just as limited, hovering around four servings a day, and that figure is vastly inflated by pota-toes. A recent national survey showed that fewer than one in three of us gets five servings of fruits and vegetables a day. This limited consumption is a pity, given the clear-cut benefits of eating fruits and vegetables.

FRUITS AND VEGETABLES PREVENT CARDIOVASCULAR DISEASE . . .

A diet that includes plenty of fruits and vegetables can help control or even pre-vent two of the main precursors of heart disease and stroke, high blood pres-sure and high cholesterol. Even better, investing in a plant-rich diet pays off in terms of lower chances of developing several forms of heart disease and stroke.

The protective benefit, while not huge, is well worth the small effort of adding more fruits and vegetables to your diet. By combining the results of sev-enteen large, long-term studies, researchers estimated that people in the top

Presidential Passion for Olive Oil and Vegetables

Olive oil drizzled over cooked carrots, roasted eggplant, or grilled peppers conjures up images of Mediterranean cooking. Yet it's as all-American as the founding fathers. Here's what Thomas Jefferson had to say about the olive tree and olive oil in a letter to William Drayton, a South Carolina lawyer, congressman, and planter: "The olive is a tree the least known in America, and yet the most worthy of being known. Of all the gifts of heaven to man, it is next to the most precious, if it be not the most precious. Perhaps it may claim a preference even to bread, because there is such an infinitude of vegetables, which it renders a proper and comfortable nourishment."

Our third president knew something that cooks and chefs are beginning to rediscover—that olive oil can perk up vegetables. Jefferson, a curious naturalist and ardent horticulturalist, repeatedly tried to cultivate olive trees in South Carolina and Georgia, but with little success. He ultimately had to rely on imported olive oil for his table.

Jefferson's enthusiasm for the marriage between olive oil and vegetables was driven by taste. Follow his example and you, too, may discover intense new flavors and a new appreciation for vegetables. And your heart may silently thank you.

tier of fruit and vegetable consumption (about thirty-five servings a week, or your basic five a day) are 15 percent less likely to have a heart attack or other problem caused by restricted blood flow to the heart muscle than those in the bottom tier. Among more than one hundred thousand men and women participating in the Nurses' Health Study and the Health Professionals Follow-up Study, we found that eating about thirty servings of fruits and vegetables a week (or just under five a day) was associated with a 30 percent lower risk of the most common type of stroke (ischemic stroke), the kind caused by a blood clot blocking an artery in, or to, the brain. We calculated that eating one extra serving of fruits or vegetables a day decreases the chances of having an ischemic stroke by about 6 percent. In this study, most of the benefit seemed to come from eating broccoli, spinach, kale, romaine lettuce, and citrus fruit or juice.

High blood pressure often sets the stage for stroke, heart attack, and other kinds of circulatory problems. Formally known as hypertension, high blood pressure affects more than fifty million Americans and a staggering one billion people worldwide. It's increasingly common with age, affecting less than 10 percent of U.S. adults between the ages of twenty and thirty-four and more than 75 percent of those over age seventy-five. Sometimes called the silent killer, high blood pressure causes no real symptoms. That's one reason at least one-third of people with high blood pressure don't know they have it. Of those who are well aware they have high blood pressure (also known as hypertension), many have a hard time keeping it under control.

As a pill-oriented culture, we tend to rely on medications to control blood pressure. But two of the best ways are losing weight, if you are overweight, and increasing your daily physical activity. Eating more fruits and vegetables can also lower blood pressure without the side effects and cost of medications. Even better, eating plenty of fruits and vegetables may help prevent high blood pressure in the first place.

An innovative study called DASH, short for Dietary Approaches to Stop Hypertension, clearly showed that eating more fruits and vegetables can substantially lower blood pressure, especially as part of a diet low in animal fat. DASH wasn't your garden-variety nutrition study but a full-blown clinical trial, much like those done to test a new drug. All 457 of the DASH participants, some with high blood pressure, some without, were randomly assigned to one of three diets: a control diet that mirrored the typical American diet (about three servings of fruits and vegetables a day, nearly 40 percent of calories from fat, and one dairy product daily); a fruit-and-vegetable diet similar to the control diet but with eight servings of fruits and vegetables a day; and a combination diet that included nine servings of fruits and vegetables a day plus three servings of low-fat dairy products. The beauty of the DASH method was that all of the volunteers' meals during the study were specially prepared in hospital kitchens, a strategy that minimized variation from person to person.

After eight weeks, the combination diet (fruits and vegetables plus three servings of dairy) substantially lowered blood pressure among the volunteers who had high blood pressure. So did the fruit-and-vegetable diet, though not quite as much. For both experimental diets, the reductions were about as large as what drug therapy can do for mild high blood pressure. Both the combination diet and the fruit/vegetable diet also lowered blood pressure in people without hypertension, suggesting that this may be an easy, side-effect-free way to prevent this condition. A second DASH trial showed that a low-salt version of the DASH diet can subtract a few extra points from blood pressure (see chapter 10).

Many components of the DASH diet contribute to its ability to lower blood pressure. A follow-up study showed that the single most important factor is the extra potassium provided by the fruits and vegetables.

Cholesterol levels also seem to respond to a diet with plenty of fruits and vegetables. This may be one of the ways that fruits and vegetables reduce the risk of heart disease and stroke. No one knows for sure how fruits and vegetables lower cholesterol. Since eating more plant foods often means eating less meat and dairy products, lower cholesterol levels may come from eating less saturated fat. They could also be due to the ability of soluble fiber to block the absorption of cholesterol from food. In spite of what food companies are claiming, though, soluble fiber's effect on cholesterol is relatively small.

. . . AND EYE DISEASES . . .

Eating plenty of fruits and vegetables also keeps those portals to your soul healthy, clear, and focused. This goes way beyond the common admonition to eat carrots for better vision (actually better night vision). A number of studies now show that people who regularly eat dark green leafy vegetables like spinach and collard greens are less likely to develop two common aging-related eye diseases, cataract and macular degeneration. Together, these two afflict millions of Americans over age sixty-five. Cataract is the gradual clouding of the eye's lens, a disk of protein that focuses light on the light-sensitive retina. Like clear floor wax that turns dull and cloudy from the pounding and scuffling of feet, decades of "insults" damage and cloud the lens. Macular degeneration, the leading cause of blindness among older people, is caused by cumulative damage to the macula, the center of the retina. It starts as a blurred spot in the center of what you see. As the degeneration spreads, vision shrinks.

In both diseases, free radicals are believed to be responsible for causing much of the damage. Free radicals are highly reactive and out-of-control substances generated inside the eye by bright sunlight, cigarette smoke, air pollution, and infection. Dark green leafy vegetables contain two pigments, lutein and zeaxanthin, that accumulate in the eye. These two can snuff out free radicals before they can harm the eye's sensitive tissues.

. . . AND BOWEL TROUBLE

What you can't digest of fruits and vegetables is as healthful as what you can. Fiber, or what some call roughage, is essential for healthy bowel function. Without enough indigestible material in the diet, stools can become hard and difficult to pass. Fiber sops up water like a sponge and expands as it moves through the digestive system. This can calm the irritable bowel. By triggering regular bowel movements, fiber can relieve or prevent constipation. The bulking and softening actions of fiber also decrease pressure inside the intestinal tract and so may help prevent diverticulosis (the development of tiny, easily irritated pouches inside the colon) and diverticulitis (the often painful inflammation of these pouches).

BUT DO THEY PROTECT AGAINST CANCER?

Twenty-five years ago, two eminent epidemiologists estimated that "dietary factors" accounted for 35 percent of cancer deaths in the United States, or roughly the same amount as were chalked up to smoking at the time. Major reports from the U.S. National Academy of Sciences *(Diet and Health)* and the World Cancer Research Fund *(Food, Nutrition, and the Prevention of Cancer)*, among others, have echoed this conclusion. While 35 percent may be overly optimistic, the basic message that better diets—heavy on the plant foods, please—can help guard against a variety of cancers is perfectly sound.

So far, more than two hundred studies have looked at the connection between diets high (or low) in fruits and vegetables and the development of cancer. Initially, they estimated a 50 percent reduction in most major cancers if everyone got at least five servings of fruits and vegetables a day. That was the basis of the National Cancer Institute's ongoing 5-a-Day program.

Most of the early studies were case-control studies (see page 31). In a nutshell, these involve comparing differences in diet, habits, and other possible causes of cancer between a group of people with a particular cancer and a group without it. Such comparisons aren't always fair or without bias. People with cancer, for example, tend to be seeking reasons for why they were stricken and may be more apt to find fault with their diets than those without the disease. The consistency of results from case-control studies created a deceptively strong idea that eating plenty of fruits and vegetables helped ward off cancer.

Cohort studies, in which information on diet and other lifestyle factors are collected *before* cancer, heart disease, and other conditions occur, tend to give more reliable and durable results. Not long ago, our team at the Harvard School of Public Health combined information on fruits and vegetables and cancer from our two large cohort studies (the Nurses' Health Study and Health Professionals Follow-up Study) after the 110,000 participants had been followed for almost twenty years. During this time, 9,100 had developed some type of cancer. Those who averaged eight or more servings of fruits and vegetables a day developed cancer at about the same rate as those who ate fewer than one-and-a-half servings a day.

Does this mean that eating fruits and vegetables has no impact whatsoever on cancer? No. Although they don't have a blanket anticancer effect, fruits and vegetables may work against specific cancers. The International Association for Research on Cancer commissioned an exhaustive review of the hundreds of case-control and cohort studies that have looked at fruit and vegetable consumption and cancer over the years. The expert panel concluded that higher intake of fruit *probably* reduces the risk of esophageal, stomach, and lung cancer and *possibly* reduces the risk of mouth, throat, ovarian, kidney, bladder, and colorectal cancer, while higher intake of vegetables *probably* reduces the risk of esophageal and colorectal cancer and *possibly* reduces the risk of mouth, throat, stomach, lung, ovarian, and kidney cancer.

Drill down a bit into the data and there's some evidence that certain types of fruits or vegetables work against specific cancers. Examples include the following:

- *Bladder cancer.* Eating cruciferous vegetables like broccoli has been linked with lower rates of bladder cancer.
- *Colon and rectal cancer.* There is strong evidence that the vitamin folic acid (sometimes called folate) helps protect against colon and rectal cancer. Vegetables such as spinach and beets are good sources of folic acid and so once helped fight these cancers. Today, with so many foods fortified with folic acid, the contribution of fruits and vegetables to protection against colon and rectal cancer may be dwindling.
- *Prostate cancer.* Lycopene from tomatoes and cooked or processed tomato products, such as tomato sauce or ketchup, seems to be involved in the prevention of prostate cancer. In the Health Professionals Follow-up Study, for example, men who consumed several servings of tomatoes, tomato sauce, or tomato juice a week were less likely to develop prostate cancer and advanced prostate cancer than those who ate one to two servings a week.

Although the anticancer effects of fruits and vegetables isn't quite what it was thought to be a few years ago, every little bit helps. The genes you inherited from your parents play a role in determining whether or not you will get cancer. So do habits like smoking cigarettes, drinking too much alcohol, getting too much sun, and not exercising. Your occupation may also play a role. Still, a nutritious diet—and that includes fruits and vegetables—is an important part of any stay healthy strategy.

FIBER—PRAISE FOR THE INDIGESTIBLE

From a health standpoint, one of the wonderful things about eating fruits and vegetables is that they contain much you can't digest. Many of the substances that give plants their strength and flexibility aren't broken down by the acids and enzymes in the human stomach or intestines. These substances, generically called fiber, include cellulose, pectin, and gums. There are two classes of fiber—soluble and insoluble. Both pass through the digestive system largely untouched. The big difference is that soluble fiber dissolves in the intestinal fluid, while insoluble fiber doesn't.

Soluble fiber is plentiful in peas, apples, and citrus fruits, as well as in oats and other grains and seeds. It forms a sticky, gooey, Jell-O-like mass as it passes through the intestines. This gummy substance traps cholesterol-rich bile acids and carries them out of the body in the stool. The more cholesterol you excrete, the less is available for transfer into the blood and the lower your serum cholesterol. The lower your cholesterol, the lower your risk of heart disease and other circulatory problems.

Insoluble fiber comes from the cell walls of plants. The main component is cellulose, a long string of glucose molecules linked in a way the human digestive system can't separate and that can't dissolve in the intestine's fluids. Thirty years ago, research among the Bantu people of South Africa suggested that their high-fiber diet was responsible for their low rate of colon cancer. As insoluble fiber passes unchanged through the intestine, so the thinking went, it carries along partly digested food, and by speeding the passage of food through the digestive system, it may reduce the intestine's exposure to toxic or cancer-causing substances found in food. After a few small studies showed much the same thing, the fiber craze was on. Media reports prompted many of us to start crunching through bran flakes or bran muffins for breakfast, and food manufacturers began adding fiber to cereals, breads, and pastries. In reality, though, most studies did not show lower colon cancer risks among persons who ate higher amounts of fiber from grain products. In a detailed look at this issue, women in the Nurses' Health Study were followed for up to sixteen years. Those who consumed the most fiber, no matter what the sources, did not have lower risks of colon cancer or colon polyps, which are tiny growths from which most cancers arise. This larger study was followed by two randomized trials in which fiber supplements and a high-fiber/low-fat diet were compared with control groups. In neither case did the higher fiber intake reduce the recurrence of new polyps. Taking these findings together, high-fiber diets do not appear to be an effective way to reduce colon cancer risk.

Despite the disappointments for colon cancer, don't throw out the All-Bran and stock up on Wonder Bread. By dragging partly digested food through the intestine, insoluble fiber delays the absorption of sugars and starch. This helps blunt the spikes in blood sugar and insulin that occur after eating foods that are easily converted into glucose and a similar spike in triglycerides, particles that ferry fat from the intestine to the tissues. Consistently high levels of insulin and triglycerides in the blood increase the chances of having a heart attack, and the repeated demand for large amounts of insulin can increase the risk of developing type 2 diabetes.

PHYTONUTRIENTS AT WORK

How fruits and vegetables protect the human system from certain cancers, heart disease, gastrointestinal problems like diverticulitis, or age-related eye diseases is still something of a mystery. Although we've been eating plants for aeons and seriously studying them for decades, what we know today is the proverbial tip of the iceberg.

Identifying the benefits of fruits and vegetables has been a challenging job, especially since plants have tremendous nutritional variability. A single type of plant, say, a Best Boy tomato, isn't a stable, well-defined entity. Instead its chemical composition varies with the season, the soil in which it grew, the amount of water it got, what pests it had to withstand, how ripe it was when picked and eaten, and under what conditions it was stored. What's more, the nutrients it delivers depend on how it is processed or cooked.

It will be decades before we have identified all of the complex compounds in food and even longer before we truly understand how they interact with one another and what they do in our bodies. Even so, scientists have isolated a number of substances that plants make or store that may play critical roles in keeping us healthy. These include the following:

• *Vitamins.* The first set of phytochemicals discovered were what we call vitamins today. By definition, vitamins are carbon-containing compounds that the body needs in small amounts to maintain tissue and keep metabolism humming. Vitamins have traditionally been defined by studying diseases of deficiency, things like rickets (too little vitamin D), pellagra (not enough niacin), and beri-beri (not enough thiamine). More and more it looks as though cancer, heart disease, stroke, diabetes, osteoporosis, and other chronic diseases are, in part, diseases of deficiency. Exactly what the deficiencies are is the focus of intense research. Inadequate intake of folic acid is emerging as a potential risk factor for heart disease and some cancers. Low consumption of a special class of vitamins known as antioxidants, which capture and neutralize free radicals, appears to be involved in the early stages of heart disease, cancer, aging-related eye disease, dementia, and possibly aging itself. (See chapter 10.) Perhaps some of the known or yet to be discovered phytochemicals will earn vitamin status for preventing these diseases. Or perhaps we should just consider whole fruits and vegetables as vitamins, given their already proven ability to prevent these new diseases of deficiency.

• *Essential elements.* Plants are excellent sources of potassium, magnesium, and other elements the body needs for a host of critical tasks. Magnesium and potassium help control blood pressure and may reduce the risk of fatal rhythm disturbances of the heart.

• *Plant hormones.* The Food and Drug Administration has given food manufacturers the go-ahead to claim in ads and on packages that eating protein from soybeans lowers the risk of heart disease. One group of compounds found in soy, the isoflavones, can mimic or inhibit the hormone estrogen. (See chapter 6.) Another group, the phytosterols, can influence the absorption and metabolism of cholesterol.

OUR HEALTH DEPENDS ON PLANTS

The diet we eat today doesn't look a thing like the diet our hunter-gatherer ancestors ate over hundreds of thousands of years. They probably relied on a wide variety of fruits and vegetables, scrabbling to pick and eat whatever edible morsels they could find. It is very possible that, over time, humans became metabolically dependent on dozens, if not hundreds, of compounds made by plants. These phytochemicals help detoxify the harmful chemicals found in plants; help some of our enzymes fight cancer, infection, and other cellular disruption; and help others repair cellular damage. So far, only a small number of these compounds have been labeled as essential nutrients.

"Vegetables and fruits contain the anticarcinogenic cocktail to which we are adapted," writes noted cancer researcher John Potter. "We abandon it at our peril."

PUTTING IT INTO PRACTICE

There isn't any magic daily number or combination of fruits and vegetables for optimal health. Instead, I offer two words of advice: *more* and *different*.

• *Aim high.* Use five servings a day as a minimum goal and shoot for more. In the DASH study described on page 138, the target of nine servings a day was definitely beneficial.

• *Eat for variety and for color.* On most days try to get at least one serving from each of the following fruit and vegetable categories:
  • dark green, leafy vegetables
  • yellow or orange fruits and vegetables

- red fruits and vegetables
- legumes (beans) and peas
- citrus fruits

• *Cook your tomatoes.* Treat yourself to tomatoes, processed tomatoes, or tomato products cooked in oil on most days. Tomatoes are rich in lycopene, a powerful antioxidant that has been linked with lower rates of a variety of cancers, particularly lung, stomach, and prostate cancer. Because lycopene is tightly bound inside cell walls, your body has a hard time extracting it from raw tomatoes. Cooking breaks down cell walls, and oil dissolves lycopene and helps shuttle it into the bloodstream.

• *Fresh is better.* Eat several servings of fresh, uncooked fruits and vegetables each week because cooking damages or destroys some important phytochemicals. Vitamin C and folic acid, for example, are sensitive to heat. Otherwise the physical state of the fruits and vegetables you eat doesn't much matter. Frozen fruits and vegetables are nearly as good as fresh ones and may even be more nutritious than "fresh" fruits and vegetables that have been stored for weeks or months under conditions that prevent ripening. Canned fruits and vegetables are usually fine, though many come loaded with salt and added sugar.

Fresh Fruits and Vegetables

Truly fresh fruits and vegetables add enormously to the pleasure of eating a healthy diet. The freshest produce is what you grow yourself and pick just before you eat it. You don't need a farm plot or a big suburban backyard to do this. My backyard is only about 40 feet by 20 feet. Yet in that space, not far from busy Harvard Square, my wife and I have a peach tree that yields several bushels of fruit a year, a pear tree, raspberries that bear fruit in both June and October, blueberries, and four varieties of grapes, as well as garden space for tomatoes, cucumbers, greens, and herbs. Our garden gives us something fresh and tasty for at least four months of the year. By placing the trees near the edge of the yard and growing the grapes on an overhead arbor, this still leaves enjoyable outdoor living space.

CHAPTER EIGHT

You Are What You Drink

"To your health." That traditional toast captures what we are only now beginning to learn—that what and how much you drink may be just as important as what and how much you eat.

More than half of your body weight is made up of a briny fluid that is much like the oceans that nurtured primordial life. This fluid bathes, cushions, and lubricates cells, tissues, and organs. It gives cells their shape and provides their substance, and it forms the watery highways that transport nutrients, wastes, hormones, and other substances throughout the body.

When it comes to fluids, the constant struggle for survival can be reduced to this: You dry, you die. Your skin, kidneys, a number of hormones, and even your nasal passages work together to keep the fluid part of you from drifting off into dry air. But preventing water loss isn't enough. You need to take in enough fluid to carry out a variety of critical metabolic tasks, things like making enough urine to flush away toxic by-products of digestion and metabolism and other wastes, maintaining blood volume, preventing body salts from getting too concentrated, and replenishing whatever water you lose.

The average person needs about a milliliter of fluid for every calorie burned. That's about eight 8-ounce glasses for a 2,000-calorie-a-day diet. Exactly how much fluid you need depends on you. An individual's needs are partly genetically programmed and largely determined by diet, the environment, and activity.

- *Diet.* If you eat lots of fruits and vegetables, which are mostly water, you may not need to drink as much as someone who eats a lot of meat or bread. In western Tanzania, people drink much less water than they do elsewhere because they satisfy much of their daily fluid needs from cooked bananas, which make up a large part of the diet.

- *Environment/weather.* When the temperature is perfectly comfortable, you lose about four pints of water a day through your skin, the moist air you exhale, and urine. When it's "too darn hot," as Ella Fitzgerald croons, you lose even more. You can also lose extra fluid in the winter, when the relative humidity plummets and the dry air seems to draw water out of your skin.

• *Activity.* The more active you are, the more fluid you need. As your muscles burn glucose, they generate heat. As you sit and read these words, some of that waste heat helps keep your body temperature up near 100° F. Start scraping old wallpaper off a wall or running around a track and you quickly make more heat than you need. This extra heat must be vented or you literally risk cooking the temperature-sensitive proteins that make you you. That's what sweat does. As sweat forms on your skin and evaporates, it carries heat away from your body.

When you are giving your body a real workout, you can lose up to a quart of fluid an hour. Because your body doesn't have an easy-to-read gauge that tells you when your fluid level is low, several rules of thumb are often offered: Drink when you are thirsty. Drink before you are thirsty. Drink enough so your urine is consistently clear or pale yellow rather than bright or dark yellow.

Thirst, unfortunately, isn't a very good guide—by the time you feel thirsty, your fluid level can already be low. That's especially true when you are working or playing hard and losing water quickly. In addition, aging tends to uncouple the sense of thirst from the body's fluid level, and many older people can become dehydrated without realizing it. Also, urine color by itself is not a perfect guide because it is also influenced by what you eat and some vitamin supplements. An easy guideline is to drink at least one glass of your beverage of choice with each meal and one in between meals. Boost your fluid consumption if you are physically active or if you find yourself urinating infrequently.

The consequences of not taking in enough fluid each day range from the life-threatening to the merely irritating. Extreme dehydration, which can be deadly, is relatively uncommon, occurring mostly among children and older people during very hot weather and among endurance athletes. Minor dehydration can make you feel grumpy and tired and make it hard to concentrate. Chronic minor dehydration is a cause of constipation, especially among older people. It may also lead to the development of kidney stones and bladder cancer.

So far I have been deliberately general in talking about fluid intake rather than specifying any specific beverage. Plenty of things fit the bill, including water, juice, soda, milk, coffee, tea, and alcohol. Some are better than others, especially as routine thirst quenchers. Let's take a look at each one. The "healthy" list might surprise you.

WATER

For plain old topping off your tank, water is hard to beat. It has 100 percent of what you need—pure H_2O—and no calories or additives. And when it comes from the tap, water costs a fraction of a penny per glass.

You may have heard or read that you need to drink eight 8-ounce glasses of water a day in addition to whatever other beverages you drink. That's actually a medical urban legend, one of those "facts" that is repeated so often it gains the ring of truth. It probably comes from the fact that someone who eats two thousand calories' worth of food a day needs about sixty-four ounces of fluid. Some of this fluid comes from food, and the rest must come from beverages. Almost any will do.

Many people feel strongly that bottled water—or water from specific springs—is better than tap water. Scientists have raised the possibility that the chlorine-based chemicals used to rid tap water of disease-causing bacteria can react with organic matter to create potentially cancer-causing compounds. Carcinogens can also leach into water supplies from leaking gasoline and other underground storage tanks, from factories and other business (this scenario was the basis of the best-selling book *A Civil Action,* by Jonathan Harr), from landfills and garbage dumps, and from a variety of other sources. In the United States, though, it is doubtful that actual increases in cancer risk have been connected with contaminated water supplies. In the case profiled in *A Civil Action,* for example, the homes of some of the families with children who developed leukemia didn't get their water from the allegedly contaminated wells. The other problem is that bottled water supplies aren't always regulated and aren't necessarily different from public water supplies. In fact, some bottled water comes straight from the tap, not from the pristine mountain springs conjured up by their names or the illustrations on their labels.

The bottom line is that our public water supplies are generally very safe and that chlorination has saved countless lives by blocking the spread of infectious diseases. If there are risks to drinking tap water, they are very low compared with other "hazardous" habits. That said, the levels of chlorine in some city water can make it taste pretty bad. In this case, drinking bottled water is an inexpensive and healthy alternative to drinking soda, juice, or other beverages in place of tap water.

SODA

Imagine dumping seven to nine teaspoons of sugar onto a bowl of cereal. Too sweet to eat? That's how much sugar is in a twelve-ounce can of Coca-Cola, Pepsi, Orange Crush, or most other sugared soft drinks, and we drink the stuff by the gallon. According to the National Soft Drink Association, the industry makes the equivalent of almost six hundred 12-ounce cans of soda, pop, tonic, or whatever you call it *per person* each year. The vast majority of this is the full-sugar variety. Carbonated soft drinks make up more than 25 percent of what Americans drink. That's a huge proportion for a beverage that has absolutely no nutritionally redeeming value.

I say this because soda delivers pure calories completely divorced from the healthful nutrients you might get from real fruit juices, things such as vitamins, minerals, other phytochemicals, and maybe some fiber. That's a problem on several levels:

- Most Americans already take in too many calories and struggle to lose weight. One can of soda a day doesn't seem like a big deal, especially if you manage to cut back on food calories. If you don't, though, an extra 150 calories a day can translate into a fifteen-pound weight gain over a year! The danger of drinking sugared sodas and juices instead of water is that many people treat "liquid calories" as somehow different from "food calories" and often don't make up for the calories in soda or juice by eating less.
- High-sugar diets make the pancreas pump out more and more insulin, which may lead to diabetes. The simple sugars in soda trigger rapid and intense increases in blood sugar and insulin levels. When this happens several times a day on top of the increases that occur after eating, it can cause problems, especially for people who are growing more and more resistant to insulin's ability to ferry glucose inside cells. Women in the Nurses' Health Study who drank one soda a day nearly doubled their risk of diabetes. Also, in people who are insulin-resistant, taking in lots of carbohydrates raises the blood level of triglycerides, a kind of fat-carrying particle that increases the chances of heart disease.

What about calorie-free sodas? As a beverage, they are better than the sugared versions, although they're an expensive way to get water. As a weight-loss gambit, don't count on this approach all by itself. Instead, you have to keep your eye on extra calories from all sources.

Alarms have been sounded about the artificial sweeteners in calorie-free sodas. The FDA has approved five sugar substitutes for use in foods and beverages—saccharin, aspartame, acesulfame-K, sucralose, and neotame. Despite what you might read on the Internet or hear in the popular press, these probably do not pose a health hazard. No one knows, though, how they affect children who may down large amounts of these over a lifetime. Why bother with the uncertainty when plain water or water with a twist of lemon or a dash of juice are better options?

JUICE

A glass of real juice gives you a glass of water plus some vitamins, minerals, maybe some fiber, and a delightful taste. As a morning eye-opener or as a small part of your total fluid requirement, real juice (as opposed to juice-flavored sugar water) can be an important part of a healthy diet. In fact, the tradition of having a small glass of orange juice with breakfast has helped eliminate scurvy—a disabling condition caused by a deficiency of vitamin C—from the United States. But as a regular beverage, fruit juice can slyly add a hefty daily dose of calories. A twelve-ounce bottle or can of orange juice, for example, gives you 150 calories or so, or the equivalent of three chocolate-chip cookies. That's an awful lot of calories if you just need something to quench your thirst. If you prefer juice, dilute it with regular or sparkling water. Start with two parts juice to one part water and gradually work your way to one part juice to three or four parts water. Another trick for putting some zest into plain water is adding a squeeze of fresh lemon or lime. Vegetable juices tend to have fewer calories than fruit juices, but check the label to be sure, and look up the sodium content as well.

The biggest problem with drinking fruit juice instead of water is that many people don't eat less to adjust for the extra calories in juice. That's a surefire recipe for gradual weight gain.

Among the many types of juices, grapefruit juice stands out from the pack because it changes the way some people absorb and metabolize certain drugs. For example, grapefruit juice can reduce the absorption of the allergy medication fexofenadine (Allegra); digoxin, which is used to treat congestive heart failure; losartan (Cozaar), used to control blood pressure; and the anticancer drug vinblastine. By altering their metabolism, grapefruit juice can also *boost* the blood levels of other drugs, sometimes to dangerous heights. Drugs in this category include calcium channel blockers such as felodipine (Plendil), nifedipine

(Procardia), and nisoldipine (Sular), which are used to control high blood pressure; carbamazepine (Carbatrol, Tegretol), used to control epilepsy; some widely used cholesterol-lowering medications such as lovastatin (Mevacor), atorvastatin (Lipitor), and simvastatin (Zocor); cyclosporine, an immunosuppressant taken mainly by people who have had an organ transplant; and buspirone (BuSpar), used to fight alcohol abuse, depression, panic disorder, and a variety of other problems.

Second, something in grapefruit juice may create conditions that help form kidney stones. In the Nurses' Health Study and the Health Professionals Follow-up Study, every eight ounces of grapefruit juice a day appeared to increase the chances of developing kidney stones by 44 percent. While more research is needed to confirm this finding, it's a good reason not to have grapefruit juice every day.

MILK

As described in chapter 9, there are more reasons not to drink milk in large amounts than there are to drink it. I don't recommend it as a beverage for adults and believe you should think of milk as an optional food, not one you need two or three times a day.

COFFEE

Here's something you may not have expected me to say: Coffee is a remarkably safe beverage. Its dubious health reputation, which stretches back hundreds of years, is more image than substance.

Over the years, dozens of studies have been done on the health effects of coffee. A few early ones linked the bitter brew with breast cancer, pancreatic cancer, and heart disease. Many of these had a major flaw. They didn't take into account a key habit—cigarette smoking—that once went hand in hand with coffee drinking. More carefully controlled studies eventually showed that it was the smoking, not the coffee drinking, that accounted for the health problems. In fact, some new research shows that coffee may actually be good for a few things that ail us.

I don't mean to imply that coffee is as innocuous as water. It isn't. The caffeine in coffee (and tea, many sodas, and chocolate) has definite druglike activity. The pep and mild euphoria that caffeine offers is probably why most people drink coffee and other caffeine-containing beverages. As with any drug, there are downsides to caffeine. Drinking too much coffee can give you the shakes, make you irritable, and keep you from sleeping. It's also addictive. Regular caffeine consumers tend to get nasty headaches if they miss their morning cup(s). Drinking espresso, French press, or other coffee that doesn't drip through a paper filter can increase your cholesterol a few points. And people who drink a lot of coffee may be more at risk for developing osteoporosis or breaking a bone. In moderation, though, coffee is low on the totem pole of health risks and even has a number of benefits. In addition to the gentle pick-me-up, these include the following:

- *Lower chance of developing kidney stones.* Few afflictions are as painful as kidney stones. These nuggets of calcium and other substances such as oxalate and phosphate afflict hundreds of thousands of adults in the United States alone. Stones form for a variety of reasons: not drinking enough water, chronic urinary tract infections, diseases such as gout, and as a side effect of some medications. Among the men and women of the Health Professionals Follow-up Study and the Nurses' Health Study, coffee drinkers were less likely to develop these stones than non–coffee drinkers. While we aren't certain why this is so, caffeine's activity as a diuretic—a substance that stimulates the body to excrete more water—helps flush out the plumbing and may make urine that is too dilute to form kidney stones.
- *Lower chance of developing gallstones.* About one million people a year are diagnosed with gallstones, solidified chunks of cholesterol or bile salts that can be as small as a grain of sand or as large as a golf ball. People who drink coffee aren't as prone to gallstones as those who don't partake of the bean. Exactly how coffee does this isn't exactly clear. It stimulates the gallbladder to contract regularly, and this churning may stir things up enough to prevent stone formation. Caffeine also interferes with cholesterol crystallization, a key step in stone formation.
- *Lower risk of type 2 diabetes.* The Stockholm Diabetes Prevention Program is a study that includes almost 8,000 Swedish men and women, half with a family history of diabetes and half without. In this study, those who drank five or more cups of coffee a day were less likely to have diabetes than those who drank two or fewer cups. Results from the Nurses' Health Study and Health Professionals Follow-up Study show a similar connection between regular coffee drinking and reduced risk of type 2 diabetes.

- *Fewer suicides.* Coffee (and other caffeinated beverages) may act like mild antidepressants. Both the Nurses' Health Study and a study from a large California HMO have shown that suicide rates are as much as 50 percent lower among coffee drinkers than non–coffee drinkers.

One lingering concern about coffee is its potential for increasing bone loss and the risk of broken bones. Increased risks with four or more cups per day have been seen in several studies, but the final answer is not in. Given the body of research on coffee, it's safe to say that there aren't any major health hazards lurking in the murky depths of your cup. In short, when drunk in moderation, coffee is no threat to your health.

TEA

According to Chinese mythology, Emperor Shen Nung discovered how to make tea in 2737 B.C., using the leaves of the plant known today as *Camellia sinensis.* Nearly five thousand years later, tea ranks as the second-most-drunk beverage in the world, right behind water. The health-promoting properties long ascribed to tea are only now receiving the careful scientific scrutiny they deserve.

Some of the benefits attributable to coffee also apply to tea, such as a gentle mental and physical pick-me-up and lower risk of kidney stones and gallstones. Some studies have suggested that drinking green tea may protect against heart disease and some cancers, particularly stomach cancer. Substances in tea called flavonoids might be involved. In the laboratory, tea and/or flavonoids improve cholesterol levels and artery function and inhibit early steps leading to cancer. In real life, though, the evidence is mixed and often contradictory. In worldwide surveys, increasing tea consumption has been associated with an increased risk of heart disease in the United Kingdom and Australia but a decreased risk in continental Europe and other regions. Ongoing cancer research is also pointing toward little anticancer effect, if any.

Flavonoids aren't limited to tea. Other good sources include berries, apples, tomatoes, broccoli, carrots, and onions. It may be necessary to look at all their contributions simultaneously to determine whether or not the current enthusiasm for flavonoids is warranted. For now, don't count on tea to bring any special benefits besides a reduced risk of kidney stones and a pleasant way to begin, enjoy, or end the day.

ALCOHOL

In the United States, public health campaigns have traditionally urged people to cut back on their drinking or avoid alcohol altogether. Concerns about alcohol are definitely justified. Alcohol is implicated in about one-third of all fatal traffic accidents. Heavy drinking is a major cause of preventable deaths in the United States. It contributes to liver disease, a variety of cancers, high blood pressure, so-called bleeding strokes, and a progressive weakening of the heart and other muscles. Too much alcohol can dissolve the best of intentions and the closest relationships.

Alcohol in moderation, though, is probably good for most people. A drink before a meal can improve digestion or offer a soothing respite at the end of a stressful day; the occasional drink with friends can be a social tonic. These physical and psychic effects may improve health and well-being. Drinking alcohol helps raise levels of HDL, the protective form of cholesterol, and also reduces the formation of clots that can block arteries in the heart, neck, and brain and ultimately cause heart attacks and the most common kind of stroke. There is good evidence that these and other effects of moderate alcohol consumption translate into protection against heart disease and ischemic strokes, and mounting evidence that it protects against diabetes and gallstones.

Exactly how many drinks is moderate? That's a tricky question and a topic that is the focus of intense research. For men, study after study has shown that men who have one or two alcoholic drinks a day are 30 to 40 percent less likely to have heart attacks than men who don't drink alcohol at all. That's about the same as seen for the powerful cholesterol-lowering drugs known as statins. For men with diabetes, who are at very high risk of developing heart disease, a drink or two a day has similar benefits. More than two drinks a day further increases the heart and stroke protection, but also increases the chances that the dark side of alcohol will emerge. (See Figure 18.)

For women, it is tougher to define moderate. Women, too, benefit from alcohol's ability to raise HDL and prevent clot formation. But the Nurses' Health Study and others have shown that two drinks a day increases the chances of developing breast cancer by 20 to 25 percent. This doesn't mean that 20 to 25 percent of women who have two drinks a day will get breast cancer. Instead it is the difference between about 12 of every 100 women developing breast cancer during their lifetimes—the current average risk in the United States—and 14 to 15 of every 100 women developing the disease. But it is still enough of an increase to be worrisome.

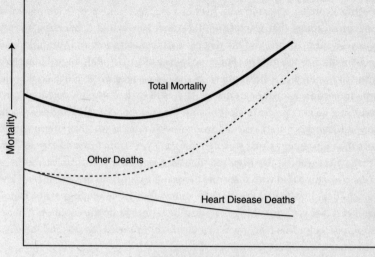

FIG. 18 Alcohol and Death. Alcohol has different effects on different causes of death. As alcohol intake increases, deaths from heart disease gradually decline, while deaths from accidents, liver disease, and other causes increase, slowly at first and then sharply at high levels of consumption. The result is a J-shaped curve, with the lowest mortality associated with moderate alcohol consumption and higher mortality associated with no drinking and with excessive drinking. The optimal range for an individual depends on age, sex, folic acid intake, and other factors, but is generally considered to be one to two drinks a day for men and no more than one drink a day for women.

New evidence from large prospective studies of women show that the increased risk of breast cancer linked to drinking alcohol is seen mostly in women who get insufficient amounts of the B vitamin known as folic acid in their diets. The same applies to colon cancer: The increased risk with alcohol consumption seems mainly to occur among persons with lower intakes of folic acid. So, as discussed in chapter 10, taking a multivitamin that contains folic acid is especially important for those who drink alcohol.

For both men and women, even moderate drinking carries some risks. Alcohol can disrupt sleep. Its ability to disrupt judgment is legendary. Alcohol, particularly in higher amounts, interacts in potentially dangerous ways with a variety of medications, including acetaminophen, antidepressants, anticonvulsants, painkillers, and sedatives. It is also addictive, especially among people with a family history of alcoholism.

So who might benefit from a daily alcoholic drink? Alcohol offers little benefit and potential risks for a pregnant woman and her unborn child, a recovering alcoholic, a person with liver disease, and some people taking one or more medications that interact with alcohol. Nor would it benefit a twenty-eight-year-old man, because his risk of heart disease is low and you can't bank the benefits for the future. For a sixty-year-old man with high cholesterol whose father died of a heart attack at age sixty-one, a drink a day could offer some protection against heart disease that is likely to outweigh potential harm (assuming he isn't prone to alcoholism). The risk-benefit calculations are a bit more difficult for a sixty-year-old woman with a sister who has breast cancer. More than ten times as many women die each year from heart disease as from breast cancer—about five hundred thousand women a year from cardiovascular disease, compared with forty-one thousand a year from breast cancer. However, studies show that women are far more afraid of developing breast cancer than heart disease, something that must be factored into the equation. There's a sound basis for this fear, given that deaths from breast cancer tend to be at a younger age than those from heart disease.

From the early studies suggesting that moderate alcohol consumption could prevent heart attacks and other heart disease emerged the so-called French paradox—the unexpectedly low rate of heart disease in France despite a typically high-fat diet. Some researchers suggested that red wine was the answer, something the wine industry heavily and heartily endorsed. Red wine alone isn't the reason for the low heart disease rates. The overall diet and lifestyle in parts of France, especially the south, have much in common with other Mediterranean regions, and these may account for some of the protection against heart disease. What's more, a number of recent studies have shown that any alcohol-containing beverage offers the same benefits. Red or white wine, beer, cordials, or spirits such as gin or Scotch whiskey all seem to have the same effect on cardiovascular disease. Claims that the small amounts of resveratrol and other antioxidants found in red wine and grape juice prevent heart disease have yet to be proved; if they do indeed offer any extra benefit, it is likely to be small.

One's drinking pattern seems to be more important than the type of alcoholic beverage. My colleagues and I looked at drinking habits among more than almost forty thousand men whose health and lifestyles we had been following for twelve years. When compared with men who drank less than once a week, those who drank at least three days a week were 30 percent less likely to have had a heart attack. The type of alcoholic drink and whether or not it was consumed with meals had little effect on this association.

When the alcohol–heart disease connection was in its early days, the standard caution most of us used in our scientific papers and when talking to reporters or the public was that no one should start drinking alcohol just for the heart benefits. Now that these benefits are well proven and durable, I offer these more concrete guidelines:

- If you don't drink alcohol, don't feel compelled to start—you can get similar benefits by beginning to exercise (if you don't already) or boosting the intensity and duration of your activity.
- If you already drink alcohol, keep it moderate.
- A drink a day three or more times a week is far, far better for you than three or more drinks one day a week.
- If you are a man with no history of alcoholism who is at moderate to high risk for heart disease, a daily alcoholic drink may help reduce that risk.
- If you are a woman with no history of alcoholism, benefits of a drink a day may be counterbalanced by a small increase in your chances of developing breast cancer. Getting enough folic acid (at least 400 milligrams per day) can prevent this increase in risk (see chapter 10).
- Alcohol may be particularly beneficial if you have low HDL (good) cholesterol that just won't budge upward with a healthy diet and plenty of exercise.
- Talk with your health care provider to help you weigh decisions about alcohol.

CHAPTER NINE

Calcium: No Emergency

YOU'VE SEEN THE ADS—CELEBRITIES like pop star Britney Spears, home-run king Mark McGwire, former New York City mayor Rudy Giuliani, film director Spike Lee, and television's Buffy the Vampire Slayer, each sporting a gleaming white milk mustache. They are supposed to be making you aware of the dangers of not getting enough calcium in your diet while urging you to drink three glasses of milk a day to combat our country's "calcium emergency."

I hope you can resist the genial, folksy allure of this slick but misleading campaign, sponsored by the National Dairy Council. For starters, there isn't a calcium emergency. When it comes to calcium in the diet, the United States is near the top of the list of average calcium intake per person, second only to some Scandinavian countries and parts of Latin America (where calcium is used to make tortillas). More important, while there's no question that calcium is an essential part of a healthy diet, there are other major questions. Some of the most important include the following:

- *How much calcium do we really need each day?* It depends on whom you ask. In the United States, the official currently recommended intakes are 1,000 mg/day from ages nineteen to fifty and 1,200 mg/day after that. In the United Kingdom, everyone over age nineteen is urged to get 700 mg/day. The World Health Organization says 400–500 mg of calcium a day are needed to prevent osteoporosis. In Canada, the target for adults is 1,000 mg/day up to age fifty and then 1,500 mg/day after that.

Why the differences? Different types of studies yield different answers about how much calcium people need, so reliance on one type rather than another leads to the range of recommendations. The kinds of studies used to set the current daily calcium requirements have some serious flaws. What's more, there's no good evidence that merely increasing the amount of milk in your diet will protect you from breaking a hip or wrist or crushing a backbone in later years.

- *How much calcium or milk is safe?* Nutrition experts have long assumed that calcium is a lot like vitamin C—your body merely excretes what it can't use. But it's beginning to look as though too much calcium might be a bad thing. For men, a high calcium intake seems to increase the odds of developing fatal prostate cancer. For women, drinking a lot of milk has been linked with higher rates of ovarian cancer. In both cases the evidence isn't conclusive, but it is enough to sound a warning about possible negative effects of getting too much calcium and drinking too much milk.

• *Is milk, or are dairy products in general, the best source of calcium?* Milk is clearly a highly efficient way to get calcium from food, since it delivers almost 300 mg per eight-ounce glass. (See table, page 160.) But milk delivers more than just calcium, and some of its other components—like extra calories, saturated fat, and the sugar known as galactose—aren't necessarily good for you. What's more, as many as fifty million adults in the United States can't completely digest the milk sugar known as lactose. Nor can most of the world's population.

The main reason for all the concern about too little calcium is the frightful prospect of osteoporosis, the gradual and insidious loss of bone that often comes with old age. In the United States alone, osteoporosis affects ten million women and men. Each year osteoporosis leads to more than 1.5 million fractures, including 300,000 broken hips. Breaking a hip in old age can be disabling, even deadly—almost one-quarter of older people who break a hip die in the following year, often from complications caused by their injury.

Unfortunately, there's little evidence that just boosting your calcium intake to the high levels that are currently recommended will prevent fractures. And all the high-profile attention given to calcium is distracting us from strategies that really work—like exercise, getting enough vitamin D, avoiding too much vitamin A, and taking certain medications.

As I will describe in the next few pages, dairy products shouldn't occupy a prominent place in our diet, nor should they be the centerpiece of the national strategy to prevent osteoporosis. Instead, the evidence shows that dietary calcium should come from a variety of sources and, if more calcium is really needed, from cheap, no-calorie, easy-to-take supplements. Then you can look at dairy products as an optional part of a healthy diet and take them in moderation, if at all.

WHY YOU NEED CALCIUM

Your body contains roughly two pounds of calcium, about 99 percent of which is locked into bone. Think of calcium as the mortar that cements and solidifies the components that give bone its substance and strength. The rest is dissolved

Calcium and Magnesium in Foods

FOOD	AMOUNT	CALCIUM		MAGNESIUM	
		MG	% DR*	MG	% DR**
Total cereal	3/4 cup	1104	92	39	12
Tofu	1/2 cup	861	72	73	23
Yogurt, low-fat	1 cup	448	37	42	13
Orange juice, calcium-fortified	6 ounces	350	29	19	6
Milk, skim	1 cup	306	26	27	8
Cornbread	1 two-ounce piece	162	14	16	5
Collard greens, cooked	1/2 cup	133	11	19	6
Soybeans	1/2 cup	130	11	54	17
Spinach	1/2 cup	122	10	78	24
English muffin, whole wheat	1	100	8	22	7
Navy beans	1/2 cup	63	5	48	15
Figs, dried	4	54	5	23	7
Mustard greens	1/2 cup	52	4	10	3
Orange	1 medium	52	4	13	4
Black turtle beans, boiled	1/2 cup	51	4	45	14
Swiss chard, boiled	1/2 cup	51	4	75	23
Kale, boiled	1/2 cup	47	4	12	4
Vegetarian baked beans	1/2 cup	43	4	33	10
Sweet potato, baked	1 medium	43	4	31	10
Butternut squash, baked	1/2 cup	42	4	30	9
Chickpeas, cooked	1/2 cup	40	3	39	12
Raisins	1/2 cup	36	3	23	7
Broccoli, boiled	1/2 cup	31	3	16	5
Green beans, boiled	1/2 cup	29	2	16	5

| Food | Amount | Calcium | | Magnesium | |
		MG	% DR*	MG	% DR**
Brussels sprouts, cooked	¹/₂ cup	28	2	16	5
Chocolate bar	1¹/₂ ounces	10	1	46	14
Pearled barley, cooked	¹/₂ cup	9	1	17	5
Bulgur, cooked	¹/₂ cup	9	1	29	9

* DR: Daily requirement based on 1,200 milligrams for a man or woman aged 50 years or older

** DR: Daily requirement based on 320 milligrams for a woman aged 50 years or older

Source: U.S. Department of Agriculture, National Nutrient Database for Standard Reference, Release 17, 2004, www.nal.usda.gov/fnic/foodcomp

More detailed lists of foods rich in calcium or magnesium are available from the USDA Nutrient Data Laboratory's Web site, www.nal.usda.gov/fnic/foodcomp/Data/SR17/wtrank/wt_rank.html.

in your blood and the fluid inside and outside cells. That dissolved calcium helps conduct nerve impulses, regulates your heartbeat, and controls other cell functions.

Like an obsessive remodeler, your body constantly builds up and tears down bone. Early in life, building up dominates. Throughout midlife, the two processes generally balance out. Later on, though, demolition may outpace construction and lead to weak or broken bones. Many factors influence bone remodeling. Putting a bone under repeated stress—say, the stress of lifting a weight or carrying a body at a trot—triggers growth. Lack of stress—meaning little or no physical activity—leads to degeneration. Sex hormones such as estrogen and testosterone stimulate bone-building activity. It is the chaotic rush of these hormones during puberty that sets off an adolescent's growth spurt. Their loss later in life—a gradual ebbing away in men, a more abrupt cessation in women—shifts the balance toward bone loss, a shift that can be sudden and dramatic in women. The amount of calcium available to bone-building cells (called osteoblasts) also influences bone remodeling, as do the amounts of vitamin D and vitamin K. But as I will describe shortly, exactly how much calcium you need each day is a very open question.

Osteoporosis is usually portrayed as a woman's disease. But it also affects men. Men enter adulthood with stronger, denser bones than women, and they never face the sudden bone-draining loss of estrogen that occurs with menopause. This gives men a five-to-ten-year hedge against osteoporosis, but not lifetime protection.

BEYOND BONE

Although calcium's main activity is related to bone, it plays other roles in maintaining good health.

• *Colon cancer.* Over the past two decades, studies of different types and sizes have indicated that increasing intake of calcium from milk or supplements offers modest protection against colorectal cancer. Megadoses aren't necessary—most benefits accompany the intakes seen in a reasonable diet, around 700–800 mg of calcium per day.

• *Blood pressure.* A calcium-rich diet, or taking calcium supplements, can lower blood pressure. Although the effect is relatively small for most people, it may be enough to forgo medication or reduce the risk of having a heart attack or stroke. Getting enough calcium may also help stave off the gradual rise in blood pressure that tends to come with aging.

• *Weight loss.* Ads for the "got milk?" campaign have touted milk's ability to help people shed pounds. "Drinking three glasses of milk daily when dieting," they say, "can help you lose body fat while maintaining muscle mass." That's a bit misleading. Scientific studies in rats and people link consuming dairy products with weight loss—*if* calories are scaled back, too. It's the eating less, not the calcium, that's important. Not surprisingly, calcium supplements don't affect weight.

CALCIUM REQUIREMENTS ARE UNCLEAR

Although you'd never know it from the "got milk?" milk-mustache ads, no one really knows the healthiest, safest amount of dietary calcium. Different scientific approaches yield different estimates, so it's important to consider *all* the evidence.

One good starting place is to look at the connection between calcium intake and fractures in different countries. Around the world there's a huge variation in average daily calcium intake, from 300 mg/day in India, Japan, and Peru to 1,300+ mg/day in Finland and some other Scandinavian countries. Curiously, countries with the highest average calcium intakes tend to have higher, not lower, hip fracture rates (Figure 19). There are also important differences

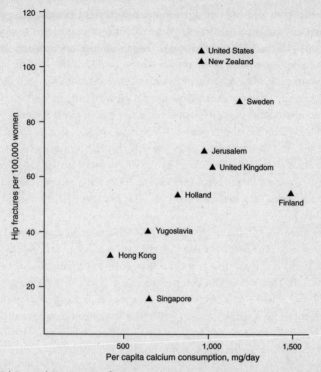

FIG. 19 Calcium and Fractures. Hip fractures tend to be more common in countries with high average calcium intake, such as the United States and New Zealand, than in those with low calcium intake, such as Singapore and Yugoslavia.

in physical activity levels, sunlight, and other dietary factors that could obscure the real relationship between calcium and fractures.

Daily calcium requirements are traditionally calculated using a balance study. This is a relatively straightforward test—you assemble a group of volunteers, put them on a diet or supplements containing different amounts of calcium for a few days or a few weeks, then measure the amount of calcium they excrete in their urine and stool. The balance point is the level at which calcium in equals calcium out. Balance studies show that about 550 mg of calcium a day is an optimal level for the mythical average adult. Another route to estimating daily calcium requirements is called the maximal retention study. This type, too, usually lasts only a few weeks. By giving volunteers high doses of calcium, it tries to determine the highest amount of calcium that the body (mainly the bones) can grab and hold on to. Yet another piece of evidence comes from measurements of bone density using special X-ray machines before and after a year or so of calcium supplementation. These studies show a very encouraging 1 to 2 percent increase in bone density. If you could increase the density, and thus the strength, of your bones by 1 to 2 percent a year for five or ten years, you would certainly fortify your skeleton against future damage.

The expert panel that established the latest (1997) dietary reference intake (DRI) for calcium used information from these kinds of studies to set the target at 1,000 mg/day for adults up to age fifty and 1,200 mg/day for those over age 50. This "overrecommendation" is one way to make sure that 95 percent of people are covered by the recommendation. (The DRIs replace the old RDAs, or recommended dietary allowances, you may have seen listed on food or vitamin labels.)

But there are two big related problems with the studies on which the standards are based. The first has to do with the nature of bone itself. A small part of bone, essentially the part that is most able to grow and change, usually contains little calcium. This is called the remodeling space. If you were to greatly increase your calcium intake—by adding several glasses of milk a day or taking calcium supplements—for a year or so, this space would sponge up extra calcium. Your bone's calcium content would increase by a small amount, about 2 percent, but only temporarily. After the first year, the filled-up remodeling space couldn't hold any more calcium, so continued calcium supplementation or a high-calcium diet would have little further effect on bone density. What's more, any gains in bone mass would be lost when the higher calcium intake stops. The second problem is that most studies last just one or two years and so observe only what is happening in the remodeling space and not what is really happening in the big picture of overall bone strength.

What these short-term studies fail to capture is the body's remarkable capacity to adapt. A unique study of Scandinavian prisoners, all men, shows that their bodies were still adapting after several years on a lower-calcium diet (500 mg/day), mainly by excreting less calcium and using calcium more efficiently.

In real life, broken bones are a better test of desirable calcium levels than the short-term flow of calcium in and out of the body or measurements of bone density. Studies comparing people who have broken their hips or wrists because of osteoporosis with people who haven't broken bones have yielded mixed results. Some show that getting extra calcium protects against fractures, and others show no benefit of getting extra calcium. More important, the results from seven long-term prospective studies done in the United States, England, and Sweden that have followed large groups of people for long periods don't show any important reduction in risk of broken bones with increasing calcium intake. In the Nurses' Health Study, for example, women who drank two or more glasses of milk a day were at least as likely to break a hip or forearm as women who drank one glass or less a week. The same was true for men participating in the Health Professionals Follow-up Study.

When the evidence from several different sources doesn't add up, the best answer usually (though not always) comes from a randomized trial. That would mean assembling a large group of volunteers and asking half of them to take a calcium supplement and half to take an identical placebo. Because osteoporosis takes a long time to develop, a trial like this must last for years. It isn't clear what would be the best age at which to do it—adolescence and early adulthood, when bone building is at its peak; middle age; or later in life, when dwindling physical activity and hormone levels combine to weaken bone.

So far, there's no clear proof from such trials. They have either been too small to generate solid results or have used a combination of calcium and something else, usually vitamin D, that make it impossible to tell if the reduction in fractures is due to calcium or to the something else. The typical high-dose calcium supplementation trial (1,000–2,000 mg/day) can't say much about required intake—if it shows a benefit, it is possible that a much smaller dose could have done the same thing.

The National Institutes of Health started the ongoing Women's Health Initiative, a long-term, large-scale study to test a variety of promising but unproven strategies for preventing the leading causes of death and disability among older women—chronic diseases such as heart disease, stroke, cancer, and osteoporosis. In one component of the Women's Health Initiative, more than twenty thousand women take daily calcium (1,000 mg) and vitamin D (400 IU) supplements and another twenty thousand take placebo pills. While this seven- to eleven-year experiment should soon tell us something about the effect of the calcium/vitamin D combination on fractures, it won't say much about calcium alone.

THE DARK SIDE OF CALCIUM AND DAIRY PRODUCTS

If no one really knows the best daily calcium target, then why not play it safe and boost your calcium by drinking three glasses of milk a day? Here are six good reasons: lactose intolerance, saturated fat, extra calories, unneeded hormones, a possible increased risk of prostate cancer, and a possible increased risk of ovarian cancer.

- *Lactose intolerance.* All babies are born with the ability to digest milk. Some, especially those of northern European ancestry, keep this trait for life. Most children, though, gradually lose it as their bodies stop making an enzyme called lactase that breaks down milk sugar (lactose). In fact, only about a quarter of the world's adults can fully digest milk. In the United States, as many as fifty million Americans aren't equipped to digest milk. Half of Hispanic Americans, 75 percent of African Americans, and more than 90 percent of Asian Americans can't tolerate a lot of lactose. For them, drinking a glass of milk can have unpleasant consequences, such as nausea, bloating, cramps, and diarrhea.

A lot of effort has gone into helping lactose-intolerant people drink milk or eat cheese or ice cream. The U.S. Agriculture Research Service touts its development of the lactose-modified milk known as Lactaid as one of its top fifteen accomplishments in the last fifty years. A variety of lactose-digesting powders or tablets that can be added to milk or taken before eating dairy products are available over the counter. And dairy proponents point to a number of studies showing that people who have trouble digesting lactose can tolerate small amounts throughout the day, especially when taken with other food. But because there are easier ways to get enough calcium, I don't believe that people who have trouble digesting lactose need to spend the extra money or time to drink milk or eat dairy products. It is perfectly fine if you want to do that. But you shouldn't force yourself to do it or feel guilty if you don't. After all, you're in good company, with three-quarters of the world's adults.

- *Saturated fat.* An eight-ounce glass of whole milk contains almost 5 grams of saturated fat, or about 20 percent of the recommended 20-gram daily limit. Drinking three glasses a day would be the equivalent of eating twelve strips of bacon or a Big Mac and an order of fries. Cheese is another way to get calcium. A one-ounce serving of cheese made from whole milk delivers about two-thirds of the calcium as a glass of milk and the same amount of saturated fat. If you enjoy milk, low-fat and skim are certainly better choices than whole milk.

If enough people make the switch to low-fat or skim milk, you might expect that lower rates of heart disease would follow. They won't, at least not at the population level. That's because once a cow is milked, the fat from that milk is in the food supply, and someone ends up drinking or eating it. Much of the fat skimmed from milk resurfaces in premium ice cream, buttery pastries, and high-fat snack foods. Many of the same people who have switched to skim milk have a bowl of high-fat Ben & Jerry's or Häagen-Dazs ice cream before going to bed, and people who drink whole milk or don't drink milk at all—often poorer, less educated, or less health-savvy people—are eating more and more high-fat products made with milk fat.

• *Extra calories.* Three glasses of whole milk a day add 450 calories to your diet—about one-quarter of your daily intake allowance. Low-fat milk, at 330 calories, adds a bit fewer, but that is still a lot if the main goal is just to get more calcium.

• *Extra hormones.* Cows make most of the same hormones that humans make. Before farming turned into agribusiness, the hormone levels in milk weren't an issue. Today, though, they may well be a cause for concern.

Over the years, dairy cattle have been bred to produce more milk. Since 1960, American Holstein cows' genetic potential for milk production has increased nearly *seven thousand pounds* for each period of lactation. Cows are also routinely milked while they are pregnant, which also keeps milk production high. This is great for cattle farmers and milk producers, and it helps keep the price of milk relatively low. But it also means that today's milk contains a more concentrated hormonal stew than it did years ago. Naturally occurring hormones in milk include estrogens and progestins, androgens, and insulinlike growth factors, to name just a few. Estrogens and progestins can stimulate breast cancer, androgens promote prostate cancer, and elevated levels of insulinlike growth factor have been linked with breast, prostate, and colon cancer.

Almost ten years ago, my colleagues and I started the Growing Up Today Study among children of women in the Nurses' Health Study. The more than sixteen thousand volunteers complete forms on diet, exercise, lifestyle factors, and health much as their mothers do. In this group, the largely hormone-driven condition of teenage acne is more common among milk drinkers. This is important because it suggests that the hormones in milk are strong enough or abundant enough to stimulate glandular tissue such as the sebaceous glands in the skin—and possibly mammary glands in the breast.

• *Prostate cancer.* A diet high in dairy products has been implicated as a risk factor for prostate cancer. In nine separate studies, the strongest and most consistent dietary factor linked with prostate cancer was high consumption of milk or dairy products. In the largest of these, the Health Professionals Follow-up Study, men who drank two or more glasses of milk a day were almost twice as likely to develop advanced or metastatic (spreading) prostate cancer as those who didn't drink milk at all.

At first, researchers thought that the connection between dairy products and prostate cancer was due to the saturated fat in dairy products. But results from the Health Professionals Follow-up Study, as well as more careful analyses of other data, suggest that calcium might be the main culprit. In this study, men who took in more than 2,000 mg of calcium a day from food and supplements combined were almost three times as likely to develop advanced prostate cancer and more than four times as likely to develop metastatic prostate cancer than men who got less than 500 mg/day.

There's a plausible explanation for this. Inside the prostate (and elsewhere), the active form of vitamin D may act like a brake on the growth and division of cancer cells. Too much calcium slows or even stops the conversion of inactive vitamin D to its biologically active form and so may rob the body of a natural anticancer mechanism.

To be on the safe side, men should try to keep their daily calcium intake below 1,000 mg.

• *Breast cancer.* Early-onset breast cancer (cancer that appears before menopause) seems to be associated with high intake of full-fat dairy products. This is especially the case for estrogen-receptor positive (ER+) breast cancer, in which estrogen stimulates cancer cells to grow and divide.

• *Ovarian cancer.* About fifteen years ago, Harvard Medical School researchers suggested that high levels of galactose, a simple sugar released by the digestion of lactose in milk, could damage the ovary and possibly lead to ovarian cancer. Since then a number of studies have tested this hypothesis. While the evidence isn't conclusive (some studies have supported this notion and others haven't), a positive link between galactose and ovarian cancer shows up too many times to ignore the possibility that it may be harmful.

The ideal prevention strategy is one that stops something bad from happening without causing any other bad things to happen. Consuming plenty of dairy products is being portrayed as a key way to prevent osteoporosis and broken bones. But not only does this fail to fit the bill as a proven prevention strategy, it doesn't even come close. The totality of evidence doesn't support the claim that just getting more calcium prevents fractures over the long term, and there is plenty of evidence that drinking two or three glasses of milk a day does little to reduce the chances of breaking a bone. What's more, dairy products pose several proven and potential problems. So if you are worried about osteoporosis, other prevention strategies make better sense.

IF NOT CALCIUM, WHAT?

Complex processes are often influenced by a host of different factors. That is certainly true for bone building. In addition to calcium, some of the

Nutrient Content of 1 Cup of Whole Milk

NUTRIENT	AMOUNT	PERCENT DAILY VALUE*
Water	215 grams	-
Energy	146 calories	7
Protein	8 grams	17
Total lipid (fat)	8 grams	13
Carbohydrate	11 grams	8
Fiber	0	0
Calcium	276 milligrams	23
Iron	0.1 milligrams	1
Magnesium	24 milligrams	7
Phosphorus	222 milligrams	32
Potassium	349 milligrams	7
Sodium	98 milligrams	8
Vitamin C	0	0
Vitamin B_6	0.1 milligrams	7
Folate	12 micrograms	3
Vitamin B_{12}	1 microgram	42
Vitamin A	249 IU	36
Vitamin E	0.2 milligrams	1
Vitamin D	99 IU	16
Saturated fats	4.5 grams	20
Monounsaturated fats	2 grams	—
Polyunsaturated fats	0.5 grams	—
Cholesterol	24 grams	8

* Daily recommended intake, as set by the Institute of Medicine, for a woman 51–70 years old who eats 2,000 calories a day.

Source: U.S. Department of Agriculture, Agriculture Research Service, National Nutrient Database for Standard Reference, Release 17, 2004 (www.nal.usda.gov/fnic/foodcomp).

things you can tinker with that influence bone growth are exercise, the sex hormones estrogen and testosterone, and nutrients such as vitamin D, vitamin K, and fluoride. The amount of protein in your diet also might make a difference.

• *Exercise.* A bone bends when some force is applied to it. Apply a large force and the bend turns into a break. Apply a small one and the bend is minuscule but physiologically important, especially if the force is repeated over and over. Cells inside bone sense physical strain or stress and orchestrate a silent symphony of activity that remodels the bone to make it more dense and stronger. Among children and young adults, vigorous physical activity sketches the blueprint for the growing skeleton. The more activity and healthy stress on bones, the more bone is built and the larger the bone reservoir upon which to draw during adulthood and old age. During adulthood, exercise helps maintain the balance between bone-building and bone-dissolving processes. During old age, exercise limits bone loss.

Keep in mind that activity doesn't build or strengthen *all* bones, just those that are stressed, so you need a variety of exercises or activities to keep all your bones healthy.

While the impact of exercise on bone health is widely accepted, experts haven't yet defined the best way to maintain strong bones. Some combination of weight-bearing exercises (like brisk walking) and muscle-strengthening exercises will probably turn out to be the ideal combination. Not only would this combination continually stimulate bone growth, but it would also strengthen muscles and improve balance and so help prevent bone-breaking falls.

• *Hormones.* Two potent members of this class of compounds are estrogen and testosterone. Estrogen is sometimes called the female hormone, and testosterone the male hormone, even though women and men make both. Numerous studies have shown that these two hormones are important for building new bone early in life and for keeping it strong over the next seventy years or so. That's a problem because production of sex hormones plummets after menopause in women and falls off more gradually in men.

Hormone replacement therapy, usually with estrogen plus a progestin, was once the first-line treatment for preventing osteoporosis in older women. It is an effective way to control the hot flashes that often accompany menopause. It was also thought to help prevent heart disease. Widespread use of hormone replacement therapy ended when results from the federally funded Women's Health Initiative showed a large increase in breast cancer and a small but significant increase in the risk of heart disease and stroke among women who used estrogen with a progestin. Alternatives to estrogen include drugs called bisphosphonates, such as alendronate (Fosamax), etidronate (Didronel), and ibandronate (Boniva); selective estrogen receptor modulators such as raloxifene (Evista); and calcitonin.

The slowdown in sex hormone production in men isn't as abrupt or as predictable as it is in women. If there are warning signs of osteoporosis, a testosterone check is a good idea for men over age sixty-five. If levels are low, then daily testosterone gel or patches or biweekly shots of testosterone might be considered.

For women or men, the decision to begin hormone therapy isn't something to take lightly. It is a complicated issue with rapidly changing options. Weighing the benefits and risks and sorting through these options is best done with a trusted health care provider.

• *Vitamin D.* This fat-soluble vitamin's best-known function is helping the digestive system efficiently absorb calcium and phosphorus. It helps build and maintain healthy bones in other ways, too (see chapter 10). Several studies have shown that vitamin D deficiencies are more common among older people with broken bones than those without them. In the Nurses' Health Study, older women who got at least 500 International Units (IU) of vitamin D a day were one-third less likely to have broken a hip than women who got under 200 IU a day. Results from randomized trials of vitamin D and fractures have been mixed, but all that used 800 IU per day showed a benefit, while those using lower daily doses did not.

The current official target for daily vitamin D intake is 200 IU (5 mcg) between the ages of nineteen and fifty; 400 IU (10 mcg) between the ages of fifty-one and seventy; and 600 IU (15 mcg) after age seventy. Yet many lines of evidence point to a higher level—at least 800 IU per day—to get the full benefits of vitamin D.

Few foods naturally contain vitamin D, so you need to get most of yours from either sunlight or supplements. A tablespoon of cod-liver oil delivers more than 1,200 IU. Standard multivitamins carry 400 IU of vitamin D. Don't take two of these to get extra vitamin D, since a double dose of preformed vitamin A (retinol) might counteract vitamin D's effects. Some calcium supplements come with added vitamin D, which is a good idea since there is actually better evidence for benefits from vitamin D supplements than for calcium. In addition, the two substances may have a synergistic effect.

Can extra vitamin D help prevent osteoporosis-related fractures? Although the evidence isn't totally consistent, extra vitamin D may be an effective way to prevent bone loss. I certainly agree with an editorial in the *New England Journal of Medicine* that succinctly concluded, "A widespread increase in vitamin D intake is likely to have a greater effect on osteoporosis and fractures than many other interventions." For most people, the easiest way to do this is to take supplements that contain vitamin D. More on this in chapter 10.

- *Vitamin K.* Until recently, vitamin K was thought to be necessary mostly for the formation of proteins that regulate blood clotting. It turns out, though, that this fat-soluble vitamin also plays one or more roles in the regulation of calcium and the formation and stabilization of bone. So too little vitamin K may help set the stage for osteoporosis. In the Nurses' Health Study, women who got more than 109 mcg of vitamin K a day were 30 percent less likely to break a hip than women who got less than that amount. The current recommended daily intake for vitamin K is 90 mcg for women and 120 mcg for men. Vitamin K is found mainly in green vegetables such as dark green lettuce, broccoli, spinach, Brussels sprouts, and kale. Eating one or more servings of these foods a day should give you enough vitamin K. If you take warfarin (Coumadin) or other medications to prevent blood clots, talk with your doctor first before boosting your daily intake of vitamin K.

- *Fluoride.* The same substance that is added to drinking water and toothpaste to fight cavities can also fight osteoporosis. Fluoride therapy is already used in many countries, and the Food and Drug Administration is considering its use in the United States. While low-dose fluoride pills aren't being eyed as a way to *prevent* osteoporosis and late-in-life fractures, a fluoride-calcium combination could be a safe, effective way to help treat existing osteoporosis. Fluoride supplements aren't something to try on your own, though. Early enthusiasm for high-dose fluoride supplements evaporated when later studies showed that the dense bones they helped build were sometimes more brittle and more likely to break. While the amounts of fluoride added to drinking water are perfectly safe, stay away from fluoride supplements unless they are prescribed by your physician.

- *Protein.* As your body digests protein, it releases acids into the bloodstream. Calcium, drawn mostly from the skeleton, helps neutralize these acids. A number of studies have shown that the more protein consumed, the more calcium excreted in the urine. When it comes to leaching calcium from bone, animal protein is somewhat more powerful than vegetable protein. The connection between protein and calcium loss may explain part of the high rate of broken bones in meat-eating countries such as the United States and those in northern Europe, though the link between protein and bone health is far from settled.

PUTTING THIS INTO PRACTICE

How much calcium we need is one of the major unsettled issues in human nutrition. It is abundantly clear that active, healthy people who get only low to moderate amounts of calcium can have low fracture rates. It is unclear whether getting more will further lower this risk, but the evidence doesn't look promising. Because a small benefit can't be ruled out, and because calcium seems to help fight colon cancer, a reasonable strategy for women in middle age and beyond is to get an extra 500–1,000 mg/day. Calcium supplements are the best way to do this, though low-fat dairy products are an alternative for those who really like milk. For men, the balance of benefits and risks tips against a lot of extra calcium.

There are four things proven to reduce the chances of developing osteoporosis that almost everyone can do:

- Be as physically active as possible. Engage in a variety of activities to keep your bones healthy and your muscles strong.
- Take 800–1,000 IU of vitamin D a day. Only a few vitamin brands contain this much.
- Get enough vitamin K by eating at least one serving of green leafy vegetables a day.
- Don't get too much extra preformed vitamin A (retinol) unless prescribed by your doctor. Keep your daily dose from supplements under 2,000 IU.

CHAPTER TEN

Take a Multivitamin for Insurance

ONCE UPON A TIME, VITAMINS were thought of only as nutrients needed in small amounts to prevent diseases with exotic-sounding names like beri-beri, pellagra, scurvy, and rickets. So nutritional guidelines for vitamins were based on the amount needed to avoid these diseases. Because they were becoming rarer and rarer, it seemed that the vast majority of Americans was getting enough vitamins. Getting more than the amounts needed to prevent those deficiency diseases, from either food or supplements, was a waste, so the thinking went. Or as one critic of vitamin supplements was fond of saying, they are good for nothing more than giving America the "richest urine in the world."

Some innovative thinking and the wonderful, logical conversation of science has been changing the way we think about vitamins, minerals, and other micronutrients. The biggest shift has been the realization that many cases of chronic diseases such as some cancers and heart disease could be partly due to nutrient deficiencies, just like beri-beri and scurvy. The new findings suggest that some people—probably many people—don't get enough of these essential micronutrients. By increasing the amount we get, mostly from food but maybe from supplements as well, we could substantially improve our long-term health.

What really blew the cover off the old vitamin-deficiency disease connection was the discovery of a direct link between inadequate intake of the B vitamin folic acid (or folate) and birth defects such as spina bifida and anencephaly. Both of these, collectively called neural tube defects, happen when the tissues destined to become the spinal cord, the bony tube that protects it, and the brain don't develop as they should during the first twenty-eight days of pregnancy. Spina bifida can cause paralysis and other disabilities. Children with anencephaly are born without most of the brain and spinal cord; they are either stillborn or survive for only a short time after birth. Worldwide, about three hundred thousand babies are born with neural tube defects each year.

Clinical observations that neural tube defects were most common in poor populations with poor diets prompted a search for nutritional causes. In 1976 a British team found that mothers of children with neural tube defects had relatively low levels of micronutrients. The realization that drugs that interfered with folic acid increased the risk of having a child with a neural tube defect helped focus on folate. After the not uncommon scientific seesaw—some studies implicated low folic acid in these birth defects, others didn't, some small trials showed a benefit for folic acid supplements, others didn't—two large trials gathered conclusive proof that women who didn't get enough folic acid were more likely to have a child with spina bifida or anencephaly and that taking folic acid supplements could prevent these birth defects.

At first, the recommendations on folic acid were cautious. Initial guidelines from the Centers for Disease Control (CDC) in 1991 were aimed only at women who had already had a child with a neural tube defect. A year later the CDC broadened its message, recommending that all women who could become pregnant get 400 micrograms of folic acid a day. That was more than double what had been recommended before. Because many women were not heeding this advice, the U.S. Food and Drug Administration now requires that folic acid be added to most enriched breads, flours, cornmeals, pastas, rice, and other grain products along with the iron and other B vitamins that have been added for years. This boosts the average intake of folic acid by about 100 micrograms per day.

This extra folic acid—which many experts believe is too little—is already reducing the number of children born with neural tube defects. The number of neural tube defect-affected pregnancies in the United States fell from four thousand in 1995–1996, before folic acid fortification, to three thousand after fortification had been in effect for two years. It is too soon to tell if it will have an unintended but extremely welcome side effect—less heart disease and cancer. As described below, low folic acid has been implicated in both of these.

This chapter doesn't exhaustively review all vitamins and minerals. Instead it touches on those with newly recognized (or suspected) roles beyond the classic deficiency diseases starting with antioxidants, a group of vitamins and minerals implicated in everything from Alzheimer's disease to poor circulation in the legs. Along the way, it points out how to get more vitamins and minerals in your diet and which ones you might want to, or need to, get from a supplement. The table on pages 205–207 lists the current recommended daily intake of vitamins and minerals.

WHAT ARE VITAMINS?

The classic definition of vitamin is this: a carbon-containing compound essential in small quantities for normal functioning of the body. In plainer English, vitamins are a type of nutrient your body can't make and must get from somewhere else. Vitamins are usually classified as either fat-soluble or water-soluble. Fat-soluble vitamins like vitamin A tend to accumulate in the body, while water-soluble vitamins like vitamin C don't.

ANTIOXIDANTS

On a list of the biggest nutritional buzzwords from the last decade, antioxidant would be near the top. Before 1990, this pack of electron-donating compounds was of interest mostly to chemists and food researchers. Today they are touted in books with titles like *The Antioxidant Miracle* or *Antioxidants Against Cancer.* They are promoted in herbal pharmacies and mainstream magazines as wonder substances that can prevent cancer, heart disease, memory loss, and cataracts and even reverse the aging process.

The antioxidant hoopla is a classic case of good science that has been co-opted and overstated. We have every reason to believe that taking extra antioxidants may do some of the things attributed to them, but little solid proof that they really do. We know with near certainty that the package of antioxidants, minerals, fiber, and phytochemicals found in fruits and vegetables can help prevent heart disease, strokes, diverticular disease, cataracts, and a host of other chronic ills. But whether or not the single antioxidants that Americans gobble up in increasing numbers can do this is an open question.

Let's back up for a second to define antioxidants and why they are essential for good health. Antioxidants are a group of substances that protect tissues, cells, and important compounds like proteins and DNA against the destructive power of oxygen and its relatives. You thought oxygen was only beneficial? Think again. It's turning out to be a dangerous friend. Oxygen-using reactions like those needed to burn fats and carbohydrates generate many oxygen-based by-products called free radicals. These electronically unfulfilled molecules are so desperate for electrons that they scavenge them from whatever is handy. All too often the donor is DNA, important structural or functional proteins, LDL cholesterol particles, even cell membranes. The simple loss of electrons can subtly alter the function of, or even outright damage, these substances or cell parts. Over time, this damage adds up—free radicals are thought to play roles in cancer, heart disease, arthritis, cataract formation, memory loss, a to name just a few.

Free radicals and oxidizing agents also come from the environment. They are in the air you breathe, the food you eat, and the water you drink. They are plentiful in cigarette smoke, yours or someone else's. Sunlight hitting the skin or beaming into the eye also generates free radicals.

Bruce Ames, a noted molecular biologist at the University of California, Berkeley, has estimated that the genetic material in each cell of the human body gets about ten thousand "oxidative hits" a day. Multiply this by the several trillion cells in your body and factor in the other cellular components that can be damaged by free radicals and oxidizing agents and you get an idea of the magnitude of the attack.

Like marines, antioxidants stand ever ready to neutralize free radicals. Deployed strategically throughout all cells and tissues, antioxidants do one thing exceptionally well—generously, even aggressively, give up electrons to free radicals without turning into electron-scavenging substances themselves.

Today the term *antioxidant* usually encompasses vitamin C, vitamin E, beta-carotene and other related carotenoids, as well as the minerals selenium and manganese, which are needed by several free-radical-destroying enzymes in order to work properly. In reality, there are probably hundreds of antioxidants in the foods we eat. Given the intense interest in these substances, it won't be a surprise when new ones are added to the list. Actively investigated antioxidants include glutathione, coenzyme Q_{10}, lipoic acid, flavonoids, phenols, polyphenols, and phytoestrogens.

We tend to think of antioxidants as an interchangeable group of chemicals. That's misleading. Each antioxidant has a unique set of chemical behaviors and biological properties. This diversity is important and valuable and allows antioxidants to work together as parts of an elaborate network, with each different substance (or family of substances) playing a slightly different role. For example, beta-carotene sits upright in cell membranes, poking out like little flags from the cell surface. Lycopene insinuates itself into the middle of the cell membrane, while other carotenoids and antioxidants end up completely inside or outside the cell.

Understanding this chemical minuet carries a very practical message. No single antioxidant can do the work of the whole crowd. Taking high-dose beta-carotene or vitamin E pills, then, is like listening to a single violin play a Mozart symphony—you get a little something, but not the full, glorious effect. It's also possible that the imbalance that occurs by taking too much of any one antioxidant may be like listening to an orchestra in which one section is playing at eardrum-shattering volume.

• *Antioxidants and heart disease.* Heart disease often begins with the quiet transfer of electrons from LDL (bad) cholesterol to free radicals.

When LDL is abundant in the bloodstream—say, from a diet high in saturated and trans fats—it latches on to cells lining the inner surface of artery walls. After oozing inside these cells, LDL is attacked by free radicals and surrenders some electrons. This transforms the otherwise sluggish and inactive LDL into a more reactive substance that starts damaging the artery lining. Repair cells flock to the injury, penetrate the artery wall, and begin gorging on the oxidized LDL particles just as they would gorge on infective bacteria. The repair cells swell into white, puffy cells called foam cells. All this activity stimulates smooth muscle cells lining the artery wall to grow and thicken. If this process goes on long enough, the resulting narrowed arteries cut down blood flow to the heart and brain. Narrow arteries are also fertile grounds for the formation of artery-blocking clots.

If free-radical oxidation of LDL kicks off this potentially deadly chain reaction, then diets high in antioxidants should help prevent cardiovascular disease, or at least limit its extent or severity. Several lines of evidence suggest that this antioxidant hypothesis might be true. Laboratory studies show that a variety of antioxidants do indeed protect LDL from oxidation. Long-term cohort studies, including a study of 1,300 elderly Massachusetts residents, the Nurses' Health Study, the Health Professionals Follow-up Study, and the Iowa Women's Health Study, all found that people whose diets were high in antioxidants or who took antioxidant supplements (usually vitamin E) tended to have less heart disease.

Yet several recent randomized trials haven't shown that taking antioxidant supplements prevents heart disease in people at high risk for developing it or limits heart disease once it has been diagnosed.

How to explain this disconnect between the observational evidence and what is presumably the more rigorous experimental evidence? It's possible that the people who take vitamin supplements or eat lots of fruits and vegetables (and who had less heart disease in the observational studies) also do other healthy things—keep a healthy weight, reduce stress, get more exercise. But most studies have statistically adjusted for differences in these and other lifestyle factors. It's possible that single agents just aren't as effective as fruits and vegetables, which deliver a whole antioxidant package. It's also possible that randomized trials are too short and that it takes longer than a few years to see what antioxidants can do, especially when someone already has heart disease. One thing is clear—eating plenty of fruits and vegetables is an excellent way to get antioxidants (including many that haven't been discovered yet) as well as fiber, minerals, and other good things important for keeping your heart and blood vessels healthy.

- *Antioxidants and cancer.* Cancer is a betrayal on the most intimate level. Responding to some signal from within or without, one of your own cells turns against you. It stops living by the rules set out for all your other cells and starts playing by its own. It grows and divides at will, unchecked by nearby cells or lack of food, and gladly piles into great disorganized masses. These renegade cells no longer need the same highly regulated brew of nutrients and growth factors that normal cells depend on. They may even break their moorings, travel to new parts of the body, put down new roots, and begin to grow and divide.

There isn't a single trigger for cancer. One fundamental change common to all cancers, though, is damage to DNA, the helical megamolecule that stores the instructions for all cellular activity. DNA is a favorite target for free radicals and oxidizing agents. Antioxidants are part of the protective shield that minimizes DNA damage. They also block the formation of several nitrogen-based compounds that act as carcinogens.

The evidence that supplements containing specific antioxidants prevent cancer, though, has been generally disappointing. Take beta-carotene, which ten years ago was being heralded as a blockbuster nutrient that would prevent cancer, not to mention heart disease and cataracts, and possibly even slow the aging process. A number of prospective studies in the 1970s and 1980s, including one with 250,000 participants, showed lower rates of heart disease and cancer among people who ate lots of fruits and vegetables. Based on the rather long-shot possibility that beta-carotene might be the protective factor in these foods, four large randomized trials were started to test the effect of beta-carotene supplements. Only one of the four showed any benefit for beta-carotene, and that one was done using a cocktail of different antioxidants in a rural part of China where nutrition was poor and people suffered from several dietary deficiencies. The next two to be published, one in 29,000 Finnish smokers and another in 18,000 U.S. smokers and workers exposed to asbestos, actually found a slightly *increased* risk of lung cancer among those taking beta-carotene supplements for four to eight years. The fourth, a

Harvard-affiliated twelve-year study of U.S. physicians, found no benefit or harm from beta-carotene.

One of the newest studies, though, still holds out some promise for antioxidants as cancer fighters. In the French Supplementation en Vitamines et Mineraux Antioxydants (SU.VI.MAX) study, more than 13,000 men and women took either a daily capsule containing vitamin C (120 mg), vitamin E (30 mg), beta-carotene (6 mg), selenium (100 mcg), and zinc (20 mg), or an identical placebo, for more than seven years. By the study's end, overall rates of cancer, heart disease, and death were the same in the two groups. When the researchers looked at the results by sex, the antioxidant cocktail had a protective effect for men but not for women, who had higher levels of antioxidants (especially beta-carotene) in the bloodstream at the study's start than did men.

- *Antioxidants and vision.* Two common aging-related eye problems are partly due to free radicals. Cataracts form when damage from sunlight and free radicals clouds the clear proteins that make up the lens of the eye, much as heat clouds the clear protein in egg white. Cataract is the leading cause of vision problems among older people. It affects more than twenty million Americans over age forty; more than half of those over age eighty have cataracts. At least one million cataract extraction operations are done in the United States each year, at a cost of more than $3 billion.

A number of studies suggest that plenty of antioxidants sponge up free radicals before they have a chance to wreak havoc in the eye. While most research has focused on vitamin C, it looks as though two carotenoids may also be involved. Lutein and zeaxanthin are the only two carotenoids found in the eye's macular region, and some studies have shown a connection between higher intakes of these two and lower rates of macular degeneration.

Two trials have tested whether supplements can stave off cataract or macular degeneration or at least prevent them from getting worse. The Age-Related Eye Disease Study (AREDS) tested a daily cocktail that included 500 mg of vitamin C, 400 IU of vitamin E, 15 mg of beta-carotene, 80 mg of zinc, and 2 mg of copper. It wasn't a wonder drug. The supplement didn't help people with cataract or early macular degeneration. But it did slow the progression of macular degeneration in some people and kept an intermediate case from becoming an advanced one. Zinc alone did much the same thing. The Lutein Antioxidant Supplementation Trial (LAST) tested 10 mg of lutein alone or lutein plus other antioxidants, vitamins, and minerals against a placebo among people with macular degeneration. Visual function improved in both groups taking lutein.

As is true for the link between antioxidants and other chronic diseases, we still don't know if antioxidant supplements can prevent cataract, macular degeneration, or other vision problems. But because good sources of lutein and zeaxanthin such as spinach, kale, and dark green lettuce appear to be helpful for all-around good health, it makes sense to include more plants in your diet.

• *Antioxidants and aging.* Almost fifty years ago, a newly minted M.D. named Denham Harman with an interest in physics and free radicals saw many similarities between how radiation and aging affect cells. Those observations led to the free-radical theory of aging in 1956. This hypothesis holds that the gradual accumulation of DNA mutations and other end products of oxidative damage slows down cells and interferes with their activity. This, in turn, is believed to lead to cancer, cardiovascular disease, a decline in the activity of the immune system, arthritis, eye disease, and cognitive problems such as memory loss and Alzheimer's disease.

It may be a stretch to blame lack of antioxidants for all of this. It's also a difficult theory to test. But it raises the possibility that healthy eating can stave off some of what we used to think of as the inevitable consequences of aging.

VITAMIN A

A key lesson in virtually every high school biology course covers the role that vitamin A plays in vision—transforming light that hits the eye's retina into electrical impulses the brain interprets as images. That's certainly an interesting and important part of this vitamin's activity, but it accounts for less than 1 percent of your body's vitamin A. Its other vital roles include helping maintain the cells that line the body's interior surfaces, boosting the production and activity of white blood cells, and helping direct bone remodeling. Vitamin A also helps regulate cell growth and differentiation, the processes by which cells split and specialize. This suggests that vitamin A may be one of the ways the body keeps normal cells from turning into cancer cells and keeps cells that do become cancerous from dividing and spreading. Preliminary studies suggest that getting too little vitamin A may lead to a modest increase in cancer risk. They also show that once you reach a certain threshold level of vitamin A in your system, there's no benefit in getting more.

That threshold appears to be in the range of the current recommended daily intakes—900 mcg of retinol for men (the equivalent of 3,000 IU) and 700 mcg for women (the equivalent of 2,333 IU).

Getting much more than this may harm your bones. High intakes of retinol, the active form of vitamin A, stimulates cells called osteoclasts that break down bone. Several studies have shown that intakes of preformed vitamin A (retinol) above 5,000 IU (1,500 mcg) increase the chances of losing bone density, breaking a hip or other bone, or increasing the risk of cancer. Why would too much preformed vitamin A pose problems? In high amounts, vitamin A can block the effects of vitamin D, which is good for bones and muscles and has a calming effect on cancer cells.

It is relatively easy to get too much vitamin A from supplements. I recommend avoiding special vitamin A supplements unless you have a specific medical reason for needing them. When shopping for a multivitamin, look for one that gets all or most of its vitamin A activity from beta-carotene. Try to keep your intake of preformed vitamin A (retinol) from supplements under 2,000 IU per day.

Food gives you either preformed, ready-to-go vitamin A or provitamin A that your body can readily convert to active vitamin A. Good sources of preformed vitamin A—liver, fish liver oil, eggs, and dairy products—often deliver things you don't particularly need, like extra calories and saturated fats. Provitamin A comes from several carotenoids (see below), including alpha-carotene, beta-carotene, and beta-cryptoxanthin. Good fruit and vegetable sources of provitamin A include carrots, yellow squash, red and green peppers, spinach, kale, and other green leafy vegetables.

BETA-CAROTENE, LYCOPENE, AND OTHER CAROTENOIDS

Plants make hundreds of different pigments. Some trap sunlight and transform it into chemical energy, others prevent sun damage. Some advertise ripeness to the animals that will disperse their seeds, others warn hungry critters of nasty or poisonous contents.

One large group of plant pigments is the carotenoid family. You probably know a number of carotenoids by sight, if not by name. Beta-carotene is the pigment that gives carrots and sweet potatoes their characteristic orange hues. Lycopene is responsible for the tempting red of a juicy tomato or the cool pink of watermelon flesh. Other well-studied carotenoids include lutein and zeaxanthin (the only carotenoids found in the eye's retina), alpha-carotene, and beta-cryptoxanthin. These six are just a drop in the bucket of five hundred or so known carotenoids.

We use carotenoids for two main functions—some of them are turned into vitamin A, and others act as powerful and adaptable antioxidants. Given the intense research on this family of biological compounds, other important functions are just waiting to be discovered.

There's a widely held notion that carotenoids in general, and several carotenoids in particular, prevent a variety of chronic ills. Dozens of observational studies show that people who choose to eat more fruits and vegetables high in carotenoids have less cardiovascular disease; cancers of the prostate, lung, stomach, colon, breast, cervix, and pancreas; memory loss; and cataract formation and macular degeneration. Unfortunately, randomized trials in which volunteers have taken specific antioxidants have not (so far) shown much reduction in risk of developing cancer or cardiovascular disease.

This seeming contradiction could be the result of weak studies that set up false hopes. It could mean that you need the whole, complex net of antioxidants delivered by fruits and vegetables, not just one or two specific ones. It could mean you need antioxidants plus the other important nutrients found in fruits and vegetables. Or it may mean that we just haven't tested the right carotenoid or carotenoid combination for long enough periods.

After two decades of research, some true benefits for specific carotenoids may be in sight. There is good evidence that lutein and zeaxanthin are important for preventing macular degeneration and cataract. And a strong report from the Harvard-based Physicians' Health Study is reviving interest in beta-carotene as a supplement that can help preserve memory and thinking skills into old age.

VITAMIN C

Do you reach for vitamin C at the first sign of a cold? If so, you aren't alone. It's an impulse nudged by a book written thirty-five years ago, *Vitamin C and the Common Cold,* by Linus Pauling, a double Nobel laureate and self-proclaimed champion of vitamin C. Pauling fervently believed that megadoses of vitamin C, between 1,000 and 2,000 mg/day (the amount in twelve to twenty-four oranges!) could prevent and abort colds and could do the same for cancer.

Vitamin C does play a role in infection control. It helps make collagen, a substance you need for healthy bones, ligaments, teeth, gums, and blood vessels. It is involved in making several hormones and chemical messengers used in the brain and nerves. Vitamin C is also a potent antioxidant capable of neutralizing many free radicals and oxidants found in the body.

We've known for almost two hundred years that citrus fruits prevent scurvy, a once feared disease that killed an estimated two million sailors between 1500 and 1800. (It wasn't until 1932, though, that vitamin C was discovered and found to be the active agent in citrus fruits responsible for fighting scurvy.) Can high doses of vitamin C fight other diseases? Not the common cold—study after study has failed to prove Pauling's proposition. There's a smattering of evidence that a little extra vitamin C, about the amount found in a typical multivitamin, at the very beginning of a cold might relieve symptoms some, but there's no support for megadoses. Prevent cancer and heart disease? The evidence is thin, and the jury is still out on those subjects. It's possible that a little extra vitamin C might help prevent cataract formation (see page 180), but here again more research is needed.

The current recommended daily intake for vitamin C is 75 mg/day for women and 90 mg/day for men, with an extra 35 mg/day for smokers. There seems to be no harm in getting more, though the latest dietary reference intake (DRI) report on vitamin C cautions against taking megadoses above 2,000 mg/day.

As the evidence continues to unfold, I suggest getting 200–300 mg of vitamin C a day. This is easy to do with a good diet and a standard multivitamin. Good food sources of vitamin C are citrus fruits or citrus juices, berries, green and red peppers, tomatoes, broccoli, and spinach. Many breakfast cereals are also fortified with vitamin C.

There's no need to overdo vitamin C. Your body can't store much of it (about 1,500–3,000 mg at a time) and flushes out the excess in bright yellow urine. What's more, there's no evidence that big daily doses help and some preliminary evidence that they may be harmful. At high concentrations, vitamin C can switch roles and act like a free radical instead of an antioxidant and could possibly cause the things you may be trying to prevent.

VITAMIN E

In some ways, the vitamin E story is like the one for beta-carotene: early curiosity, intriguing laboratory results, and promising observational studies followed by relatively disappointing clinical trials in which large groups of volunteers—mostly people already diagnosed with heart disease—were randomized to take either vitamin E or placebo pills. There are some important differences, though. Most people get between 5 and 15 IU of vitamin E a day. Yet it takes several hundred IU a day to significantly block the oxidation of LDL cholesterol, and the biggest inhibition happens at about 800 IU a day. In the Nurses' Health Study and Health Professionals Follow-up Study, we saw lower risks of heart disease in women and men who took vitamin E supplements of at least 100 IU for at least two years. This is very different from the prelude to beta-carotene studies, which focused on fruits and vegetables, not supplements.

Vitamin E supplements have been tested against heart disease in several randomized trials. In the Cambridge Heart Antioxidant Study (CHAOS), done among people with heart disease, those who took 400- or 800-IU supplements of vitamin E were less likely to have a heart attack or die from cardiovascular disease than those taking a placebo. In the Gruppo Italiano per lo Studio della Sopravvivenza nell'Infarto miocardio (known as the GISSI Prevention Trial), among 11,000 heart attack survivors, more than three years of treatment with vitamin E had no effect on the rate of heart attacks, strokes, or deaths from any cause, the main "outcomes" the study was designed to test. But it did appear to cut down on deaths due to cardiovascular disease and sudden deaths. A few months later, results from the Heart Outcomes Prevention Evaluation (HOPE) trial also showed no cardiovascular benefit after more than four years of treatment with 400 IU of vitamin E daily among more than 9,500 men and women already diagnosed with heart disease or at high risk for it.

At the end of 2004, an international team pooled the data from nine long-term cohort studies in order to tease out whether vitamin E (along with vitamin C and other antioxidants) had an impact on heart disease. According to the researchers, "The results weakly support the hypothesis that higher dietary intake of vitamin E . . . reduces the risk of coronary heart disease." At the beginning of 2005, an analysis of the results of nineteen vitamin E trials suggested that users of high-dose vitamin E (more than 400 IU per day) might have a slightly higher death rate than nonusers. Headlines screamed, "Vitamin E Death Risk," but I don't believe this is so. Most of the trials in the analysis included only volunteers with heart disease. And an exhaustive review of vitamin E by the Institute of Medicine showed it is safe at much higher doses.

Results from the Women's Health Study threw cold water on hopes that vitamin E might prevent heart disease. In this Harvard-based trial, almost 40,000 healthy middle-aged women took 600 IU of natural-source vitamin E or an identical placebo every other day for ten years. By the study's end, the number of heart attacks and strokes was virtually the same in the vitamin E and placebo groups. However, deaths from cardiovascular disease were lower in the vitamin E group. This means that the final role of vitamin E in preventing heart disease remains unsettled.

We don't know why the trial results don't square with those from observational studies. That will be grist for future research. With the information we have in hand right now, it is wise not to rely only on high doses of vitamin E to protect you against a heart attack or stroke.

Because of its antioxidant effects, vitamin E has also been proposed as an anticancer agent. However, most studies have not supported a benefit, although in a few investigations, lower risks of colon and prostate cancer were seen. Another huge trial compared a daily pill containing 600 mg vitamin E, 250 mg vitamin C, and 20 mg beta-carotene daily versus a placebo pill among more than twenty thousand people with heart disease or diabetes. The antioxidant vitamins were safe but had no impact on heart attacks, deaths, diabetes, or other measures.

Some early studies suggest that vitamin E supplements may prevent age-related dementia. Another possibly promising line of research involves vitamin E and amyotrophic lateral sclerosis (sometimes called Lou Gehrig's disease). This is a rapidly progressive, invariably fatal disease that attacks nerve cells responsible for controlling voluntary muscles. Among almost one million men and women taking part in a long-term cancer prevention study, those who regularly used vitamin E supplements for ten years or more were two-thirds less likely to have developed this disease as nonusers of vitamin E. Whether this work holds up in large studies remains to be seen.

Unlike beta-carotene, vitamin C, and other antioxidant vitamins, vitamin E is not present in food alone at the levels thought to be protective (and the level used in most studies). Getting 400 IU of vitamin E means taking a special high-E multivitamin or a vitamin E supplement along with a typical multi-vitamin.

The latest dietary reference intakes increased the recommended daily intake to 15 mg of vitamin E from food, the equivalent of 22 IU from natural-source vitamin E or 33 IU of the synthetic form. Although synthetic vitamin E is somewhat less potent than the natural form, the difference is probably not large enough to be important if one is taking 200 IU per day or more. A review by the Institute of Medicine concluded that vitamin E is safe up to doses of 1,000 mg/day (1,500 IU of natural-source vitamin E). The only documented harmful effect of too much vitamin E is the worsening of a rare eye problem known as retinitis pigmentosa. Because vitamin E can reduce the blood's ability to clot, people who take blood thinners should talk with their health care providers before starting to take vitamin E supplements.

THE THREE B'S—B_6, B_{12}, FOLIC ACID

Actually there are eight B vitamins, all of them familiar to anyone who reads the labels on cereal boxes—thiamine, niacin, riboflavin, pantothenic acid, biotin, B_6, B_{12}, and folic acid. All of these help a variety of enzymes do their jobs, ranging from releasing energy from carbohydrates and fat to breaking down amino acids and transporting oxygen and energy-containing nutrients around the body. I am focusing on just three of these because of new evidence that they may play pivotal roles in reducing heart disease and cancer.

HOMOCYSTEINE AND THE HEART

Back in 1968, the deaths of an eight-year-old boy and a two-month-old infant from massive strokes got a Boston pathologist named Kilmer McCully thinking. Both children had genetic defects in the way their bodies handled homocysteine, a by-product of eating protein. And both had damaged, cholesterol-clogged arteries. McCully wondered if the high levels of homocysteine in these children may have been the reason for their artery problems and hypothesized that the same thing might cause clogged arteries in adults. Instead of being welcomed as a new theory to explain how arteries that feed the heart become clogged with cholesterol-filled plaque, McCully's idea was initially ridiculed and ignored. Thirty years later, high levels of homocysteine are being eyed as a risk factor for heart disease.

Vitamins come into play here because three B vitamins—B_6, B_{12}, and folic acid—help recycle homocysteine into harmless amino acids. (See Figure 20.) A diet low in one or more of these vitamins leads to higher homocysteine levels and possibly an increased risk of heart disease. So getting enough folic acid, vitamin B_6, and vitamin B_{12} is one more nutritional strategy for protecting yourself against heart disease.

Since McCully first outlined the possible connection between homocysteine and heart disease, results of a number of studies support his idea. In the Physicians' Health Study, high homocysteine levels tripled the chances of having a heart attack. In the Nurses' Health Study, we have shown that women with the highest intakes of vitamin B_6 and folic acid were about half as likely to have heart attacks or die from heart disease as women with the lowest intakes. Studies also suggest that homocysteine-induced narrowing of the arteries may lead to stroke and that healthy amounts of this trio of B vitamins can keep this from happening.

As exciting and as definitive as all this sounds, the homocysteine–heart disease connection still remains a theory—one not supported by the first of several planned trials. In the two-year Vitamin Intervention for Stroke Prevention (VISP) trial, nearly four thousand stroke survivors took a high-dose or low-dose cocktail of folic acid plus vitamins B_6 and B_{12}. Although homocysteine

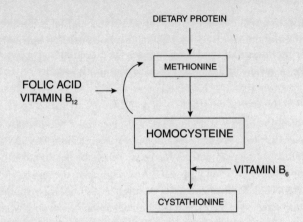

FIG. 20 Homocysteine and the Three Bs. Three B vitamins—vitamin B$_6$, vitamin B$_{12}$, and folic acid—help the body turn the protein breakdown product homocysteine into less damaging substances. A buildup of homocysteine could be involved in the artery-clogging process known as atherosclerosis.

levels fell moderately in the high-dose group, this had little effect on recurrent strokes, heart attacks, or stroke- or heart-related deaths. This trial was started after the U.S. government made food companies fortify bread and other grain products with folic acid, which also dropped homocysteine levels in the placebo group.

Even if homocysteine isn't a direct cause of heart disease, there's strong evidence to show that getting plenty of folic acid cuts the risk of developing this all-too-common condition. While ongoing research aims to solve the homocysteine puzzle, it makes excellent sense to get enough B vitamins.

Enough doesn't mean taking megadoses. For most people, it means just reaching the current recommended daily intakes of 400 mcg for folic acid, 1.3–1.7 mg for vitamin B$_6$, and 2.4 micrograms of vitamin B$_{12}$. Unfortunately, only a small fraction of U.S. adults achieves this by diet alone.

• *Vitamin B$_6$.* This vitamin is really a group of six related compounds. They are mostly involved with making and breaking down amino acids, the building blocks that are used to make proteins. The classic signs of too little B$_6$ are dermatitis (an inflammation of the skin), anemia, depression and confusion, and convulsions. Even without these signs, too little B$_6$ may also mean too much homocysteine and an increased risk of heart disease.

Many people take vitamin B_6 to treat a variety of diseases and conditions, sometimes without much backing from scientific evidence. It is promoted as a remedy for premenstrual syndrome at doses far exceeding the recommended daily intake. A review in the *British Medical Journal* shows that 50–100 mg of vitamin B_6 a day may improve both the physical symptoms and depression that are part of premenstrual syndrome, and that there is no justification for higher doses. Vitamin B_6 has been used off and on to treat carpal tunnel syndrome. Although there's little proof that this works, some people seem to get relief with doses of 100–200 mg.

One form of vitamin B_6 helps convert the amino acid tryptophan into serotonin, an important chemical messenger used by the brain and nervous system. Because of this connection, B_6 has been tested as a treatment for depression, attention deficit disorder, and other serotonin-related problems. Again, there's no solid evidence to show whether it works or doesn't work for these conditions.

We tend to get much of our daily ration of vitamin B_6 from fortified breakfast cereals. Other good sources are meat, nuts, and beans. Very high B_6 intake that can be reached only by high-dose supplements—250 mg/day—can cause neurologic damage.

- *Vitamin B_{12}.* Early in the twentieth century, pernicious anemia was a grim and inevitably deadly disease. It sometimes started with paleness and fatigue, which were gradually accompanied by tingling and numbness of the arms and legs, memory loss, disorientation, and even hallucinations. In some cases, memory loss, disorientation, and hallucinations were the *only* symptoms. In 1934, three American researchers won the Nobel Prize in medicine for their discovery that injections of liver extract effectively treated pernicious anemia. These extracts worked because liver contains large amounts of vitamin B_{12}, which is an essential ingredient for making red blood cells.

Today, full-blown pernicious anemia is uncommon. But getting too little vitamin B_{12} can still cause an array of problems, including memory loss and dementia, muscle weakness, loss of appetite, and tingling in the arms and legs. It can also lead to the accumulation of homocysteine, since vitamin B_{12} is involved in converting homocysteine into the amino acid methionine.

Because vitamin B_{12} is found only in animal products, deficiencies tend to crop up in strict vegetarians, also called vegans. In addition, as many as one in six older Americans has low blood levels of B_{12}. Most of the time, the problem isn't a low-B_{12} diet. Instead it is an inability to absorb the B_{12} in food. The form of B_{12} in fortified food or multiple vitamins can still be absorbed even when B_{12}

from food is not. Fortunately, by age fifty most of us have accumulated enough B_{12} in our lives to keep us going for years, even if our capacity to extract it from food declines. People with inflammatory bowel disease or AIDS can have problems absorbing vitamin B_{12} from food, and drinking too much alcohol interferes with this vitamin. So do a number of drugs, including some of the acid-neutralizing drugs used to treat ulcers; colchicine, used to treat gout; and Dilantin, used to treat seizures.

The current recommended daily intake for vitamin B_{12} is 2.4 mcg. Liver is clearly the most efficient food source of B_{12}, delivering about 23 mcg per ounce. Other good sources include tuna, yogurt, cottage cheese, and eggs.

*   *Folic acid (Folate)*. In 1998, the Institute of Medicine's Food and Nutrition Board set the recommended dietary allowance for folic acid at 400 mcg per day. That's more than double the previous recommendation, set in 1989 before the explosion of interest in folic acid.

As described earlier in this chapter, folate helps guide the development of the embryonic spinal cord. Pregnant women who get too little folic acid increase the chances that their baby will be born with spina bifida or anencephaly.

It also does a lot more. Like vitamins B_6 and B_{12}, folate helps the body get rid of homocysteine and so may help protect against homocysteine-related heart disease. A study from the USDA Human Nutrition Research Center on Aging in Boston showed that, following the federal regulation that all grain products be enriched with folic acid beginning in 1998, average blood folate levels among participants in the Framingham Offspring Study (a follow-up of the famous Framingham Heart Study) more than doubled, and average homocysteine levels fell by 7 percent.

Folate's key role in building DNA means that it probably has a hand in cell division and so may help prevent cancer. Getting plenty of folic acid seems to decrease the risk of developing colon cancer and breast cancer. One of the interesting things we have seen in the Nurses' Health Study, and other researchers have seen in other populations, is that folic acid may temper the increase in breast cancer seen in women who average more than one alcoholic drink a day. The same is true for colon cancer, another disease that is more common among alcohol drinkers than nondrinkers. People who drink alcohol *and* get 600 mcg or more of folic acid each day, though, aren't at increased risk. This makes sense, because alcohol blocks the absorption of folic acid and also inactivates circulating folic acid.

There are many excellent sources of folic acid other than that old standby, liver (see the table on page 191). Most breakfast cereals now contain 100 mcg

Good Sources of Folic Acid

Food	Serving	Folic Acid (micrograms)	% Daily Value*
Chicken liver, cooked	3¹/₂ ounces	560	140
Total cereal	³/₄ cup	477	120
Centrum multivitamin	1	400	100
Cheerios	1 cup	200	50
Lentils, cooked	¹/₂ cup	179	45
Chickpeas, canned	¹/₂ cup	141	35
Spinach, cooked	¹/₂ cup	131	33
Black beans, cooked	¹/₂ cup	128	32
Spaghetti, cooked	1 cup	108	27
Sunflower seeds, dry roasted	1¹/₂ ounces	101	25
White rice, cooked	1 cup	92	23
Broccoli, cooked	¹/₂ cup	84	21
Orange juice	6 ounces	82	21
Lima beans, cooked	¹/₂ cup	78	20
Beets, cooked	¹/₂ cup	68	17
Potato	1 medium	66	17
Romaine lettuce	1 cup	64	16
Peanuts, dry roasted	1¹/₂ ounces	62	16
Peas, frozen, cooked	1/2 cup	59	15
Wheat germ	2 tbsp.	49	12
Orange	1 medium	39	10
Tofu	¹/₂ cup	37	9
Tomato juice	6 ounces	36	9
Baked beans	1 cup	30	8
Sweet potato	1 medium	7	2

* Based on a daily value of 400 milligrams of folic acid for a 2,000-calorie-a-day diet.

Source: U.S. Department of Agriculture, Agriculture Research Service, National Nutrient Database for Standard Reference, Release 17, 2004, www.nal.usda.gov/fnic/foodcomp

per serving, and some contain 400 mcg, a full day's requirement. Beans are another good source, with lentils, chickpeas, and black beans delivering 20 to 50 mcg per serving. Spinach, pasta, and orange juice are other good sources. As mentioned earlier, folate-fortified flour adds about 100 mcg per day to the average American's diet.

VITAMIN D

We are only now beginning to understand the widespread importance of vitamin D. Once known solely for its ability to help the body absorb and hold on to calcium and phosphorous, it is turning out to be far more versatile.

Vitamin D isn't exactly a vitamin. Instead, it is a hormone made by a rather unusual gland—your skin. Sunlight striking the skin turns a cousin of cholesterol into pre–vitamin D. This is first processed by the liver and then activated by the kidneys, or by cells in the heart, immune system, breast, or prostate. Very few foods naturally contain vitamin D. Coldwater fish such as mackerel, salmon, sardines, and bluefish contain plenty of this fat-soluble vitamin; their livers contain very high levels. Most of what we get from food comes from dairy products (which by law must be fortified with vitamin D); vitamin-fortified breakfast cereals; and eggs from hens fed vitamin D.

Although calcium usually gets all the credit for building bones and preventing fractures, vitamin D should get equal billing. It helps on several levels. Vitamin D ensures that calcium and phosphorus (another integral part of bone) are absorbed as they pass through the digestive system. It signals the kidneys to hang on to these minerals so they aren't lost in urine. It also inhibits the breakdown of bone and boosts bone-building activity.

In chapter 9, I mention a study showing that many women who break a hip have an unsuspected vitamin D deficiency. A growing body of research suggests that the large majority of Americans could reduce bone loss by getting extra vitamin D. In fact, doing this more effectively reduces hip and wrist fractures in older women and men than does dramatically increasing calcium consumption.

There are other reasons besides strong bones for getting more vitamin D. Stronger muscles and fewer falls, for one. Less cancer, for another, as well as the possibilities of better blood pressure, a stronger heart, and protection against multiple sclerosis.

• *Muscles and falls.* Vitamin D signals muscle cells to make new protein. This may strengthen muscle and improve stability, especially in older people. Several large trials show that vitamin D supplementation reduces the risk of falling by 20 percent or so among relatively healthy older people. Falls are the single largest cause of injuries among older people. They can lead to permanent disability, loss of independence, and even death.

• *Cancer.* In test tubes, vitamin D strongly inhibits the growth and reproduction of a variety of cancer cells, including those from the breast, ovary, colon, prostate, and brain. New studies using measurements of vitamin D intake or blood levels of the vitamin suggest that the same thing happens in our bodies. This means vitamin D could stifle new cancer cells much like a blanket on a small fire, snuffing out their progression to life-threatening tumors.

• *Heart disease.* Several small studies suggest that getting more vitamin D, especially from sunlight, helps lower blood pressure. Getting too little may contribute to heart failure and peripheral artery disease (blocked blood flow in the legs) and may be implicated in the artery-clogging process known as atherosclerosis.

• *Multiple sclerosis.* This disease, which occurs when the immune system mistakenly attacks the protective covering of nerves, is more common in areas where people have low vitamin D levels. In mice, vitamin D prevents or slows the course of experimentally induced multiple sclerosis. It may do much the same thing in humans. In the Nurses' Health Study, women who took vitamin D supplements were almost half as likely to develop multiple sclerosis as those who didn't take vitamin D.

People who can bask in strong sunlight for a few minutes on most days year-round make plenty of vitamin D. That rules out everyone living north of San Francisco, Denver, Indianapolis, and Philadelphia. During the winter months, the amount of ultraviolet light hitting those northern regions (above forty degrees latitude) isn't enough to generate vitamin D. It also rules out people who work inside all day and can't, or don't, get out for a fifteen-minute walk when the sun is high in the sky; those whose ability to get outside is limited by arthritis or other chronic diseases; and those who live in nursing homes. In other words, millions of people. Two in three Americans between the ages of fifty-one and seventy fall short of the current target for vitamin D; older people fare even worse, with nine in ten not meeting the daily requirement.

The darker your skin color, the less effectively your body converts sunlight to vitamin D. In a national survey of Americans, blacks had about half the vitamin D in their blood as whites.

The gradual loss of skin pigmentation as humans migrated northward from the so-called cradle of mankind in Africa was probably an evolutionary adaptation to capture more vitamin D from less sunlight. Yet even the near complete loss of melanin in the skin in very fair Scandinavians isn't enough to compensate for the lack of strong sunlight, and thus many have low levels of vitamin D. Many northern populations compensated for this by eating plenty of fatty fish, including the vitamin D–rich livers, or taking cod liver oil. The loss of such traditions may have major impacts on health.

The current dietary reference intake for vitamin D is 200 IU (5 mcg) between the ages of nineteen and fifty; 400 IU (10 mcg) between the ages of fifty-one and seventy; and 600 IU (15 mcg) after age seventy. But mounting evidence points to a higher level—800–1,000 IU per day—in order to get the full benefits of vitamin D.

Unless you live in the South and get out in the sun most days of the week, the only way to achieve this is by taking a supplement. Most multiple vitamins contain only 400 IU. Don't take two a day, because the extra preformed vitamin A may work against vitamin D. Some calcium supplements contain 220 IU of vitamin D along with 500 mg of calcium. So one option for women is to take a standard multiple vitamin and two of these calcium pills. I don't recommend this for men, though, because of the possible connection between high calcium intake and fatal prostate cancer. A standard multivitamin plus a specific vitamin D supplement is another option. Your best bet is to find a multivitamin that delivers 800–1,000 IU of vitamin D. A few of these are on the market, and I hope more will be coming soon.

VITAMIN K

This fat-soluble vitamin helps make six of the thirteen proteins needed for blood clotting. Recent research showing that some of these same proteins are involved in building bone suggests another possible function—maintaining bone health. Low levels of circulating vitamin K have been linked with low bone density, and supplementation with vitamin K shows improvements in biochemical measures of bone health. A report from the Nurses' Health Study suggests that women who don't get much vitamin K are twice as likely to break a hip as women who get plenty. We estimated that eating a serving of lettuce or other green leafy vegetables a day cut the risk of hip fracture in half when compared with eating one serving a week.

According to conventional wisdom, most adults get enough vitamin K because it is found in so many foods, especially green leafy vegetables and commonly used cooking oils. That wasn't entirely backed up by a 1996 survey of vitamin K in the American diet, which showed average intakes hovering slightly under the recommended daily intake of 120 mcg for men and 90 mcg for women. It also showed, though, that a fair number of Americans, particularly young ones, aren't getting the vitamin K that they need, mainly because they don't eat enough green leafy vegetables.

CALCIUM

The role of calcium, and the controversial need for it, is explored in detail in chapter 9. In a nutshell, no one really knows how much calcium adults need each day. Given the inconsistent and sometimes misleading data on calcium and bone health, the current recommended daily intakes for adults (1,000 mg/day for adults up to age fifty and 1,200 mg/day after that) are probably more than enough. You certainly need some calcium each day—it's a good idea to get at least 500 mg—but 1,200 mg is probably more than enough, especially for men.

Contrary to the catchy milk-mustache campaign, dairy products aren't the best way to get plenty of calcium. If you feel you need to get more, try a calcium supplement. They contain no calories and no saturated fat and are far cheaper than several daily servings of dairy products. Chewable calcium-based antacids such as Tums are a cheap and efficient way to get calcium. A supplement that also includes vitamin D is even better.

IRON

Half of the earth's inhabitants don't get enough iron. Too little of this mineral makes it hard for red blood cells to ferry oxygen from lungs to tissues. Iron-poor blood can leave a person pale, fatigued, and mentally dull. Lack of iron stunts the growth and development of children and can damage long-term thinking skills. It accounts for 20 percent of mothers' deaths during childbirth.

Iron deficiency isn't a major problem in the United States, thanks to our penchant for eating meat and to iron-fortified grain and other products. Two groups in which anemia isn't surprising are infants and women in their childbearing years. That's why infant formulas contain extra iron, why pregnant women are encouraged to take a multivitamin supplement with extra iron, and why menstruating women are urged to get enough iron in their diets.

Older people are also prone to anemia. It affects up to one in eight older Americans, sapping energy, causing cardiovascular problems or making them worse, impairing memory and thinking skills, hampering function and self-care, and contributing to depression.

People who need extra iron are often advised to eat lean red meat. Meat is certainly a great source of this mineral, but it is also high in calories, saturated fat, and cholesterol. Another drawback is that your body doesn't regulate the absorption of iron from meat as carefully as it does from grains, fruits, vegetables, and supplements. If your iron storehouse is well stocked, the kind of iron in plants and supplements passes through your body. The iron in meat, though, seems to slide under this mineral radar and add to the stockpile even if your body already has plenty of iron.

This could be a problem if, as some research has shown, iron acts as a powerful generator of free radicals. A controversial "iron hypothesis" for heart disease was first floated in 1981 and suggests that the higher the iron store, the greater the risk of heart disease. However, the evidence supporting this idea was weak to begin with and has gotten weaker with further studies. A similar hypothesis has been raised for cancer, and for this the jury is still out.

The current daily target for iron is 8 mg for men, 18 mg for women up until menopause, and then 8 mg after that. Healthy men and postmenopausal women rarely run low on iron. In fact, low iron levels in these groups are usually a tipoff of internal bleeding. A generally healthy diet with plenty of green vegetables, beans, and moderate amounts of poultry or red meat provides plenty of iron. Menstruating women need extra iron, either from eating more red meat or iron-rich vegetables or by taking a daily multivitamin, multimineral supplement.

No matter what your gender, don't take supplements that contain more than the recommended level of iron found in a standard multivitamin, multimineral pill unless you first talk with your health care provider and have your iron levels checked.

MAGNESIUM

This common element is essential for hundreds of biological processes, from building substances such as DNA and proteins from scratch to releasing the energy in food, and from contracting muscles to sending signals along nerves. Your heart, muscles, nerves, bones, and reproductive and other cells all depend on having enough magnesium.

In the United States, relatively few people are truly magnesium deficient. That said, Americans get less magnesium today than they did a century ago. Fewer fruits and vegetables in the diet are one reason; fewer whole grains are another. Whole-wheat bread and brown rice, for example, contain four times more magnesium than white bread or white rice.

Current nutrition guidelines recommend that men get 420 mg of magnesium a day and women get 320 mg. Few do, with average intakes hovering about 100 mg below these targets among whites and even lower among blacks and Hispanics. Less-than-healthy magnesium levels are common among older people, who may not be getting enough in their diets or who may have trouble absorbing what they get. Magnesium deficiency can also be a problem for people taking diuretics (a type of high blood pressure medication) and for heavy drinkers. Diabetes speeds the loss of magnesium. So does drinking alcohol or caffeinated beverages. Caffeinated soft drinks represent a double whammy, because the phosphates found in carbonated drinks also wash magnesium from the system.

Lack of magnesium can make the body work harder to accomplish even low-intensity activities. It can also prompt abnormal heart rhythms. Some studies show that people with lower levels of magnesium are more likely to develop type 2 diabetes or heart disease than those who get plenty. Other studies don't show a link between low magnesium and these chronic conditions.

It's fairly easy to meet your magnesium needs by food alone if you eat plenty of fruits and vegetables and whole grains. Cold breakfast cereals, which are often fortified with magnesium, are also a decent source. Cold cereals that are mostly whole grains are even better. Multivitamin, multimineral tablets usually contain about 100 mg of magnesium, which can help make up for shortfalls.

POTASSIUM

Potassium is the most abundant positively charged particle inside your cells. Your body regulates the concentration of potassium very carefully, because too much or too little can cause problems. A drop in potassium can make you feel weak and tired, trigger extra heartbeats (especially in people who already have heart disease), and cause muscle cramps or pain. Too little potassium combined with too much sodium may also cause high blood pressure, a condition shared by fifty million Americans.

Adults should get almost 5 grams of potassium a day. Most Americans don't get nearly this much in their diets. Low potassium is a special problem for people who take diuretics to control high blood pressure and for those who drink a lot of coffee or other caffeinated beverages, because diuretics and caffeine increase the amount of potassium lost in urine.

Getting extra potassium in your diet, from food, from potassium salt, or from supplements, can lower blood pressure. In so doing it also reduces the

Potassium Content of Some Foods

Food	Serving	Potassium (Milligrams)	% Daily Value*
Beet greens, cooked	1/2 cup	654	14
Baked beans	1 cup	551	12
Lima beans	1/2 cup	478	10
Yogurt	8 ounces	475	10
Spaghetti sauce	1/2 cup	470	10
Winter squash	1/2 cup	448	10
Cantaloupe	1 cup	427	9
Banana	1 medium	422	9
Spinach, cooked	1/2 cup	419	9
Tomato juice	6 ounces	417	9
Milk, skim	1 cup	407	9
Orange juice	6 ounces	355	8
Avocado	1/2 cup	354	8
Almonds	1 1/2 ounces	317	7
Prunes	1/4 cup	311	7
Potatoes, mashed	1/2 cup	311	7
Tofu	1/2 cup	299	6
Peanuts, dry roasted	1 1/2 ounces	280	6
Raisins	1/4 cup	272	6
Beets, cooked	1/2 cup	259	6
Orange	1 medium	237	5
Broccoli, cooked	1/2 cup	229	5
Tomatoes, raw	1/2 cup	213	5
Bran flakes	3/4 cup	185	4
Wheat germ	2 tbsp.	134	3
Coffee	1 cup	116	2
Collards, cooked	1/2 cup	110	2
Figs, dried	6	86	2

* Based on a daily value for potassium of 4,700 milligrams in a 2,000-calorie-a-day diet.

Source: U.S. Department of Agriculture, Agriculture Research Service, National Nutrient Database for Standard Reference, Release 17, 2004, www.nal.usda.gov/fnic/foodcomp

chances of having the kind of stroke caused by the blockage of blood flow to the brain. Bananas are famous for the amount of potassium they contain. But many other fruits and vegetables are also good sources. These include apricots, dates, kidney beans, oranges, and spinach (see the table on page 198). Although the best way to ensure an adequate potassium intake is by eating lots of fruit and vegetables, potassium salt can be helpful to people with hypertension, those who take diuretics, or heavy coffee drinkers. Don't take potassium supplements unless you have discussed this with your physician, because they can be deadly when the kidneys aren't working properly.

SODIUM

Most of us get more sodium than we need. It's hard not to. Prepared foods are often loaded with table salt, which is one-third sodium. A cup of boxed macaroni and cheese or an order of Burger King salted French fries can deliver more than 1,000 milligrams of sodium. And it's often found where you least expect it—a cup of pasta sauce can have almost half of a healthy daily salt allotment. (See the table on page 200.)

Although the "Daily Value" for sodium listed on food labels is 2,300 mg, the average person needs less than 1,000 mg/day to keep systems in good working order. That's less than $^1/_2$ teaspoon of salt. The average American *gets* 3,500–4,000 mg of sodium. The excess is excreted, but not always before it can do some damage. Excess sodium mainly pulls water from cells and thus increases blood pressure, especially in people whose genes make them more sensitive to salt.

While scientists agree that too much salt promotes high blood pressure in some people, there has been curiously little agreement over whether reducing dietary sodium lowers high blood pressure. Cutting back on sodium is often one of the first things that health care providers suggest to people who have just been diagnosed with high blood pressure, along with stopping smoking and getting more exercise. The results of salt reduction studies have been inconsistent, but the Dietary Approaches to Stop Hypertension (DASH) II study, which carefully controlled the amount of salt in diets, showed that aggressively cutting back on salt had an important impact on blood pressure. As described in chapter 7, the first DASH trial clearly showed that eating more fruits and vegetables can substantially lower blood pressure. Thus, the most effective means of keeping blood pressure low combines weight loss, abundant intake of fruits and vegetables rich in potassium, and avoiding foods high in salt.

Hidden Salt in Food

FOOD	SERVING	SODIUM (MILLIGRAMS)	% MAXIMUM RECOMMENDED DAILY LIMIT (2,300 MILLIGRAMS)
Kung pao chicken with rice	2 cups	2,610	113
Ham sandwich with mustard	9 ounces	2,340	102
Lasagna	2 cups	2,060	90
Canned sauerkraut	1 cup	1,560	68
Tuna salad submarine sandwich	6 inches	1,293	56
Baked beans, canned	1 cup	1,106	48
Chicken noodle soup, canned	1 cup	1,106	48
Macaroni and cheese, canned	1 cup	1,061	46
Pasta sauce	1 cup	1,030	45
Corned beef brisket	3 ounces	964	42
Burger King Whopper	1	900	39
Chicken pot pie	1 small	857	37
Dill pickles	1 (3 ounces)	833	36
Chicken bouillon	4-gram cube	743	32
Ham	2 slices	739	32
Vegetable juice cocktail	1 cup	653	28
KFC Biscuit	1	560	24
Cottage cheese	1/2 cup	457	20
American cheese	1 slice	422	18
McDonald's French fries	Super size	390	17
Waffle, frozen	1	383	17
Raisin Bran cereal	1 cup	361	16
Canned green beans	1 cup	354	15
Cheese pizza	1 slice	336	15
Lobster	1/2 cup	323	14
Light tuna, canned	1/2 can	301	13
Frozen peas	1 cup	115	5

Sources: U.S. Department of Agriculture, National Nutrient Database for Standard Reference, Release 17, 2004, www.nal.usda.gov/fnic/foodcomp, and Center for Science in the Public Interest.

The bottom line is that a salty diet doesn't do you any good and may be harmful, so cutting out unnecessary salt makes sense.

SELENIUM

Although the metal selenium is a potent antioxidant, there isn't enough of it in our bodies to act as a direct antioxidant. Instead, selenium sits at the active site of several enzymes that break down peroxides, potent oxidizing agents that are made throughout the body. So far, though, there is no convincing evidence to show that too little selenium increases the risk of cancer or that selenium supplements prevent cancer. Of the few studies done on selenium and chronic disease, some show a reduction in cancer, others don't. In the 1980s, selenium was added to fertilizer in Finland, where the soil levels (and thus intake) were low. Although blood levels of selenium rose dramatically, cancer rates didn't budge. In contrast, the Nutritional Prevention of Cancer Study showed some hard-to-interpret benefits. This study included more than 1,300 elderly volunteers, half of whom took 200 mcg of selenium a day for just over four years. Selenium had no effect on what the study was designed to examine, skin cancer, which occurred in the same percentage of selenium takers and placebo takers. But fewer of those taking selenium died from cancer during the study, and fewer developed lung, colorectal, and prostate cancer. The investigators themselves called for a larger trial to confirm these results. One such trial, called SELECT, is examining whether 200 mcg of selenium and 400 mg of vitamin E, either alone or together, help prevent prostate cancer. Its results aren't expected until 2012 or so.

The level of selenium used in these trials is almost quadruple the current recommendation of 55 mcg/day for women and men for this trace element. It is also an amount that is hard to get from food, because soil selenium levels vary from region to region. While selenium is safe at levels up to 400 mcg/day, there's currently no convincing evidence you need that much. The results of SELECT and other trials could change that, but for right now there isn't enough evidence that you should seek out extra selenium.

ZINC

Ignore those strategically placed racks near the checkout counter of your local pharmacy or grocery store displaying packs of zinc lozenges to fight or prevent colds. Little, if any, zinc from these sweets reaches your nasal passages. And an overview of six studies of people just developing colds, some of whom took zinc and some of whom didn't, found that the cold sufferers who popped the unpleasant-tasting zinc lozenges were just as likely to still have a cold at seven days as those taking placebo lozenges.

There's no question that zinc plays a key role in keeping the immune system healthy. It also acts as an antioxidant, is needed for proper vision, and is involved in blood clotting, wound healing, and the normal development of sperm cells. Does all this mean you should reach for a zinc supplement? No. Despite the fact that most U.S. residents actually get less than the recommended daily amount of zinc—11 mg for men and 8 mg for women—there's little evidence that these levels cause health problems. Studies looking at colon cancer, prostate cancer and prostate inflammation (prostatitis), macular degeneration, and colds have not shown a clear link with zinc.

Pregnant and lactating women need extra zinc, for themselves and the child they are carrying or feeding. Children also need enough zinc. A number of studies have shown that too little zinc may be one of the ways that undernourishment slows brain development and motor skills, contributes to hyperactivity, and causes problems with attention. Older people need extra zinc for several reasons. They tend to consume less zinc than younger people. They often have trouble absorbing zinc from food. The medications they take, especially diuretics for high blood pressure, can increase zinc excretion. And the extra fiber and calcium they may take can bind zinc and make it unavailable to the digestive system. Heavy drinkers, people with digestive problems such as Crohn's disease and ulcerative colitis, and those with chronic infections may also need extra zinc.

Red meat is a major source of zinc in our diets. The high zinc content of meat is sometimes used to justify eating one or more servings a day. Poultry is another good source. Yet vegetarians seem to do just fine with their lower-zinc diets. The advantage of getting your zinc from food, not from supplements or lozenges, is that it's hard to get too much from food.

Overdosing on zinc is easy—symptoms of zinc overload can begin appearing at just a little over the recommended amount of 15 mg/day. These include a depressed immune system, poor wound healing, problems with taste and smell, hair loss, and skin problems. High zinc intake may also promote the development or growth of prostate cancer. In the Health Professionals Follow-up Study, men who took supplements containing 100 mg/day or more of zinc had nearly twice the risk of prostate cancer compared with men who didn't take zinc.

PUTTING IT INTO PRACTICE

You pay top dollar to insure your home and your car. You may even have the kind of life insurance you'd rather not have a loved one collect. A far cheaper and more personally gratifying kind of life insurance comes from a daily multivitamin.

Research is pointing ever more strongly to the fact that several ingredients in a standard multivitamin—especially vitamins B_6 and B_{12}, folic acid, and vitamin D—are essential players in preventing heart disease, cancer, osteoporosis, and other chronic diseases. A year's supply costs under $40, or about a dime a day—it's the best nutritional bang for your buck.

I use the term *insurance* for good reason. A multivitamin can't in any way replace healthy eating. It gives you barely a scintilla of the vast array of healthful nutrients found in food. It doesn't deliver any fiber. Or taste. Or enjoyment. The only thing it can do is offer a nutritional backup or fill in the nutrient holes that can plague even the most conscientious eaters. For example, eating more fruits and vegetables is great, but it won't give you much in the way of vitamin D. Adding more whole grains to your diet is also wonderful, but it won't net you much vitamin B_6. Older people and those with digestive problems may not be able to absorb enough vitamin B_{12} from food. Anyone who regularly drinks alcohol needs extra folic acid to make up for alcohol's folate-reducing effects. So taking a daily multivitamin is a safe, rational plan that *complements* good eating but can never replace it.

The five vitamins that many people don't get enough of from their diets are

- Folic acid
- Vitamin B_6
- Vitamin B_{12}
- Vitamin D
- Vitamin E

Should you take a multivitamin plus minerals? You certainly can if you want to or if you feel you need an extra safety net. But it probably isn't necessary if you follow healthy eating strategies like the ones described in this book. For menstruating women, especially those who eat little or no red meat, a multivitamin, multimineral supplement will provide iron lost through menstruation.

You don't need a designer vitamin, a name-brand vitamin, or an "all natural" formulation. A standard, store-brand, RDA-level multivitamin plus some single supplements is a perfectly fine place to start. Look for labels that say the product meets the standards of the United States Pharmacopeia (USP). This organization sets manufacturing standards for medications and supplements sold in the United States. The single supplement extras include vitamin E, vitamin D, and calcium for women.

The less preformed vitamin A (retinol) in the multivitamin and the more beta-carotene, the better. Choose a supplement that contains no more than 2,000 IU of preformed vitamin A.

For most men and women, an extra vitamin E supplement makes sense. Even though the ending hasn't yet been written to the vitamin E story, at least 400 mg/day, and possibly more, may be needed for optimal health. Standard multivitamins contain only 30 IU.

Extra vitamin D is definitely worth pursuing. Standard multivitamins offer 400 IU, half of what's needed for optimal health. You can make up the other 400–600 IU by taking a combined calcium/vitamin D supplement or a separate vitamin D tablet or capsule.

A few companies are making supplements that replace most of the preformed vitamin A with beta-carotene and contain adequate doses of vitamin D. One example is the Basic One multivitamin formulated by Dr. Kenneth Cooper, founder of the Cooper Clinic in Dallas. It contains plenty of vitamin A (3,000 IU), all in the form of beta-carotene and other carotenoids, along with 800 IU of vitamin D and 400 IU of vitamin E.

When there's contradictory evidence for an intervention—changing a diet, taking a pill, or even using a new gadget in heart surgery or cancer therapy—and there are hints of possible harm, it makes good sense to wait for more evidence before urging that it be used. The same caution is warranted when a new intervention is expensive.

So far, there's no consensus on ideal vitamin intakes because scientific knowledge about them is still evolving. We could definitely use more evidence about the true benefits of the commonly used vitamins. At the same time, harm isn't likely when they are taken in reasonable doses, and the cost is minimal. In this situation, it seems to be a bit foolish to demand that all the evidentiary i's be dotted and t's be crossed before acting.

Recommended Daily Intake of Vitamins and Minerals (Established by the Institute of Medicine)

VITAMIN (COMMON NAMES)	RECOMMENDED DIETARY ALLOWANCE (RDA) OR DAILY ADEQUATE INTAKE (AI)		UPPER LIMIT (UL)
	Women	*Men*	
Vitamin A (preformed = retinol; beta-carotene can be converted to vitamin A)	700 micrograms (2,333 IU)	900 micrograms (3,000 IU)	3,000 micrograms (about 10,000 IU)
Thiamin (vitamin B₁)	1.1 milligrams	1.2 milligrams	Not known
Riboflavin (vitamin B₂)	1.1 milligrams	1.3 milligrams	Not known
Niacin (vitamin B₃, nicotinic acid)	14 milligrams	16 milligrams	35 milligrams
Pantothenic acid (vitamin B₅)	5 milligrams	5 milligrams	Not known
Vitamin B₆ (pyridoxal, pyridoxine, pyridoxamine)	19–50: 1.3 milligrams 51+: 1.5 milligrams	19–50: 1.3 milligrams 51+: 1.7 milligrams	100 milligrams
Vitamin B₁₂ (cobalamin)	2.4 micrograms	2.4 micrograms	Not known
Biotin	30 micrograms	30 micrograms	Not known
Vitamin C (ascorbic acid)	75 milligrams* * Smokers: Add 35 milligrams	90 milligrams*	2,000 milligrams
Choline	425 milligrams	550 milligrams	3,500 milligrams
Vitamin D (calciferol)	19–50: 5 micrograms (200 IU) 51–70: 10 micrograms (400 IU) 71+: 15 micrograms (600 IU)	19–50: 5 micrograms (200 IU) 51–70: 10 micrograms (400 IU) 71+: 15 micrograms (600 IU)	50 micrograms (2,000 IU)

Vitamin (Common Names)	Recommended Dietary Allowance (RDA) or Daily Adequate Intake (AI)		Upper Limit (UL)
	Women	Men	
Vitamin E (alpha-tocopherol)	15 milligrams (15 milligrams equals about 22 IU from natural sources of vitamin E and 33 IU from synthetic vitamin E)	15 milligrams	1,000 milligrams (nearly 1,500 IU natural vitamin E; 2,200 IU synthetic)
Folic acid (folate, folacin)	400 micrograms	400 micrograms	1,000 micrograms
Vitamin K (phylloquinone, menadione)	90 micrograms	120 micrograms	Not known

Mineral	Recommended Amount (Daily RDA or Daily AI)		Upper Limit (UL)
	Women	Men	
Calcium	31–50: 1,000 milligrams / 51+: 1,200 milligrams	31–50: 1,000 milligrams / 51+: 1,200 milligrams	2,500 milligrams
Chloride	19–50: 2.3 grams / 51–70: 2.0 grams / 70+: 1.8 grams	19–50: 2.3 grams / 51–70: 2.0 grams / 70+: 1.8 grams	Not known
Chromium	31–50: 25 micrograms / 51+: 20 micrograms	31–50: 35 micrograms / 51+: 30 micrograms	Not known
Copper	900 micrograms	900 micrograms	10,000 micrograms
Fluoride	3 milligrams	4 milligrams	10 milligrams
Iodine	150 micrograms	150 micrograms	1,100 micrograms

Iron	31–50: 18 milligrams 51+: 8 milligrams	31–50: 8 milligrams 51+: 8 milligrams	45 milligrams
Magnesium	19–30: 310 milligrams 31–70+: 320 milligrams	19–30: 400 milligrams 31–70+: 420 milligrams	350 milligrams from supplements
Manganese	1.8 milligrams	2.3 milligrams	11 milligrams
Molybdenum	45 micrograms	45 micrograms	2,000 micrograms
Phosphorus	700 milligrams	700 milligrams	31–70: 4,000 milligrams 71+: 3,000 milligrams
Potassium	4,700 milligrams	4,700 milligrams	Not known
Selenium	55 micrograms	55 micrograms	400 micrograms
Sodium	19–50: 1,500 milligrams 51–70: 1,300 milligrams 70+: 1,200 milligrams	19–50: 1,500 milligrams 51–70: 1,300 milligrams 70+: 1,200 milligrams	Not determined
Zinc	8 milligrams	11 milligrams	40 milligrams

RDA: the average daily dietary intake sufficient to meet the nutrient requirement of 97–98 percent of healthy individuals in a particular group according to stage of life and gender.

AI: a recommended intake when an RDA can't be determined.

CHAPTER ELEVEN

Putting It All Together

A S I HAVE TRIED TO SHOW you in the preceding chapters, much of the nutrition advice you commonly hear is steering you in the wrong direction. The road to good health needn't be one of blandness and deprivation. Instead it can be paved with hearty, tasty, and satisfying foods.

This book presents a new pyramid built with the best available nutrition science as a blueprint. The healthiest nutritional strategy, summarized in the Healthy Eating Pyramid, includes

- maintaining a stable, healthy weight;
- replacing saturated and trans fats with unsaturated fats;
- substituting whole-grain carbohydrates for refined-grain carbohydrates;
- choosing healthier sources of protein by trading red meat for nuts, beans, chicken, and fish;
- eating plenty of vegetables and fruits;
- using alcohol in moderation; and
- taking a daily multivitamin for insurance.

At first glance it looks as though I am just promoting the widely esteemed Mediterranean diet. While the Mediterranean diet would fit this description, and is an excellent place to start, what I suggest isn't limited to the culinary experience of just one place or time. Instead this strategy is a science-based, multicultural approach to healthy eating.

BENEFITS OF THIS EATING STRATEGY

Part of the payoff from following this strategy comes immediately. By opening up a new world of foods, flavors, and textures, it will make eating a healthy pleasure. It can help you break out of the often unsatisfying and not-so-healthy mealtime ruts you can fall into when following a low-fat or low-carb diet. As you gain control of your appetite and eating habits, not to mention your weight,

The New Healthy Eating Pyramid

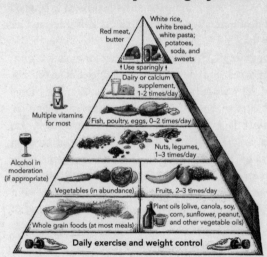

Red meat, butter

White rice, white bread, white pasta; potatoes, soda, and sweets

↑ Use sparingly ↑

Dairy or calcium supplement, 1-2 times/day

Multiple vitamins for most

Fish, poultry, eggs, 0–2 times/day

Nuts, legumes, 1–3 times/day

Alcohol in moderation (if appropriate)

Vegetables (in abundance)

Fruits, 2–3 times/day

Plant oils (olive, canola, soy, corn, sunflower, peanut, and other vegetable oils)

Whole grain foods (at most meals)

Daily exercise and weight control

cholesterol levels, and maybe even your blood pressure, you'll gain a sense of achievement and pride that may affect other areas of your life.

The other part of the payoff—protection against chronic disease—comes later. A healthy eating strategy like the one I suggest is an important part of protecting yourself against a long list of common diseases. These include heart disease, stroke, several common cancers, cataract formation, other age-related diseases, and even some types of birth defects. When combined with not smoking and regular exercise, this kind of healthy diet can reduce heart disease by 80 percent, type 2 diabetes by 90 percent, and stroke and some cancers by 70 percent, compared with average rates in the United States.

To borrow a phrase from the financial world, that's not a bad return on investment, especially when the investment is a more flavorful and less restrictive version of what you may be eating today.

THE ROMANCE AND REALITY OF TRADITIONAL DIETS

The term *traditional diet* once meant a plain, none-too-varied regional diet that was the standard fare of farmers and laborers. Today it conjures up images of heart-healthy, cancer-free, long-lived people who understand the land, eat wonderful meals brimming with taste, and dance, drink, laugh, and love. Think Zorba the Greek meets Julia Child.

A lot of popular writing on traditional diets implies that the foods that go into them have been carefully chosen over the years to promote good health. That's not the whole story. People eat what they can grow, gather, kill, or buy, and their choices are dictated by weather, geology, geography, economics, and even politics. Given these constraints, various cultures have developed many different combinations of healthy (and sometimes not so healthy) foods. Keep in mind that virtually all of these choices were for short-term health, not for prolonging life into old age. Also keep in mind that diets that seem to be good for people whose days are full of hard physical labor aren't necessarily good for people who toil at a desk all day.

In northern Europe, for example, the short growing season makes it difficult to eat fruits and vegetables year-round. It is, though, a fine climate for raising livestock, and meat and dairy products made a good match for the energy needs of people who had to survive long, cold winters. In the small island nation of Japan, the main components of the diet are fish, naturally, and rice, a plant that can yield large amounts of grain from small plots of land. In both these cases, the traditional diet kept people healthy for long enough to reproduce and raise children and also to develop complex societies. Yet their successes don't imply that these either of diets would yield the best health for contemporary people whose main occupation involves sitting for most of the day.

Comparison of Life Expectancy and Disease Rates in the 1960s of Three Countries in the Seven Countries Study

LIFE EXPECTANCY AND DISEASE RATES	GENDER	U.S.	GREECE	JAPAN
Life expectancy at age 45* (1960s)	M	27	31	27
	F	33	34	32
Heart disease[†]	M	189	33	34
	F	54	14	21
Stroke[†]	M	30	26	102
	F	24	23	57
All cancers[†]	M	102	83	98
	F	87	61	77
Colorectal cancer[†]	M	11	3	5
	F	10	3	5
Breast cancer[†]	F	22	8	4

*Years. [†]Cases per 100,0000.

Source: Keys, A., *Seven Countries*, Harvard University Press, 1980.

Characteristics of Diets in the 1960s of Three Countries in the Seven Countries Study

Diet	U.S.	Greece	Japan
Total fat (% energy)	39	37	11
Saturated fat (% energy)	18	8	3
Fruits and vegetables (grams/day)	504	654	232
Legumes (grams/day)	1	30	91
Breads, cereals (grams/day)	123	453	481
Meat and poultry (grams/day)	273	35	8
Fish (grams/day)	3	39	150
Eggs (grams/day)	40	15	29
Alcohol (grams/day)	6	23	22

Source: Keys, A., *Seven Countries*, Harvard University Press, 1980.

THE MEDITERRANEAN DIET AND BEYOND

In the 1950s and 1960s, pioneering nutrition researcher Ancel Keys and his colleagues looked at eating patterns in sixteen different populations in seven countries—Greece, Finland, Italy, the Netherlands, Yugoslavia, Japan, and the United States. This landmark work, known today as the Seven Countries Study, was the first major investigation of the link between diet and heart disease. One of the more intriguing findings was that people living in Crete, other parts of Greece, and southern Italy had very high adult life expectancies (the number of years the average forty-five-year-old can expect to live) and very low rates of heart disease and some cancers, all in spite of relatively limited medical systems. (See the tables below and on page 211.)

At the time, the traditional diet in these Mediterranean countries was mostly plant-based foods—fruits, vegetables, breads, a variety of coarsely ground grains, beans, nuts, and seeds—and olive oil was the main source of dietary fat. People ate dairy products (mostly cheese and yogurt) regularly, but not in large amounts. Fish, poultry, and red meat were eaten on special occasions, not as part of the daily fare. People (usually men) often drank wine, but typically with meals.

Keys concluded that the Mediterranean diet was an important reason for the low rates of heart disease in that region. Alarmed at the epidemic of heart disease that was hitting its peak in the United States in the 1960s, Keys and his wife, Margaret, began popularizing and promoting the Mediterranean diet in a series of best-selling books.

The Seven Countries Study certainly raised the possibility that the Mediterranean diet could cause long life and good health. But it couldn't prove that this was so. Other things such as the physically active lifestyle common throughout the region, the relatively low rates of overweight and obesity, or the low rates of smoking that prevailed until the late 1960s could have been among the causes. It was also possible that some genetic trait common among people in the Mediterranean region provided them with protection against heart disease and cancer, but studies showing that migrants to high-incidence countries lose their protection discounts this explanation.

Many detailed studies have since shown that Keys and his colleagues were on the right track. For example, our research group has documented that the main elements of the Mediterranean lifestyle are connected with lower risks of many diseases, even when practiced by people living in the United States. Results from the Nurses' Health Study document that heart disease rates could be reduced by at least 80 percent by moderate diet and lifestyle changes. The Lyon Diet Heart Study, described in chapter 4, showed that a group of heart attack survivors randomly assigned to a Mediterranean-type diet were 70 percent less likely to die over a two-year period than those assigned to a low-fat American Heart Association diet. Today the Mediterranean diet is often held up as a prime example of healthy eating that should be adopted by all.

But the Mediterranean diet isn't necessarily perfect. It evolved out of agricultural necessities imposed by a warm and semidry climate that by chance favored the growth of olive trees. Nor is the Mediterranean diet the only healthy culture-based diet. As you can see from the table on page 211, the traditional Japanese diet can also be quite healthy in some ways. Latin American diets, which emphasize corn, beans, and vegetables, are another model of healthy eating. Along with some other colleagues, I helped Oldways Preservation and Exchange Trust create a series of food pyramids that try to capture the traditional healthy diets of these regions (www.oldwayspt.org).

While researchers are still trying to refine what is known about the benefits of a Mediterranean diet, one thing we are sure of is that it is safe. The low rates of heart disease and cancer among people who eat this type of diet are solid proof of that. The high stroke rates in Japan, on the other hand, suggest that some aspect of this traditional diet, possibly high carbohydrate and salt intake combined with low consumption of fat, protein, fruits, and vegetables, may not be so safe.

TRADITIONAL DIETS *CAN* TRANSPLANT WELL

While traditional diets may have health benefits for the cultures that shaped them, a big question is whether they offer similar benefits when transplanted somewhere else—for example, to a modern society with relatively low levels of physical activity. If traditional diets are like weeds that can grow anywhere, then an Iowa accountant should get the same benefit from a Mediterranean diet as a Greek farmer. But if traditional diets are more like painstakingly bred orchids that grow only in carefully controlled environments, then adopting a traditional diet without also taking on the other aspects of the traditional culture won't necessarily make a dent in rates of heart disease, cancer, and other chronic diseases.

Fortunately, evidence from different types of studies done in many countries shows that the components of the Mediterranean diet offer major benefits even for people living modern "Western" lifestyles. It remains to be seen whether dining leisurely with a view of the Aegean Sea or taking a siesta after a midday meal adds an extra topping of good health.

Scientists, nutrition experts, and writers have often tried to condense the benefits of the Mediterranean or other traditional diets to one or two key elements, like olive oil or fiber or antioxidants. That's a dangerous proposition. While we know that the Mediterranean diet helps prevent chronic disease, and that olive oil is one of the reasons why, just loading up on olive oil or taking high-dose antioxidant supplements isn't a substitute for a comprehensive healthy eating strategy.

Most important, taking advantage of the Mediterranean diet isn't an all-or-nothing proposition. We know enough about this diet to be sure that its elements can be safely and fruitfully incorporated into other healthy eating strategies.

COST OF HEALTHY EATING

Does it cost more to eat foods that promote good health than to eat those that don't? Many people believe nutritious foods are more expensive than less healthy alternatives. They are partly right. Fats, sweets, and refined carbohydrates deliver more calories per dollar than fish or fresh vegetables. Yet when it comes to an all-around diet, cost need not stand in the way of healthy eating.

Following a healthy eating pattern is all about choices—picking good fats and steering clear of bad ones, adding more good sources of carbohydrate and cutting back on poor ones, opting for healthier protein packages, selecting smaller portions instead of super-sizing, and so on. Cost, along with taste and convenience, is a dominant factor influencing these choices.

Foods that are filling, high in calories, and satisfying are often the least expensive. In day-to-day eating and shopping, this means that a hamburger and French fries washed down with a large soda and topped off with soft-serve ice cream is a relatively inexpensive way to get calories. Foods that pack the most calories per ounce (those with the highest *energy densities*) tend to have the lowest cost per calorie. These include oil, margarine, potatoes, and soft drinks. Healthier options, such as whole grains, fresh fruits and vegetables, and lean meats, cost more per calorie.

If you have a limited income, market forces *seem* to conspire against healthy eating. If you're at the other end of the spectrum, you can pay top dollar for out-of-season fruits and vegetables, ready-to-eat packages of salad, top-of-the-line fish, and specialty breads. In between those extremes is the vast middle ground that most of us try to navigate as we make our way through the grocery store or market. Here are some suggestions for anyone interested in making healthy choices without breaking the bank.

• *Fats.* There's no question that olive oil is more expensive than canola or safflower oil. Even so, you can find some perfectly tasty types for $8–10 a liter. At two tablespoons a day, that's less than 50 cents. Use olive oil where flavor counts, such as for drizzling on vegetables or in salad dressings. Otherwise, use canola oil for sautéing or other applications where flavor isn't as important.

• *Carbohydrates.* White rice, pasta, and potatoes are some of the least expensive sources of carbohydrate. Whole grains, such as brown rice, bulgur, wheat berries, oat groats, and others, cost more. Yet when you calculate the cost per serving, using whole grains adds relatively little to the food budget.

Whole-grain breakfast cereals aren't newcomers to the cereal aisle. You can reach for the old standbys, such as Shredded Wheat, Grape-Nuts, Wheaties, or oatmeal, or choose newer entries such as Great Grains and Kashi. Per serving, whole-grain cereals cost little more than highly refined cereals. In the fall of 2004, one of the leading cereal makers, General Mills, announced it would make all of its breakfast cereals with whole grains.

• *Protein.* When Americans think of protein, they tend to think of meat. Beef is certainly a good protein source. Turkey and chicken offer a more healthful protein package and are typically less expensive. Roasting a whole chicken has long been an inexpensive main dish, and continues to be so today. Fish is an even healthier protein source. Some types, such as swordfish and halibut, are

Healthy Eating on a Budget: Cost for a Single Day's Menu

BREAKFAST

Oatmeal, 1$\frac{1}{2}$ cups cooked (10 cents)
Walnuts, 3 tablespoons (28 cents)
Raisins, $\frac{1}{4}$ cup (12 cents)
Tangerine, 1 large (22 cents)

LUNCH

Whole wheat bread, 2 slices (21 cents)
Peanut butter, 2 tablespoons (16 cents)
Banana, 1 large (14 cents)

DINNER

Chicken & Vegetable Stir Fry:
 Canola oil, 1$\frac{1}{2}$ tablespoons (7 cents)
 Skinless dark and light chicken, 3 ounces (30 cents)
 Broccoli, $\frac{1}{2}$ cup (5 cents)
 Carrots, $\frac{1}{2}$ cup (7 cents)
 Onions, $\frac{1}{2}$ cup (9 cents)
 Soy sauce, 1 teaspoon (2 cents)
 Corn starch, $\frac{1}{2}$ tablespoon (1 cent)
Brown rice, 1 cup cooked (15 cents)
Baked apple, 1 large (25 cents)

SNACK

Pear, 1 large (32 cents)
Peanuts, $\frac{1}{4}$ cup (8 cents)

Total: 2000 calories (33 percent fat)
Total Cost: $2.64 (includes items on sale)

budget breakers or once-in-a-while luxuries. Others are more reasonably priced and often on sale. These include salmon, catfish, pollock, and many types of frozen fish. Canned tuna, salmon, and mackerel—on a sandwich, in a salad, or as part of a casserole—are inexpensive ways to put fish on your plate.

Eating even lower on the food chain may be the best for your budget and your health. Making nuts, peanut butter, beans, other vegetable sources of protein, and eggs the centerpiece of meals, instead of side dishes or garnishes, would be a boon for your budget. Don't be put off by the cost of nuts. Keep in mind that meat is two-thirds water, so nuts that cost $4.50 per pound are comparable to beef that costs $1.50 per pound.

• *Fruits and vegetables.* Even though fruits and vegetables don't deliver the cheap caloric punch of fats and sugar, they are still one of the best food bargains around. The USDA calculates that a savvy shopper can get seven servings of fruits and vegetables a day for less than 75 cents: one-half cup of apple, one-half cup of grapefruit juice, one-eighth cup of raisins, and one-half cup servings of carrots, broccoli, cabbage, and romaine lettuce. Even the most expensive fruit (blackberries) and vegetable (asparagus) cost less than 70 cents a serving. (A link to this USDA report, which is full of interesting information on produce costs, is available at www.health.harvard.edu/EDBH.) Frozen fruits and vegetables are just as nutritious as fresh ones, and often cost less.

• *What you aren't buying.* Making healthier choices usually involves cutting back or cutting out foods such as beefsteak, potato chips, ice cream, your morning doughnut, and sweetened sodas. Savings from these can add up and may even offset the cost for fish, whole grains, and fresh fruits and vegetables.

If you still think healthy eating is expensive, consider the alternative. Heart disease, stroke, diabetes, some cancers, and other diet-related chronic diseases cost far more in the long run than good nutrition. The USDA's Economic Research Service estimates that healthier eating could save Americans almost $90 billion a year in medical costs and lost productivity. That's not all "invisible money" transferred from health insurance companies to doctors and hospitals. Many people pay part or all of the cost of their medications for these chronic conditions. People who are overweight pay an average of 11 percent more in out-of-pocket medical costs than do people with healthy weights, while those who are obese have 26 percent higher out-of-pocket costs.

The bottom line. By making a few smart choices, healthy eating need not cost more than the average American diet and in the long run is a sound financial investment.

HEALTHY GLOBAL EATING

We have the good fortune to live at a time when we have seemingly unlimited choices in foods. Beside the bewildering array of junk food, grocery stores routinely carry fruits and vegetables from many countries, "new" grains are becoming easier to find, and restaurants offer an ever expanding smorgasbord of the world's cuisines. Twenty-five years ago in Boston, for example, Mediterranean cuisine typically meant spaghetti and meatballs. Today many local restaurants serve up a variety of vastly more interesting and healthy traditional dishes from that region as well as from other parts of the globe.

Given these choices, I don't advocate returning to a single humble diet or switching to a particular traditional diet. Instead, what I am suggesting is a flexible eating strategy based on a completely rebuilt food pyramid that incorporates elements of healthy eating patterns from around the world and leaves plenty of room for creativity and innovation. The Mediterranean diet offers a good blueprint for healthy eating. But there's plenty of room for fine-tuning, and other cultures also have healthy eating strategies to offer. From Japan we can incorporate the tradition of serving small portions of tasty, interesting foods instead of large helpings of the relatively bland foods that are the mainstays of U.S. and northern European diets. This approach helps keep consumption in check but doesn't make you feel deprived, as many weight loss or weight control diets do. From Latin America, the region that has given us corn and tomatoes, come interesting and healthy grains such as quinoa that are unfamiliar to most North Americans. Even from Finland, the country with the most lethal diet in the Seven Countries Study, comes a great whole-grain rye bread that is much healthier and far tastier than the spongy white bread eaten by many Americans. What's more, we are learning intriguing and appetizing ways to combine and season ingredients.

This is truly a healthy diet for a modern age. It is drawn from eating strategies from around the world that have been shown to yield benefits in different populations, including Americans from all walks of life. The science has been described in the preceding sections. The global influence is unmistakable in the ingredients and recipes that follow.

I hope the new Healthy Eating Pyramid, along with the eating strategies described earlier and the recipes that follow, will help you make both healthy and delicious food choices that will enhance and lengthen your life.

CHAPTER TWELVE

Recipes and Menus

Getting Started

EATING HEALTHFULLY, as you've learned earlier in this book, is not a complicated concept. Simply put, it involves building an eating style that is based on whole grains, fresh produce, and good fats. To get you started in the right direction, we've developed a group of sixty recipes, everything from Curried Winter Squash Soup to Fruit 'n' Spicy Nut Trail Mix, that will tempt your taste buds and renew your faith that eating for good health can be a delicious endeavor. Some of the recipes are quick fixes and can go from preparation to table in under thirty minutes. Others take a bit more time but include classic favorites like meat loaf, chili, and fried rice.

In general, these recipes are just healthy, good food and so don't require any major manipulations. But if you have special health concerns (diabetes, high blood pressure, pregnancy), we've made notations at the end of each recipe to highlight some key points you might want to consider. For folks with high cholesterol, we have broken down total fat grams into the different sorts of fat and have also given the amount of cholesterol. For people with high blood pressure who must limit sodium, we've given tips on how to lower the sodium content of recipes. For people with diabetes, there's a complete nutritional analysis after each recipe that will list the total grams of carbohydrate. If you're still working with the diabetic exchange system, we've also included information about how each recipe fits into the exchange format. And where it's appropriate, we've made general notes about some of the nutrients a recipe may contain in abundant supply or offered ways to lower calories in a recipe even further. The recipes aren't geared toward weight loss. Just the fact that they emphasize whole grains, fruits, and vegetables, though, should make it easy to work these recipes into a weight loss plan.

If you are battling with excess weight, you already know there is no quick fix. As discussed in chapter 3, you'll need to retrain your eating and exercise habits for the long term to take off pounds permanently. This section of the book is going to give you an easy, delicious way to do that. Here are four point-ers to keep in mind:

- *Play the favorites.* Losing weight isn't about deprivation. It's about moder-ation. So don't put favorite foods on a taboo list, just learn to eat them in smaller portions and less frequently. At the same time, take delight in truly good, fresh food. A just-picked juicy sweet peach. Steamed fresh green beans with a squeeze of lemon juice and a sprinkle of pepper. A hot-off-the-grill salmon steak. Your tastes may eventually start shifting away from salty, sugary, overprocessed foods and waking up to a whole wonderful world of fresh, clean flavors. Who knows, your list of favorites might just change completely.

- *Move to your own beat.* Food is only one part of the weight control equa-tion; the other half is exercise. You don't need a formal exercise program to keep active. Hiking, biking, swimming, or other outdoor pursuits, even garden-ing, can burn energy and help keep your metabolism humming at a healthy pace. Instead of trying to fit yourself into an exercise program that you hate, work to change your mind-set. Always be thinking about how you can squeeze in activity or fun active-style pursuits. If you mix and match your activities, it's unlikely you'll get bored.

- *Size it up.* America is the land of big food portions. Supersize it. Oversize it. Jumbo it. It seems we've all gotten used to seeing larger and larger portions of food on our plates. But when you eat more food than your body needs, the end result is weight gain. If you're serious about losing weight, spend a week using measuring cups and scales to get an accurate idea of what you're eating. Then work to winnow portions down to realistic amounts. At dinner, for exam-ple, fill half your plate with vegetables. Add a serving of poultry or fish the size of a deck of cards and a scoop of brown rice, bulgur, or other whole grain the size of half a tennis ball.

- *Splurge on quality ingredients.* Just because you're eating less doesn't mean that food has to be less satisfying. Learn what chefs have known all along: A lit-tle bit of a high-quality ingredient goes a long way toward boosting flavor. A good-quality flavored vinegar (balsamic, sherry) can make a potent vinaigrette. A small sprinkling of fresh grated Parmesan, rather than the powdered stuff in the can, can top off a pizza or a salad with a burst of salty, nutty flavor. An extra-virgin olive oil, a roasted peanut oil, a sesame-flavored oil—just small amounts of these high-flavored ingredients can put the finishing touches on a recipe and elevate it from average to sublime.

To learn more about this new approach to healthful eating, we've come up with mouthwatering recipes that celebrate whole grains, fresh produce, and healthy fats. There's also a week's worth of menus to help you get started planning healthful meals. (At the bottom of each day's menu is some advice about how to adapt the menu to a low-calorie plan for weight loss.) Finally, there are some general tips for improving the quality of your meals and some specific suggestions for healthful snacks.

Smart Snacking

It goes without saying that fresh fruit, vegetables, and whole grains are good snacks. The snack foods you find in the supermarket—cookies, crackers, and chips—can be a mixed bag. Many are made with partially hydrogenated oils, highly processed flours, and large quantities of sugar. To find the healthiest choices, you'll need to be a bit of a label sleuth, reading the fine print on ingredient lists and Nutrition Facts panels. The goal is to search out snacks made with healthy oils, whole grains or whole-grain flours, a respectable amount of sugar, preferably the fruit variety, and no trans fats.

Here are some questions to consider, followed by a few examples of popular snacks made with healthy ingredients.

DOES IT CONTAIN TRANS FAT?

Beginning in 2006, the Nutrition Facts label on food packages must list trans fats along with total and saturated fats. (See Figure 13, page 82.) Some food companies—mostly those whose products don't contain any trans fats—have already begun doing this. (Interestingly, this simple change in the rules is motivating many companies to reformulate how they make cakes, cookies, chips, and other foods so that they won't contain any trans fats.)

Until then, you need to scan the ingredient list for the telltale signs of trans fats. If you find any hydrogenated or partially hydrogenated vegetable oils on the list, the food contains trans fat and is best avoided. Some sly manufacturers are now using the words *vegetable shortening* or *margarine* on the ingredient list, which also means trans fat. Since ingredients are listed by order of weight (or amount used), you'll be able to get a ballpark idea of how much hydrogenated oil was used to make the snack. If partially hydrogenated cottonseed oil is at the top of the list—one of the first few ingredients—then the snack has a large percentage of trans fats. Partially hydrogenated oils that are at or near the bottom of a long list don't account for much of the end product. Some companies actually mention the percentage in the ingredient list. The label may say "contains less than 2 percent partially hydrogenated corn, cottonseed or saf-flower oil."

Another way to get an estimate of trans fat is to look at labels that divulge the type of fat in a food. If the manufacturer breaks down fats by category (saturated, monounsaturated, polyunsaturated), you can add up these amounts. If the total doesn't match the total grams of fat listed on the label, chances are most of the unaccounted-for fat is of the trans variety.

IS IT MADE WITH WHOLE GRAINS?

Labels don't always come right out and boast about the use of whole grains. Look to the ingredients list for whole-wheat flour (not wheat flour), oats, corn, rye, and so on. And look to the Nutrient Facts panel for total grams of fiber. Whole grains contain large amounts of fiber. The more whole grains used in a snack, the higher the fiber content per serving. Don't be fooled by the liberal use of wheat in a snack title. Wheat flour is not necessarily whole-grain flour.

IS IT FULL OF SUGAR?

Whole grains are great ingredients. So too are unsaturated oils like canola, saf-flower, and olive. But if you pair these ingredients with large amounts of sugars, you can negate the health benefits of the grains and healthy fats. There are two words to describe sugar: empty calories. Ingredients like granulated sugar, brown sugar, and honey provide calories to a food but nothing in the way of nutrients. That's not to say that you need to avoid every speck of sugar you encounter. But some snack foods, particularly a lot of the fat-free snacks, are loaded with empty sugar calories. Better to find a snack food made with little or no sugar: popcorn, roasted nuts, whole-grain crackers—such as Ak-Mak 100% Whole Wheat Sesame Crackers or Wasa Original Hearty Rye Crispbread—and whole-grain toast with peanut butter.

WHAT ABOUT FRUIT SWEETENERS?

To the body, calories obtained from fruit sugar aren't much different energy-wise from the calories in a scoop of white or brown sugar. But when whole fruit is used to sweeten a dish, you do gain nutritional benefits from the fruit. So a cookie sweetened with applesauce will gain some fiber and other nutrients from the applesauce. A cereal sweetened with fresh-grated apple (see the recipe for Apple Crunch Oatmeal, page 256) will have more nutrients than a cereal sweetened with granulated sugar.

The question gets a bit stickier when you talk about the use of juice con-

Snack Selections

The following information is given for each snack:

Name of food Amount, Calories, Saturated Fat (grams), Unsaturated Fat (grams),* Sodium (milligrams), Fiber (grams), Comments

Snyder's of Hanover Hard Sourdough Pretzel 1 large round——1 oz, 100, 0 g, 0 g, 240 mg, 1 g, flour not 100% whole grain, but serving contains 1 g of fiber

Garden of Eatin' Blue Corn Tortilla Chips 15 chips——1 oz, 150, 0.5 g, 6.5 g, 55 mg, 1 g, made from organic blue corn

Lady J Peanut Butter Cookies 1 cookie——1 oz, 110, 0.5 g, 5.5 g, 100 mg, 2 g, made with whole-wheat flour, oats, fruit juices

Heaven Scent Windmill Cookies 2¹/₂ cookies——1 oz, 108, 0 g, 4 g, 119 mg, 2 g, made with organic whole-wheat flour, fruit juice, canola oil

Barbara's Nature's Choice Raspberry Filled Cereal Bars 1 bar——1.25 oz, 110, 0 g, 0 g, 110 mg, 2 g, made with organic whole-wheat flour, juice concentrates, fruit

Naked Strawberry Banana Smoothie 2 cups——16 oz, 260, 0 g, 0 g, 20 mg, 4 g, contains 100 percent fruit (juice and puree)

Roasted Soybeans ¹/₄ cup——1 oz, 140, 1 g, 7 g, 0 mg, 1 g, roasted without oil; small amount of fructose (fruit sugar) and molasses

Just Corn (dried corn) ¹/₄ cup——1 oz, 100, 0 g, 1.5 g, 15 mg, 1 g, no added ingredients; contains small amount of fat and sugar found naturally in corn

Oil Roasted Mixed Nuts ¹/₄ cup——1.3 oz, 219, 3.1 g, 15.9 g, 0 mg, 3.5 g, bulk of fat is unsaturated

Popcorn, oil-popped 2 cups——0.8 oz, 110, 1.1 g, 4.8 g, 195 mg, 2.2 g, figures are for popcorn popped with healthy oils. Microwave and movie theater popcorns are typically made with partially hydrogenated oils and will contain trans fats.

Popcorn, air-popped 2 cups——0.6 oz, 61, 0.1 g, 0.5 g, 1 mg, 2.4 g, white or yellow corn popped in the microwave or popcorn popper

Smucker's Natural Style Peanut Butter 2 tablespoons——1.13 oz, 200, 2 g, 14 g, 120 mg, 2 g, made with fresh ground peanuts and salt, 2.2 grams saturated fat, bulk of fat unsaturated

Barbara's All Natural Wheatines 4 crackers——¹/₂ oz, 50, 0 g, 1.5 g, 110 mg, <1 g, saltine-style cracker made with organic whole-wheat flour; small amount molasses and honey

Sources: Food labels and ESHA Food Processor.

*Food labels are not required to list grams of unsaturated fat. But it's simple to estimate those amounts, using figures for total and saturated fat, when the ingredients list includes only healthful oils.

centrates (apple, grape) to sweeten foods. In truth, there probably isn't much difference calorie-wise between concentrates and granulated sugar. And concentrates don't contain fiber like whole fruits. But in the end, many of the fruit-sweetened snacks just contain less overall sugar than traditional snacks. And that's the point: the less sugar the better.

Deciphering Food Labels

Federal regulations require manufacturers to include information about the ingredients contained in a food, as well as the food's nutrition profile, somewhere on the food label. Both of these parts of the label offer valuable information, if you know how to use it. Here's a rundown of key points to consider.

INGREDIENT LIST

This is the most detailed accounting of what a product contains, item by item. And while it doesn't give exact amounts of each ingredient, it does list them in descending order by weight. At the top of the list is the main or most predominant ingredient. Say you're looking at a juice-drink label. The first two ingredients might be water and high-fructose corn syrup. Farther down the list, about three or four ingredients later, a fruit juice like grape or apple might be mentioned. This lets you know that the drink is mostly water and sugar with a tiny amount of fruit juice. An ingredient label on orange juice, on the other hand, will list the first ingredient as orange juice or orange juice from concentrate. Remember, this is also where you'll find information about the use of hydrogenated and partially hydrogenated oils.

NUTRITION FACTS PANEL

This section gives a detailed accounting of how a serving of the food rates nutritionally, first by providing information about calorie content and key nutrients and then by comparing that information to reference values or standard requirements.

- *Serving size.* Never lose sight of this amount. All of the other information on the panel is meaningless if you can't put portion size into perspective. Unfortunately, many times the portion size listed is far smaller than what most people might eat. For example, an oversize cookie may list the calories and fat for one-fifth of the cookie as a serving rather than list calories, fat, and nutrients for the whole cookie. Or what looks like a single-serving entrée of frozen lasagna, upon closer inspection, turns out to be 2.5 servings.

- *Calories.* Calories count. Yet the numbers may not be as important as the quality of those calories. If the energy is derived mainly from healthy fats and whole grains, then higher numbers aren't a problem, particularly if you're not trying to lose weight. If calories come mainly from added sugars and saturated fats, then the food is one that's better to pass by.

- *Total fat.* This listing provides the total grams of fat per serving. Again, the number is not as important as the type of fat. Read farther down the panel to find out how much of that fat is saturated and how much is unsaturated (monounsaturated or polyunsaturated). By 2006 this section of the label will include information on trans fats, the unhealthy fats formed when liquid oils are made into solid shortenings. In the meantime, you can still decipher where the fat is coming from or, at the very least, how much of the total fat is saturated.

- *Cholesterol.* This is one number you shouldn't have trouble with, not if you're searching out whole grains, fruits, and vegetables—all foods that are cholesterol-free. Keep in mind that the American Heart Association recommends eating less than 300 milligrams of cholesterol per day.

- *Sodium.* Look to this part of the information panel if you need to restrict salt or sodium in your diet. General guidelines encourage 1,200–1,300 milligrams of sodium per day, with an upper limit of 2,300 milligrams (about the amount found in 1 teaspoon of salt).

- *Total carbohydrates.* Rather than live by numbers, it's best to emphasize whole grains. A listing of the grams of sugar and grams of fiber helps put into context the type of carbohydrate the food contains.

- *Protein.* Most Americans, even those on vegetarian diets, eat more protein than the body requires. Don't spend much time with this number.

- *Daily values.* This section highlights how several different nutrients—vitamin A, vitamin C, calcium, iron—contribute to the daily requirements set by the Food and Nutrition Board of the National Academy of Sciences. It's all based on a person who requires two thousand calories per day. That means your needs may be different if you're eating fewer calories or your energy requirements are higher.

Healthful Substitutions

No single food will make or break good health. But the overall quality of your diet, the kinds of foods you choose to eat day in and day out, does have a major impact. Good diets, ones that promote well-being, are built mainly on nutrient-dense choices, foods that contain healthful fats, fiber, and a whole host of other nutrients. Splurge. Enjoy food. But when push comes to shove, make choices that are high in flavor but also good for health. Replace unhealthy saturated and trans fats with the more healthful unsaturated variety. And make a point to start adding more whole grains, fruits, and vegetables to meals. Here are some suggestions for achieving those goals.

REPLACING BAD FATS WITH THE GOOD ONES

Both saturated fats and trans fats are damaging to the heart and to overall health. Switch to foods or food ingredients that contain more of the healthful unsaturated fats—monounsaturated fats like olive and canola oils and polyunsaturated fats like safflower and corn oil.

INSTEAD OF . . .

. . . SAUTÉING WITH BUTTER

- *Switch to olive, canola, or other healthful oils.* Calories are similar. But oils are rich in healthful unsaturated fats and low in saturated fat. Olive oil has only 1.8 grams of saturated fat per tablespoon; butter has 7, which is close to one-half of the daily limit. In fact, each tablespoon of butter gets more than half of its calories from saturated fat.

. . . BAKING CAKES, COOKIES, AND QUICK BREADS WITH SOLID SHORTENING

- *Switch to healthful oils.* Calories are roughly the same. But again, the oils are rich in unsaturated fats. The solid shortening is made from oil that is partially hydrogenated, so it will contain unhealthful trans fats.

. . . COOKING PORK LOIN OR FATTIER CUTS OF PORK

- *Switch to pork tenderloin.* Pork tenderloin is as lean as skinless white meat chicken. A 3-ounce cooked serving contains only 4 grams of fat, just 1.4 grams of it saturated. The same-size serving of cooked pork loin contains nearly 12 grams of fat, 4.5 grams of it saturated. A good rule of thumb is that the leaner the cut of meat, the less saturated fat it contains.

. . . COOKING FATTY HAMBURGER MEAT (73 TO 80 PERCENT LEAN)

- *Switch to extra-lean ground meat.* A 3-ounce portion of a fatty hamburger meat, before it's cooked, can have nearly 23 grams of fat, 9 of it saturated. A lean ground beef, one that is labeled 91 percent lean, carries only 8 grams of fat, 3 of it saturated. Cooking, particularly if you broil or grill meat to the well-done stage, can reduce fat—but not dramatically enough to make fatty meat as lean as the extra-lean variety.

. . . USING FLOUR TORTILLAS MADE WITH PARTIALLY HYDROGENATED OILS

- *Switch to whole-grain (corn or wheat) tortillas made with oil.* Flour tortillas don't contain large amounts of fat, just a few grams per serving. But they're made with partially hydrogenated oils, so they contain trans fats. They're also void of fiber. A better choice is whole-grain corn or whole-wheat tortillas that contain no added fat or just a small amount of a healthful fat like canola oil.

. . . USING WHOLE MILK IN SAUCES OR BAKED GOODS

- *Switch to skim milk.* Each 8 ounces of whole milk contains close to 8 grams of fat, nearly 5 of it saturated. Skim milk contains less than .5 gram of fat in this same-size serving and less than .25 gram of fat. If you'd rather not use any dairy products, consider using soy milk in place of whole milk. It's not similar flavorwise, and it contains more fat than skim milk. But the fat it contains is mainly unsaturated.

. . . ADDING SOUR CREAM TO RECIPES

- *Switch to nonfat plain yogurt.* Each cup of sour cream contains 40 grams of fat, 32 of it saturated, and 200 milligrams of cholesterol. The same amount of plain skim-milk yogurt carries a mere .5 gram of fat and only 4 milligrams of cholesterol.

. . . SPREADING SANDWICHES OR CRACKERS WITH REGULAR PEANUT BUTTER

- *Switch to natural-style peanut butter.* This saves no calories, just offers a healthful switch in the type of fat. Natural peanut butter is free of trans fats. Regular peanut butters are usually made with hydrogenated oils that do not contain trans fats but do add more saturated fat.

. . . EATING CHICKEN AND TURKEY WITH THE SKIN ON

- *Consider leaving part of the skin on the plate.* Removing the skin will remove nearly 5 grams of fat and 1.3 grams of saturated fat from a cooked 4-ounce breast of chicken. A good rule of thumb: Remove the skin after cooking, since the skin keeps the meat moist during cooking.

. . . SMOTHERING PIZZA OR SALAD WITH CHEESE

- *Use a tiny amount of high-flavored cheeses like Parmesan, blue cheese, or extra-sharp cheddar.* This adds far less fat, since you're satisfied with a smaller amount of cheese. One tablespoon of Parmesan cheese contains only 2 grams of fat, 1 gram of it saturated.

EMPHASIZING NUTRITION-PACKED FOODS

While there are no super foods that contain every single nutrient needed for good health, some foods pack more nutrients per calorie than others. Learn to emphasize these nutrient-dense foods, and the overall quality of your diet will improve practically overnight. For the most part, the list of nutrient-dense foods includes all the whole grains, fruits, and most vegetables. Following are some tips to get you started. But the best strategy is to emphasize whole grains, fruits, and vegetables at every meal. Forget five servings a day for fruits and vegetables and instead aim for nine or more.

Add dark leafy greens (spinach) to salads. Dark leafy greens contain more nutrients than iceberg lettuce. Spinach, for example, contains everything from iron to folate to fiber. Iceberg lettuce, on the other hand, is mostly water. A good rule of thumb: The darker the green, the more nutrients it contains.

Sprinkle wheat germ on cereals, casseroles, or yogurt. Adding 2 tablespoons of wheat germ boosts the fiber nearly 2 grams but adds only 54 calories. Use the toasted variety for a nuttier flavor.

Serve a whole grain (bulgur, wheat berries) for your starchy side dish instead of a baked potato. Both white potatoes and grains like bulgur and wheat berries are considered starchy side dishes. But the potatoes have nowhere near as much fiber and are not as nutrient-dense as whole grains.

Try fresh fruit such as sliced strawberries for dessert instead of ice cream or cake. One cup of strawberries contains nearly a full day's supply of vitamin C, significant amounts of folate, and only 46 calories. Although it's a good source of calcium, the ice cream is full of saturated fat and sugar.

Snack on whole-grain crackers rather than those made with processed flour. The amount of fiber varies from brand to brand. Calories vary, too. But in general, whole-grain crackers such as Triscuits or Ak-Maks contain more fiber than those made with processed flour. And that fiber can add up if you're a regular snacker.

Dictionary of Whole or Intact Grains

Grains have nourished humans since early times. But somewhere along the way most of us have lost touch with their goodness. Here's a brief refresher course on whole or intact grains, a comprehensive A to Z list with everything you need to know about cooking techniques, storage guidelines, and taste. Remember, whole grains are unrefined but can be available as flour; intact grains are just that. Read on to master the lingo.

WHOLE-GRAIN COOKING AND STORAGE TIPS

Here are some general points to keep in mind when storing and cooking whole grains.

- Soaking intact whole grains, either for just a few hours or overnight, helps to reduce cooking time.
- Toasting whole grains, like toasting nuts, helps intensify their nutty flavor. Toasting can also reduce the cooking time for some grains, including barley, spelt, wheat berries, and oat groats.
- Cooking times are not carved in stone. Grains, like legumes, may cook faster or slower depending on the length of time in storage. Just-harvested grains will cook more quickly than grains that have been in storage for a long period of time. The best measure of doneness is tenderness.
- Store whole grains in airtight containers, preferably in the refrigerator. All whole grains carry small amounts of natural oils, which can spoil quickly, particularly during hot summer months.
- Cooked whole grains will keep in the refrigerator for 2 to 3 days. They also freeze well. So you might want to consider simmering large batches of grains and packaging them for the freezer. That way you can pull them out and drop them in a soup, a casserole, or a salad without investing a long time in the kitchen.

AMARANTH

Cultivated by the Aztecs, this yellow-gold seed has a crunchy texture that softens only slightly when cooked. In fact, its creamy-crunchy texture is so much like the consistency of hot cereals that this is the way the grain is most often eaten. For the adventurous, amaranth (AM-ah-ranth) can be tucked into baked goods (see Banana-Apricot Nut Bread, page 258) or mixed with other grains to make a pilaf or casserole. Also, try toasting the seeds in a dry skillet; they will expand and "pop" just like corn. Sprinkle the crunchy popped kernels on salads, vegetables, and pizza.

Cooking Rating: Easy but time-consuming.

Must be simmered in a large amount of water (1 part grain to 3 parts water) for 25–30 minutes when eaten as cereal. To use in baking, presoak in boiling water.

Nutritional Benefits: Cholesterol-free with a small amount of fat, most of it unsaturated. Rich in iron, with 60 percent of the required amount in $1/4$ cup of the dry seed. Good source of fiber—3 grams per $1/4$ cup dry—but not as high in fiber as some of the other grains. Also a good source of calcium, with small amounts of the B vitamins.

Shopping Tip: It's unlikely you will find this grain at the supermarket. It can be found at most health food stores or ordered via mail or the Internet from companies such as Bob's Red Mill or Hodgson Mill, Inc. (See addresses and Web site information in the section that follows this dictionary.)

BARLEY

This nutty-flavored whole grain is sold in many different forms: hulled, pearled, or flakes. The pearled variety is the most common and most versatile. It retains a chewy texture even after long periods of cooking. That makes it a good candidate for soups, casseroles, and even a whole-grain-style risotto (see Wild Mushroom–Barley Risotto, page 300.)

Cooking Rating: Easy but time-consuming.

Whole hulled barley: Needs to be soaked overnight and then simmered for an hour or more.

Pearled: Made from grains that are split but still contain the center, or "pearl." Comes in a fine and regular texture. Thanks to refining, you can skip the soaking step and shave 30 minutes off the cooking time. If that's not fast enough, look for quick-cooking pearl barley (marketed by Quaker Oats under the Mother's brand). It cooks in 10 minutes.

Flakes/grits: Barley flakes, which resemble rolled oats, can be made into hot cereal or soup. Barley "grits" are a fine grind of the grain used for hot cereal.

Nutritional Benefits: Cholesterol-free, with a tiny amount of fat. Good source of protein, with decent amounts of iron, potassium, and magnesium. Excellent source of fiber—about 8 grams per $1/4$ cup dry.

Shopping Tip: Pearl and instant barley are found in most supermarkets. Whole hulled barley, barley flakes, and barley grits can be found in health food stores or via the mail or Internet from companies such as Bob's Red Mill or Hodgson Mill, Inc. (See addresses and Web site information in the section that follows this dictionary.)

BROWN RICE

Brown rice gets its characteristic brown color and nutty flavor from the fact that the bran or outer layer is left on when the rice is harvested. It can be found in short, medium, or long grains, each of which has different applications. Brown basmati rice, a special type of long-grain brown rice grown in India, has a particularly nutty flavor and gives off a wonderful aroma as it cooks. Since it still contains the bran layer (which has small amounts of oil), brown rice is best used within a few weeks of purchase. Or keep it refrigerated in an airtight container.

Cooking Rating: Easy but time-consuming. Needs to simmer for 40–45 minutes.

Nutritional Benefits: Cholesterol-free and very little fat. Twice as high in fiber as white rice; rich in vitamin E and other nutrients.

Shopping Tip: Keep in mind that quality and flavors can vary with different brands. Most supermarkets have a wide variety of brown rices, including store brands and specialty blends like those under the Lundberg logo. Several companies now market instant brown rice that is typically not as flavorful or as nice in appearance as some of the specialty brown rices.

BUCKWHEAT

Buckwheat is one of the few whole grains that isn't technically a grain. It is actually a distant cousin to rhubarb. (Two other non-grain plants used as grains are amaranth and quinoa.) Buckwheat is typically roasted and then used either whole or ground. Whole or cracked buckwheat seeds (buckwheat groats), once they have been toasted, are sometimes called kasha. In Eastern Europe, kasha is routinely used in cooking in much the same way that Americans use potatoes.

Cooking Rating: Very easy.

Nutritional Benefits: Buckwheat is not as stellar a source of fiber and nutrients as most whole grains. But it can be combined with other grains to make a healthy pilaf.

BULGUR (BULGHUR)

This whole grain is actually a form of wheat. A staple in the eastern Mediterranean, bulgur (BUHL-guhr) is made by steaming or boiling kernels of wheat, called wheat berries, and then crushing them. Bulgur comes in fine, medium, or coarse grind, although the most common form is the medium grind. It can be made from either red wheat (dark brown grain) or white wheat (golden-brown grain). The grain can be used in everything from salads to soups to veggie burgers.

Cooking Rating: Very easy.

Just add boiling water to the fine or medium grain and allow it to soak for 20–30 minutes or until tender. (Coarse-textured bulgurs must be simmered instead of soaked.)

Nutritional Benefits: Cholesterol-free, high fiber (5 grams per ¼ cup dry), and relatively high protein (4 grams per ¼ cup dry).

Shopping Tip: Easy to find at most supermarkets.

CORN

This native American grain comes in many different packages. The most obvious is fresh corn on the cob. But the grain can be ground and dried and made into grits, cornmeal, flour, and pasta. The less it's processed, the more flavor and nutrients it will contain.

Cooking Rating: Very easy.

Cornmeal: Regular cornmeal is made by stripping dried corn kernels of their outer husk and the germ, which causes loss of nutrients. It is enriched with some of these lost nutrients, however. The grain is then ground into a fine, medium, or coarse texture. Polenta is made from a coarse-grain cornmeal. Finely ground cornmeal is called corn flour; masa harina is a type of corn flour used to make corn tortillas. Look for the stone-ground variety if possible, as it contains more nutrients than other varieties of cornmeal. Note that degerminated cornmeal is not whole grain.

Hominy: Corn kernels that are soaked in a weak solution of lye. Since it's degermed and hulled after soaking, hominy isn't as nutritious as fresh corn. But it still contains fiber.

Grits: This southern specialty is made from coarsely ground dried hominy.

Nutritional Benefits: Cholesterol-free and rich in fiber. A fair source of vitamin A (yellow corn only), with traces of iron and vitamin C.

Shopping Tip: Regular supermarket.

WHOLE WHEAT COUSCOUS

Technically, couscous (KOOS-koos) is not a whole grain. However, this tiny golden-colored pasta can be made from whole-grain flour and does have quite a few nutritional benefits, not to mention a superfast cooking time. Since it is precooked, you'll just need to combine it with water, bring the mixture to a boil, remove from the heat, and let stand, covered, for 5 minutes. If seasonings (salt, olive oil, herbs) are mixed into the water or the cooking liquid is flavored (chicken broth, tomato juice), the couscous will take on these flavors. One cup of prepared whole-wheat couscous has 2 grams of fiber; regular couscous has none. High in protein, with 8 grams per 1 cup cooked. Small amounts of iron.

FLAXSEED

This tiny reddish-brown seed has a wonderfully nutty flavor that works well in baked goods. In fact, in many European countries, bakers routinely use this grain in everything from cookies to cakes to bread. Be sure to grind the seed to obtain the most benefits. Left whole, the seeds will pass through the body undigested.

Cooking Rating: Very easy.

This grain has a tough outer coating that must be partly crushed or ground (in either a clean coffee grinder or blender) in order to unlock the nutritional benefits. The crushed seeds or ground meal can then be added to breads and muffins or used as a topping for yogurt or cereal.

Nutritional Benefits: Cholesterol-free. High in fiber and rich in omega-3 fatty acids, fats that may help protect against heart disease and other chronic ills.

Shopping Tip: Although flaxseeds and ground flaxseed meal are starting to show up in many large supermarkets, the grain is still easier to find in health food stores. Store whole seeds in an airtight container at room temperature for up to a year. Keep the ground seeds in the refrigerator for up to 30 days.

MILLET

Yes, this is the same tiny yellow-gold grain that's sold as bird food. But in other parts of the world, particularly in Africa and Asia, this crunchy, nutty-flavored grain is eaten by humans and highly prized for both its flavor and its strong nutritional profile. Most often cooked as a hot cereal, millet (MIHL-leht) can also be an ingredient in puddings (used like rice in rice pudding) or mixed into pilafs, pancakes (see the recipe for Multigrain Hotcakes on page 262), soups, or stews.

Cooking Rating: Easy but time-consuming.

Cooking millet is a two-step process. To shorten the cooking time, the grain is first toasted in a heavy skillet for 2–3 minutes. Then it's placed in a saucepan (1 part grain to 2 parts water) and simmered for 25–30 minutes.

Nutritional Benefits: Cholesterol-free, with a tiny amount of fat from the whole grain. Incredibly rich in thiamin and iron, providing 20–25 percent of the recommended requirement for these two nutrients, it also carries significant amounts of protein, fiber, and potassium.

Shopping Tip: You probably won't be able to find this grain in the regular supermarket (except in the pet food aisle). But it's easily purchased at health food stores and via the Internet or mail order from companies such as Bob's Red Mill or Hodgson Mill, Inc. (See addresses and Web site information in the section that follows this dictionary.)

OATS

Probably one of the world's most popular grains (half of the farmland in Ireland and one-third in Scotland is devoted to growing it), oats are valued for their flavor, versatility, and medical prowess. The latter is due to the fact that oats are one of the top sources of soluble fiber, a type of fiber that can help lower blood cholesterol levels. Oats are sold as the whole grain—oat groats. They can also be processed into oat flour, oat bran, and oatmeal.

Cooking Rating: Easy to very easy, depending on variety.

Oatmeal: Made from whole-grain oats that have been husked or stripped of their outer coat. Some varieties of oatmeal are steamed and rolled flat (old-fashioned or quick-cooking rolled oats) before being thinly sliced. Others, like Scotch oats and Irish oatmeals, are simply sliced thin with steel blades.

Rolled oats: Unless they're the instant variety, rolled oats are simmered for about 10 minutes. Instant varieties are precooked and dried to make cooking times shorter. Quick-cooking oats are more thinly sliced than old-fashioned rolled oats and cook in only 3–5 minutes.

Steel-cut oats: Firmer and nuttier tasting than the steam-processed varieties, steel-cut oats make a creamier oatmeal but require a longer cooking time, up to 40 minutes.

Oat bran: The outer coating of the oat is high in soluble fiber and many nutrients, including iron, potassium, and thiamin. Like wheat bran, this fiber can be added to baked goods or cereal. But in some recipes, oatmeal can be added, which has nearly as much fiber and most of the same nutritional benefits.

Oat groats: Whole-oat kernel that must be simmered for 30–45 minutes. The nutty-flavored groats can also be toasted and added to baked goods (see Whole-Wheat Pizza Crust on page 284).

Oat flour: Sold in many supermarkets, the flour made from husked oats can sometimes be highly refined. But most varieties are richer in fiber than white flour. While it works well in thickening sauces, oat flour lacks gluten, the protein that helps yeast breads rise. Small amounts of oat flour can be used in baked goods, but a bread, a pizza dough, or a cake made with all oat flour will turn out poorly.

Nutritional Benefits: Cholesterol-free, with small amounts of fat from the whole grain. Rich in soluble fiber. Steel-cut oats have a lower glycemic index than standard rolled oats.

Shopping Tip: Oatmeal, even the Irish steel-cut variety, is readily found in supermarkets. Oat bran and oat flour can be found in many larger supermarkets. But the more specialized products, like oat groats, are found in health food and natural food stores, or by mail order.

QUINOA

This South American grain, grown for years in the Andes mountains of Peru, has come stateside only recently. And that's good news. Quinoa (KEEN-wah), with its distinctively nutty flavor and pearly appearance, is quite the nutrition powerhouse. Fully cooked quinoa has an almost translucent quality except for the germ of the grain, which is visible as a white crescent.

Cooking Rating: Easy. Simmers for 10–15 minutes.

Nutritional Benefits: Has the distinction of being a complete protein. In other words, it is a high-quality protein comparable to the protein found in meat and eggs.

Shopping Tip: Look for quinoa at some supermarkets or at the health food store.

RYE

Once referred to as "the grain of poverty," rye is a hearty cereal grain that can grow just about anywhere. Poor soil, high altitudes, harsh climates: none of these seem to stop this grain from taking hold. In fact, rye first appeared as a weed that overran fields of wheat nearly two thousand years ago. This hearty cereal is sold in several forms. The berries, which look and can be used like wheat berries, are found mainly in health food stores. Rye flour, because it's low in gluten (the protein that helps bread to rise), makes dense loaves of bread. It's usually used in combination with a higher-protein flour like wheat or with gluten powder.

Cooking Rating: Easy but time-consuming. Simmers for 30–40 minutes.

Nutritional Benefits: Lower in protein than wheat.

Shopping Tip: Look for the whole kernels or berries at health food stores. A medium grind of rye flour is sold in many supermarkets. Dark rye flour or the more coarsely ground pumpernickel flour is usually sold mainly at health food stores.

SPELT

An ancient cousin to wheat, these large brown kernels look nearly identical to wheat berries (whole kernels of wheat) and, in fact, are pretty much interchangeable with wheat berries in recipes. Spelt, however, is slightly higher in protein than wheat and can be tolerated by people with wheat allergies. The berries or the flaked form of spelt can be used for hot cereal or in granola mixtures (see Apple Crunch Oatmeal, page 256.) They're also good cooked into soups, salads, and casseroles. Spelt flour can be used in place of wheat flour. See the cooking instructions for wheat berries.

TRITICALE

This slightly sweet hybrid of two other grains—wheat and rye—is found mainly in health food stores at the moment. You can cook the whole berries, which look and can be used much the same as wheat berries, or buy triticale (triht-ih-KAY-lee) flakes to use as cereal or for baking. Triticale flour, like the whole grain, is low in gluten, the protein that gives yeast breads their lift, so triticale flour is used in combination with wheat flour to make an acceptable-textured baked good.

Cooking Rating: Easy but time-consuming. The whole berries must be simmered 30–40 minutes.

Nutritional Benefits: Cholesterol-free, with a small amount of fat from the whole grain. Higher in protein than wheat, but lower in gluten. (Rye is low in gluten, so this hybrid has some of its characteristics.)

Shopping Tip: Look for this grain in health or natural food stores.

WHEAT BERRIES

These whole kernels of wheat contain all the goodness of the wheat grain. Wheat berries come in soft and hard varieties, but the soft and hard moniker has nothing to do with tenderness. The difference between the two varieties is gluten (protein) content. Soft wheat is low in gluten and is ground into pastry flour. Hard wheat is high in gluten and is ground into regular or hearty flours. Very nutty in flavor, these light brown kernels make a wonderful cereal or a crunchy addition to breads and baked goods. They even make a chewy-crunchy substitute for pasta in cold salads.

Cooking Rating: Easy but time-consuming. Soft berries must be simmered for 30 minutes or so. Can be toasted in the oven or a dry skillet to shorten the cooking time.

Nutritional Benefits: Cholesterol-free and high in fiber; 16 percent of calories from protein. Small amounts of minerals, including iron and zinc.

Shopping Tip: They can be found in health food or whole-food grocery stores.

WILD RICE

Technically not a rice, but the seed of an aquatic grass, this starchy side dish rates attention for its stellar fiber content, not to mention an intensely nutty flavor. Because it is so intense (and quite expensive), wild rice is often paired with milder-flavored grains (see Wild Rice–Quinoa Pilaf on page 298). Like its grain counterparts, wild rice is cholesterol-free and low in fat. Quality can vary, with the more expensive brands typically having a larger percentage of well-shaped, uncrushed grains. Use more expensive varieties in dishes where appearance is important and less expensive ones in soups or stuffings. Steer clear of instant varieties; they may save you time, but appearance is lacking.

Filling the Healthy Shopping Bag

Now that you're committed to eating more *whole* grains and fresh produce, chances are your shopping list has a few new additions. And you may have questions about where and how to find these foods. Will you need to make routine pilgrimages to the health food store? How do organic foods fit into the overall picture? Which whole-food products taste best? These questions aren't difficult to answer. But they do involve some individual preference. The organic issue, for example, has more to do with personal choice than nutrition. The evidence is lacking that organic produce and grains are nutritionally superior to produce and grains grown by traditional farming methods. The key difference, then, is farming method. Organic produce is grown without chemicals and pesticides.

If you decide to make a commitment to organic foods, keep in mind that these products are not always widely available. One of the best strategies is to consider locally grown produce. When you shop at a local farmer's market, farm stand, or small supermarket that carries local produce, you'll be rewarded by some of the best-tasting fruits and vegetables around, organic or not. Produce that is shipped from long distances, because it can take many days to reach the supermarket, may have lost some of its flavor or nutritional value. Locally grown fruits and vegetables, picked at the height of ripeness, have incredible flavors and nutrition profiles. So rather than look for asparagus to make the Asparagus, Tofu, Shiitake, and Cashew Stir-Fry (page 281) in July when it's out of season, find a vegetable that's being harvested. Green beans are a summertime crop; they can make a nice stand-in for asparagus in the stir-fry recipe. Learn to cook with the seasons. You'll be rewarded with fruits and vegetables that are at their flavor and nutritional peak.

As for whole-grain products, locating them is probably a lot easier than you might think. Many whole-grain foods are now firmly entrenched in the regular supermarket. Look for them either in a special aisle with organic and health foods or in the regular flour, cereal, and rice/pasta aisles. Owing to a burgeoning interest in whole foods, the natural-food sections of many supermarkets are growing larger. And whole-food markets are becoming a familiar option in many cities. Then there's the Internet. Many of the larger companies that market whole-grain products have comprehensive Web sites and efficient mail-order systems. Many company Web sites have a store locator or "Where To Find" button that lets you locate nearby stores that sell their products.

Just in case you're having trouble locating some of the whole grains used in our recipes, following are names and addresses of a few of the companies that market these foods. This is by no means a comprehensive list. There are many small companies that produce or import whole-grain foods, but since their availability is limited and varies from region to region, we've listed some of the national brands. If nothing else, this list should help get you started. Then you can branch out on your own, checking out local stores and ethnic markets for all kinds of wonderful whole-grain foods. Since taste is a personal thing, chances are you'll need a bit of trial and error to find the foods that suit your palate.

Arrowhead Mills, Inc.
Hereford, Texas
Web site: www.arrowheadmills.com

Product Line: Now part of the Hain Food Group. Selections are organic and range from whole grains to whole-grain cereals to whole-grain flours and pastry flours. A line of whole-grain pasta is sold under the DeBoles brand. Some products are sold in supermarkets, but for a wider variety, check health food stores.

Bob's Red Mill
Milwaukie, Oregon
1-800-349-2173
Web site: www.bobsredmill.com

Product Line: Selections include whole grains, whole-grain cereals, whole-grain flours, and whole-grain pastry flours. Some products are sold in supermarkets, but for a wider variety, check health food stores or the Internet. This company has an excellent mail-order business.

Eden Foods, Inc.
Clinton, Michigan
1-888-441-EDEN
Web site: www.edenfoods.com

Product Line: Selections range from whole-grain pastas to canned organic tomatoes, legumes, and soy milks. Most, but not all, of the selections are organic. The company also imports some specialty products, such as an udon noodle made with brown rice from Japan.

Hodgson Mill, Inc.
Effingham, Illinois
1-800-347-0105
Web site: www.hodgsonmill.com

Product Line: Whole-grain pastas, baking mixes, cereals, flours, and cornmeal. Available in many supermarkets and health food stores. Products can be ordered via the Internet.

King Arthur Flour
Norwich, Vermont
1-800-827-6836
Web site: www.kingarthurflour.com

Product Line: Specialty flours, including whole-grain flours.

Lundberg Family Farms
Richvale, California
1-530-882-4551
Web site: www.lundberg.com

Product Line: Wide assortment of whole-grain brown rice products, including brown rice pasta and brown rice blends with names like black Japonica (blend of short-grain black rice and medium-grain mahogany rice), Christmas blend, and wehani. Often sold in bulk in health food stores. Available prepackaged in many supermarkets.

Mother's
Chicago, Illinois
1-800-333-8027
Web site: www.mothersnatural.com

Product Line: The Quaker Oats Company markets a quick-cooking pearled barley, a toasted wheat germ, and a full line of hot and cold cereals under the Mother's label.

> Westbrae Natural Foods
> Garden City, New York
> Web site: www.westbrae.com

Product Line: Wide variety of organic and natural foods. Whole-grain pastas, including corn pasta, canned legumes, and other whole-grain foods.

One Week of Menus

In order to give you some idea of how meals might shape up when you're dining according to the Healthy Eating Pyramid, we've developed a sample week of menus. These Monday through Sunday food plans are meant simply as a guideline, one that illustrates how to put into practice the principles talked about in the preceding chapters. Each day's menu is based on 2,000 calories, the reference figure that health professionals and the food industry use as a benchmark for the energy needs of the average American. Granted, not every individual needs exactly 2,000 calories each day. Most of us have varying energy needs based on age, size, activity level, and how effectively we burn energy. But this figure is a good starting point. No doubt you'll want to make adjustments to these meal plans based on your own needs. In fact, an addendum at the end of each day explains how to easily convert the menus into a 1,600-calorie plan, a realistic amount of calories if you're looking to lose weight or are just a petite, less active woman. We haven't built alcohol into these daily menus; if you are drinking a heart-healthy glass of wine or beer with your evening meal, you will need to figure in an additional 100 to 200 calories a day.

Rather than agonize over daily calorie numbers, however, think about your current situation. Are you maintaining a healthy weight? If you are, then you're no doubt eating the right amount of food for you. Look to these menu plans to guide you in the direction of healthy food choices, letting your natural instincts guide portion size. If you need to lose weight, follow the 1,600-calorie plan or just begin cutting back on what you currently eat. Weight will come off naturally as you begin to cut back and become more active.

The menus run the gamut of choices. One day's lunch looks at how a fast-food restaurant meal (grilled chicken sandwich) can fit into the average day. A weekend supper suggests what you might pull together and eat at your own

Cinco de Mayo party, a meal based entirely on selections from our recipe section. There's also a day with six small meals, a style of eating that is just as healthy as three squares a day and, in fact, may be better at helping some people keep their appetite under control and blood sugar on an even keel.

All in all, with the help of these menus, and the sixty recipes that follow this section, you'll find that eating healthfully is a simple concept, one that you can put into practice from Monday through Sunday with very little effort. Recipes for italicized items can be found in the following pages. Those marked with an asterisk (*) are Fast Fix Foods.

Sunday

BREAKFAST

Fresh-Squeezed Orange Juice, 4 ounces
Multigrain Hotcakes with Warm Apple Syrup, 2 servings
Hot Brewed Coffee

LUNCH

Tex-Mex Wheat Berry Salad with Tomatillo Vinaigrette
Herb-Crusted Grilled Chicken Breast
Fresh Cantaloupe ('/4)
Sliced Strawberries ('/2 cup)

SUPPER

Double Mushroom Meat Loaf
Roasted Winter Vegetable Medley, 2 servings
Mixed Salad Greens, 2 cups
   with 1'/2 tablespoons Extra-Virgin Olive Oil
Spiced Poached Pear

ADJUSTMENTS AND VARIATIONS

For 1,600 calories: Reduce to 1 serving of hotcakes (2 hotcakes with 3 tablespoons of syrup) at breakfast; subtract 259 calories. Omit one tablespoon of olive oil at supper; subtract 126 calories.

Monday

BREAKFAST

Bran Flakes, 2 cups
Skim or Soy Milk, 1 cup
Banana, sliced

Whole-Wheat Toast
Apricot Fruit Spread, 1 tablespoon

LUNCH

*Pesto Corn Spaghetti**
Olive Swirl Roll
Fresh Orange Sections

SUPPER

Grilled Salmon Steaks with Papaya-Mint Salsa
Green Snap Beans
Steamed Whole-Wheat Couscous
Fresh-Baked Pumpernickel Roll

SNACK

Easy Peach, Pineapple, and Apricot Crisp

ADJUSTMENTS AND VARIATIONS

For 1,600 calories: Omit whole-wheat toast and fruit spread; subtract 166 calories. Omit pumpernickel roll at supper; subtract 65 calories. Omit fruit crisp at snack time; subtract 212 calories. Munch on a ripe fresh peach instead; add 60 calories.

Tuesday

BREAKFAST

("grab and go" items)
*Mango Energy Blitz**
Banana-Apricot Nut Bread, 2 slices

LUNCH

(Fast-food restaurant)
Grilled Chicken Sandwich (with Whole-Wheat Bun if possible)
Mixed Green Salad
Vinaigrette Salad Dressing
Large Apple

SUPPER

*Pork Tenderloin with Pistachio-Gremolata Crust**
Wild Rice–Quinoa Pilaf
Steamed Fresh Asparagus
Cinnamon Applesauce

SNACK

> Whole-Grain Crackers, 3
> Natural-Style Peanut Butter, 1½ tablespoons

ADJUSTMENTS AND VARIATIONS

For 1,600 calories: Omit sandwich bun at lunch; subtract 135 calories. Omit snack; subtract 249 calories. If you are hungry in the evening, munch on raw vegetables (carrots, celery, cherry tomatoes) instead.

Wednesday

BREAKFAST

> Fried Egg Sandwich
>   on Grilled Whole-Wheat English Muffin
> Ruby Red Grapefruit
> *Blackberry-Banana Smoothie**

LUNCH

> *Onion-Crusted Tofu-Steak Sandwich*
> *Seven-Vegetable Slaw,** 1 cup
> Sliced Kiwi with Fresh Blueberries

SUPPER

> *Curried Winter Squash Soup**
> Cracked Wheat Peasant Bread, large chunk
> Spinach and Mushroom Salad,
>   with Vinaigrette

SNACK

> *Fruit 'n' Spicy Nut Trail Mix,** ½ cup
> Orange Juice Spritzer

ADJUSTMENTS AND VARIATIONS

For 1,600 calories: Cut down to 1 teaspoon of oil at breakfast to cook egg (toast English muffin or grill it dry); subtract 84 calories. Cut smoothie portion in half (6 ounces); subtract 92 calories. Cut down to a small wedge of bread; subtract 65 calories. Omit night snack; subtract 182 calories.

Thursday

BREAKFAST

Whole-Wheat Toast, 2 slices
Natural-Style Peanut Butter
Strawberry Fruit Spread
Apple-Cranberry Juice

LUNCH

Chipotle Chicken Chili
Baked Tortilla Chips
Fruit Cocktail in Juice
Oatmeal-Raisin Cookie

SUPPER

(Restaurant dinner)
Crostini with Olive Oil
Oven-Roasted Sea Bass
Wild Rice Pilaf
Steamed Broccoli
Fruit Sorbet with Almond Biscotti
Espresso

ADJUSTMENTS AND VARIATIONS

For 1,600 calories: Omit apple-cranberry juice at breakfast; subtract 128 calories. Omit cookie at lunch; subtract 74 calories. Omit biscotti at supper; subtract 180 calories.

Friday

SIX SMALL MEALS

EARLY MORNING (1)

Apple Crunch Oatmeal
Chilled Pineapple Juice, 6 ounces
Fresh Brewed Coffee or Tea

MIDMORNING (2)

Carrot–Wheat Germ Muffin
Hard-boiled Egg with Coarse Salt and Pepper
Sweet Black Grapes, 12

NOON (3)

BWT Wrap
Large Banana

MIDAFTERNOON (4)

Spicy Shrimp and Peanut Noodle Salad
Celery Sticks
Sparkling Water with Lime

EVENING (5)

Lemon-Oregano Grouper with Vegetables
Chopped Romaine Lettuce Salad
    with Light Balsamic Vinaigrette
Orange Juice Sorbet

MIDEVENING (6)

Blackberry-Banana Smoothie*
Roasted Salted Cashews, 6 small

ADJUSTMENTS AND VARIATIONS

For 1,600 calories: Replace pineapple juice with 4 ounces of orange juice at breakfast; subtract 49 calories. Omit carrot–wheat germ muffin midmorning and save for evening snack; no calorie change. Cut down to a small banana at lunch; subtract 59 calories. Omit sorbet at supper; subtract 68 calories. Omit smoothie and cashews at midevening snack and eat carrot–wheat germ muffin instead; subtract 254 calories.

Saturday

BREAKFAST

Fresh-Squeezed White Grapefruit Juice, 1 cup
Scrambled Eggs, 2
    (cooked with 2 teaspoons oil)
Whole-Grain Toast, 2 slices
Pineapple Fruit Spread
Fresh Brewed Coffee or Tea

LUNCH

California Chicken Salad*
Hearty Wheat Berry–Oat Groat Bread
Iced Tea with Lemon

SUPPER

(Cinco de Mayo party)
*Avocado-Shrimp Salsa**
*Sun-Dried Tomato Dip with Oven-Roasted Corn Chips,** 2 servings
Chipotle Chicken Chili
Mexican Beer, 12 ounces
*Rum-Glazed Pineapple**

MIDNIGHT MOVIE SNACK

Popcorn Popped in Oil, 2 cups
*Fruit 'n' Spicy Nut Trail Mix**

ADJUSTMENTS AND VARIATIONS

For 1,600 calories: Use 1 teaspoon of oil to cook eggs (instead of 2); subtract 40 calories. Cut down to half a slice of bread at lunch; subtract 75 calories. Omit beer at supper; subtract 140 calories. Choose one appetizer at supper—either the salsa or the dip and chips; subtract 90 calories. Switch to air-popped popcorn instead of oil-popped (you can still include the trail mix); subtract 50 calories.

Busy Day Menu

It isn't always easy to combine healthy eating with an intense work schedule and busy family life. Here's how I try to do it on busy days, a plan that can be varied in an almost infinite number of ways.

Wake up, boil water, and dump in a packet of Kashi, a mix of intact oats, brown rice, wheat, and other grains. Add two tablespoons of flaxseed for omega-three fatty acids. Cook for 45 minutes, just about the right amount of time for some exercise (my usual is a run along the Charles River, but the Nordic Track gets the nod on rainy or icy days) and washing up. Add dried fruit or fresh fruit in season, and maybe a few nuts; milk is optional. Orange juice diluted with carbonated water provides fresh-tasting but low-calorie hydration at breakfast. With this breakfast I'm never hungry before noon, so a snack never enters my mind. (For days with early meetings, Kashi can be cooked the night before.)

Leftover Kashi provides the beginning of a lunch that can be prepared in five minutes. In a plastic container, atop a base of Kashi, add whatever sounds good. It might be a salad or a mix of fruits or leftover bits of chicken or fish. Most of the time I also add one or more types of nuts. A few generous dashes of a flavorful olive oil with vinegar or a seasoning make almost any of these endless combinations taste good. My favorite is when our peaches, blueberries, and grapes are all ripe at the same time—with roasted almonds and olive oil, this is hard to beat. Snap on a plastic cover, slip in a bag with an apple, fork, and napkin, and this is quicker than waiting in a cafeteria line. I put all this in my backpack, dash out the door with my bike, and I'm in my office at the Harvard Medical area in fifteen minutes, faster than I can get there by driving and parking.

In the evening, if I'm lucky, my wife, Gail, may have made one of the entrées from this book, or one of countless other healthy creations, for dinner. If not, a stop at the fish market provides a quick beginning for a meal. Poach or broil with some lemon, add a salad and maybe some whole-grain bread with a little olive oil for dipping, and in fifteen minutes we can have a fresh, satisfying, and healthy meal.

High Blood Pressure

As described earlier, most cases of high blood pressure (hypertension) can be prevented by staying lean and physically active, consuming generous amounts of fruits and vegetables daily, and keeping salt intake low. If you have already been diagnosed with hypertension, these same factors continue to be important because, by following these simple guidelines, many people can control their blood pressure without need for medication. Even when medication is necessary to keep blood pressure under control, the number of drugs can be minimized by a good diet and healthy lifestyle.

Of all these factors, weight control is the most important. For those who are already overweight, a 5 percent weight loss has clear benefits, even if it is difficult to get back to a youthful waistline. Fruits and vegetables are a primary source of potassium, which helps keep blood pressure under control. Five servings a day should be a minimum, and remember, potatoes don't count. Salt restriction will also aid in controlling blood pressure, and there is certainly no benefit from the relatively high salt intakes typical in the United States. A healthy upper limit of sodium intake is 2,300 milligrams, or the amount in 1 teaspoon of salt. For those with hypertension, cutting this in half is an ambitious but reasonable goal. Don't bother counting grams of salt on a meal-by-meal basis, but it is helpful to know the important sources of salt, particularly because so much salt is hidden in manufactured foods, and to minimize or modify them. For this reason, information about salt content of the recipes is included; further information is in chapter 10.

Control of blood pressure, whether by diet or drugs, is important, and regular monitoring by a health care provider is essential.

Pregnancy

Pregnancy is a nutritionally critical period because a mother's diet must provide all the essential nutrients to nurture the developing fetus. A special pregnancy diet is not necessary because the basic foods I describe for good health will do this, but extra attention to healthy eating is important. A small reward is that most women will be able to eat an extra three hundred to five hundred calories per day while they are pregnant.

Several points are worth noting. Adequate folic acid is critical during the first month of pregnancy for the prevention of birth defects; for many women the critical period has already passed before they realize they are pregnant. For this reason, all women who might possibly become pregnant should take 400 micrograms of folic acid per day. The easiest way to do this is by taking a standard RDA-level multiple vitamin. Once pregnancy is recognized, prescribing a prenatal multiple vitamin that contains iron is standard practice. This is a valuable nutritional safety net and assures that intake of folic acid, iron, and several other vitamins will be adequate, but it should not be regarded as a substitute for a good diet because it does not contain all the constituents of foods needed for optimal health. Because the multiple vitamin contains a generous amount of vitamin A, which is stored in the body, it is best to eat liver only rarely or not at all during pregnancy, as liver is very high in vitamin A. Some evidence suggests that a high intake of vitamin A might be related to specific birth defects, although the findings are not conclusive.

For overall optimal health, I recommended that a good source of omega-3 fatty acids be consumed on most days (see chapter 4). This is especially true during pregnancy and lactation, because these fatty acids are a major building block for the brain, spinal cord, and retina of the growing fetus and infant. However, some caution is warranted: large fish, such as swordfish and tuna, are some of the best sources of fatty acids, but these fish are also high in mercury, which could adversely affect the developing child if consumed in large amounts.

The U.S. Food and Drug Administration and the Environmental Protection Agency offer three recommendations for limiting mercury intake for women of childbearing age, especially those who are pregnant or lactating, and young children. (For more information, visit the Food and Drug Administration's Web site on mercury in fish, www.cfsan.fda.gov/~dms/admehg3.html.)

- Don't eat shark, swordfish, king mackerel, or tilefish (also called golden bass or golden snapper), because they contain high levels of mercury.
- Limit your fish intake to 12 ounces (2 average meals) a week. Pick varieties of fish and shellfish that are lower in mercury. Examples include shrimp, canned light tuna, salmon, pollock, and catfish. Because albacore tuna (or white tuna) has more mercury than canned light tuna, limit it to 6 ounces (one average meal) per week.

- Check local advisories about the safety of fish from local lakes, rivers, and coastal areas. If no advice is available, eat up to 6 ounces (one average meal) per week of fish caught from local waters, but don't consume any other fish during that week.

Keep in mind that fish isn't the only source of omega-3 fatty acids. You can also get them from walnuts and some vegetable oils (see page 90). On days when you don't eat fish, try to eat some other food that delivers omega-3 fatty acids.

The optimal weight gain during pregnancy has been a matter of controversy, and recommendations have changed dramatically during the last fifty years. Current recommendations depend on the starting BMI; for a woman beginning with a normal weight, a gain of about twenty-four pounds is thought to be optimal. The best weight for you should be discussed with your obstetrician/gynecologist or midwife.

Diabetes

Good nutrition and lifestyle play important roles in the management of diabetes. Central goals are the control of blood sugar and the avoidance of cardiovascular disease, which is greatly increased by diabetes. For the less common type 1 form of diabetes, which must always be treated with insulin, a delicate balance between food intake and insulin dose is required to keep blood sugar in the optimal range. Some persons with type 2, or adult-onset, diabetes will be able to control blood sugar adequately by weight loss, regular activity, and diet, but medications may still be needed.

Dietary recommendations for the management of diabetes have varied greatly over the last fifty years, emphasizing first a low-carbohydrate intake, then high-carbohydrate/low-fat consumption. In recent years, several studies have shown better control of type 2 diabetes when some carbohydrate is replaced with monounsaturated fat, and recommendations have shifted away from high carbohydrate intake. As I have described for general good health, consuming carbohydrates in a low-glycemic/high-fiber form can help in controlling diabetes, and because of the importance of preventing heart disease, the type of dietary fat (replacing saturated and trans fats with unsaturated fats) should be emphasized. Thus, the type of diet described in this book may be particularly valuable for persons with diabetes. Overall caloric intake and regularity of consumption will need extra attention. Close coordination with a physician and dietitian is important, especially for those with type 1 diabetes.

High Cholesterol

Elevated blood cholesterol, usually considered over 240 mg/dL, is common among American adults (see chapter 4 for more details). Before becoming overly concerned about an elevated cholesterol level, a check of HDL cholesterol is essential because it is the ratio of total cholesterol divided by HDL that best relates to risk of heart disease. Some lucky persons have an elevated total cholesterol due largely to high HDL and are thus actually at reduced risk of heart disease. The ratio should be less than 4.5, but the lower the better.

If your total/HDL cholesterol is elevated, your physician will check for other conditions that could be responsible, such as thyroid or kidney disease, but these are usually normal. In this case, the first line of treatment is to modify diet and lifestyle in a way that will reduce total cholesterol (mainly LDL cholesterol) and increase HDL. The usual approach recommended by the American Heart Association has been to lower total and saturated fat intake, which typically has only a modest impact on total cholesterol and lowers HDL cholesterol, leaving the ratio unchanged. All too often, diet is then declared a failure and people are simply put on drugs, usually one of the statin class.

In the chapters and recipes in this book, I have emphasized a broad approach of replacing saturated and trans fats with mono and polyunsaturated fats along with weight control, regular physical activity, and the use of whole grains instead of high-glycemic carbohydrates and sugars. With this program, the majority of Americans can control their cholesterol levels without medication and greatly reduce their risk of heart disease. Following your total and HDL cholesterol levels with your health care provider will be important, as these can tell you whether you need to be more attentive to diet, shave off a few pounds, and up your activity level. If this doesn't bring your cholesterol levels under control, a number of options are available. One is to use the new Phytosterol-containing margarines, which have beneficial effects on blood cholesterol fractions, although their long-term effects on risks of heart disease and other conditions have not been studied. Treatment with a prescription drug, usually a statin, may be appropriate for some people. Increasingly, physicians are considering not just the cholesterol level, but also other risk factors, in deciding when a cholesterol-lowering drug is warranted. Even if a drug is used, diet will remain important, in part to minimize the dose and related side effects. Also, these drugs reduce risk of heart disease only by about one-third, meaning that someone at high risk of heart disease will remain so when treated with a statin. Far greater benefits can be achieved by also taking full advantage of the many aspects of diet that we have discussed, which operate in multiple ways besides reducing blood cholesterol fractions.

APPENDIX   A N D   B E V E R A G E S

Avocado-Shrimp Salsa *(FAST FIX)*

The buttery rich texture of avocado pairs nicely with shrimp in this guacamole-style salsa. To save time, buy cooked, peeled shrimp. If all you can find are large shrimp, cut them in half or into thirds. Try this salsa with the Oven-Roasted Corn Chips (page 251) or use as a filling for a wrap-style sandwich made with shredded romaine lettuce.

- 1/2 pound medium shrimp (about 20), peeled and cooked
- 2 small avocados, peeled and coarsely chopped (about 1 1/4 cups)
- 2 plum tomatoes, seeded and chopped (about 1 cup)
- 2 tablespoons minced red onion
- 1 tablespoon fresh lime juice
- Coarse salt to taste
- 32 baked tortilla chips

1. Place all ingredients in a medium bowl. Toss gently to mix; let stand 5–10 minutes. Serve at room temperature.

Yield: 3 cups (12 servings); Serving: 1/4 cup salsa, 4 baked tortilla chips
Calories: 86; Protein: 6.5 g; Carbohydrate: 9.7 g; Fiber: 1.6 g; Sodium: 100 mg;
Fat 3.0 g (Sat: 0.38 g, Mono: 1.47 g, Poly: 0.33 g, Trans: 0 g); Cholesterol: 46 mg

General: Avocados are high in fat, but it's a healthy type of fat, the monounsaturated variety.
Diabetic: For carbohydrate counters, total is 10 grams. Equals 1/2 medium-fat meat exchange, 1/2 starch, and 1/2 vegetable.
Sodium-Restricted: Sodium profile was calculated without added salt. To lower sodium further, purchase the "no salt added" baked tortilla chips or bake your own.
Pregnant: No special considerations. Each serving contains 12.9 micrograms of folate and 1 milligram of iron.

Scallion and Roasted Pine Nut Hummus *(FAST FIX)*

This Middle Eastern chickpea dip is usually made with lots of sesame seed paste (tahini) and olive oil. We've cut down on the oil and added some roasted pine nuts and scallions for a new flavor twist. Traditionally this dip is served with pita bread, but try spreading it on cucumber slices or serving it as a dip for celery sticks and other raw vegetables.

- 3 tablespoons pine nuts
- 1 (15-ounce) can chickpeas

$^1/_2$ cup sliced green onion, divided

1–2 garlic cloves, minced

2–3 tablespoons fresh lemon juice

$^1/_2$ teaspoon ground cumin

1 tablespoon olive oil

Coarse salt to taste

4 whole-wheat pita breads, cut into 32 wedges

Green onion slices (optional)

1. Place the pine nuts in a small nonstick skillet over medium heat. Toast for 3–4 minutes or until lightly brown, stirring frequently to prevent scorching. Remove from heat and cool.

2. Drain the chickpeas through a sieve over a bowl, reserving $^1/_4$ cup of the liquid. Place the chickpeas, $^1/_4$ cup green onions, and next five ingredients in a food processor and process until mixture resembles coarse meal. Add the reserved liquid and process into a smooth paste. (If the mixture is too thick, add water until desired consistency.) Taste for seasoning and add salt if desired. Stir in the pine nuts and remaining green onions. Garnish with more sliced green onions, if desired. Serve at room temperature with the pita bread wedges.

Note: Make this dip the night before a party, if possible. Flavors will improve if left to chill overnight. And be judicious with the garlic. The flavor of the raw garlic intensifies as the dip is allowed to stand.

Yield: 2 cups; Serving: 2 tablespoons dip, 2 pita wedges
Calories: 71; Protein: 2.8 g; Carbohydrate: 10 g; Fiber: 2 g; Sodium: 81 mg;
Fat 2.8 g (Sat: 0.40 g, Mono: 1.31 g, Poly: 0.92 g, Trans: 0 g); Cholesterol: 0 mg

General: No special considerations.
Diabetic: For carbohydrate counters, total is 10 grams. Equals $^1/_2$ starch exchange, $^1/_2$ vegetable, and $^1/_2$ fat.
Sodium-Restricted: The bulk of the sodium in this recipe comes from the canned chickpeas. To lower sodium further, cook dried chickpeas from scratch or buy an organic brand of canned chickpeas, most of which tend to have less added salt.
Pregnant: Each serving contains 35 micrograms of folate and 1 milligram of iron.

Sun-Dried Tomato Dip with Oven-Roasted Corn Chips (FAST FIX)

Sun-dried tomato pieces can be found either in the produce section of the supermarket or next to the canned tomato sauces. If you can only find sun-dried tomatoes packed in oil, go ahead and use them and omit some of the oil used in the dip.

CHIPS

6 (6-inch) corn tortillas

2 tablespoons canola oil, divided

Vegetable cooking spray or canola oil

1/4 teaspoon coarse salt

DIP

1 (15-ounce) can cannellini (white kidney beans) or other white beans

1–2 garlic cloves, minced

2 tablespoons fresh lime juice

3 tablespoons sun-dried tomato pieces

Coarse salt to taste

1. Preheat the oven to 400°F.

2. To make the chips, brush each tortilla with 1/2 teaspoon oil and stack the rounds one on top of another. Cut the stack in half and then into quarters; you will have 24 large triangles. Place the triangles on the nonstick baking sheet coated lightly with cooking spray or oil, oiled side up. Sprinkle with coarse salt and bake at 400°F for 8–12 minutes or until crisp.

3. To make dip, drain the beans through a sieve over a bowl, reserving 1/4 cup of the liquid. Place the beans, remaining oil, garlic, lime juice, and sun-dried tomatoes in a food processor and process until the mixture resembles coarse meal. Add the reserved liquid and process into a smooth paste. (If mixture is too thick, add water until desired consistency.) Taste for seasoning and add salt, if desired.

Note: Make this dip the night before a party, if possible. Flavors will improve if left to chill overnight.

Yield: 1 1/2 cups dip, 24 large chips; Serving: 1 tablespoon dip and 1 roasted corn chip
Calories: 45; Protein: 1.3 g; Carbohydrate: 6.5 g; Fiber: 1.2 g; Sodium: 75 mg;
Fat 1.7 g (Sat: 0.13 g, Mono: 0.88 g, Poly: 0.58 g, Trans: 0 g); Cholesterol: 0 mg

General: No special considerations.
Diabetic: For carbohydrate counters, total is 7 grams. Equals 1/2 starch exchange.
Sodium-Restricted: The bulk of the sodium in this recipe comes from the canned beans. To lower sodium further, cook dried cannellini beans from scratch or buy an organic brand of canned white beans, most of which tend to have less added salt. You can also cook the oven-roasted corn chips without salt.
Pregnant: Each serving contains 8.3 micrograms of folate and 1/2 milligram of iron.

Fruit 'n' Spicy Nut Trail Mix (FAST FIX)

Buying preroasted soy nuts and sunflower seeds helps save some time. The dried corn adds a nice bit of sweetness and crunch to this mix. Look for it at health food stores, which have a large selection of fruits and vegetables that are dried without sugar.

SPICY NUTS

$1/2$ cup raw cashews

$1/2$ cup raw whole almonds with skin

$1/2$ tablespoon canola or olive oil

1 teaspoon chili powder

$1/2$ teaspoon coarse salt

$1/2$ teaspoon dried oregano

$1/2$ teaspoon paprika

$1/4$ teaspoon onion powder

$1/4$ teaspoon freshly ground black pepper

TRAIL MIX

1 cup salted roasted soy nuts

$1/4$ cup salted roasted sunflower seeds

1 cup unsweetened dried apricot pieces

1 cup unsweetened dried apple slices, chopped

$1/2$ cup dried corn (such as Just Corn)

1. Preheat the oven to 375°F.

2. Combine the first nine ingredients in a small bowl and toss until blended. Place the coated nuts on a small nonstick baking sheet and bake at 375°F for 7–10 minutes or until roasted, turning the nuts once about halfway through.

3. Combine the spicy nuts and remaining ingredients in a medium bowl and stir to combine. Store the trail mix in an airtight container at room temperature.

Yield: 4$1/2$ cups; Serving: $1/4$ cup
Calories: 117; Protein: 4.0 g; Carbohydrate: 15 g; Fiber: 1.7 g; Sodium: 122 mg;
Fat 5.4 g (Sat: 0.7 g, Mono: 1.33 g, Poly: 0.52 g, Trans: 0 g); Cholesterol: 0 mg

General: This filling bit of crunch and munch has no added sugar. It also has about half the calories and one-third the fat of most candy bars, not to mention small amounts of all kinds of vitamins and minerals. Keep it on hand at the office or at home for whenever the munchies strike.
Diabetic: For carbohydrate counters, total is 15 grams. Equals 1 starch exchange and 1 fat.

Sodium-Restricted: The bulk of the sodium in this recipe comes from the salted roasted soy nuts and sunflower seeds. Both of these products can be easily found in unsalted varieties. For more flavor, consider doubling the amount of spice mix and roasting the unsalted soy nuts and seeds with the nuts.
Pregnant: No special considerations.

Blackberry-Banana Smoothie *(FAST FIX)*

The flavors for a fruit smoothie are nearly limitless. But naturally sweet blackberries and bananas—a great thickener for smoothies—are a delicious match. Try raspberries, blueberries, or strawberries in place of the blackberries.

> 2 cups frozen unsweetened blackberries (about 8 ounces)
>
> 1 large banana, peeled and cut into 4 sections
>
> 1 cup vanilla soy milk (such as Edensoy)
>
> 1/2 cup apple juice
>
> 1/2 cup soft silken reduced-fat tofu (such as Mori-Nu Lite)

1. Place all of the ingredients in a blender or food processor and process until smooth. Pour into chilled glasses and serve.

Note: Leftovers will keep in the refrigerator for up to 24 hours. Be sure to use silken-style tofu. The water-packed tofu is too firm in texture to make a smooth blend.

Yield: 2 1/2 cups, 3 servings; Serving: 3/4 cup
Calories: 185; Protein: 5.9 g; Carbohydrate: 38 g; Fiber: 6.4 g; Sodium: 2 mg;
Fat 1.8 g (Sat: 0.07 g, Mono: 0.09 g, Poly: 0.43 g, Trans: 0 g); Cholesterol: 0 mg

General: This liquid refreshment has more fiber than most breakfast cereals and small amounts of many other nutrients, everything from vitamin E to calcium to phosphorus.
Diabetic: For carbohydrate counters, total is 38 grams. Equals 1 1/2 fruit exchanges, 1 starch, and 1 vegetable.
Sodium-Restricted: Since all fruits are low in sodium, you can vary the type of fruit used in smoothies without changing the sodium level significantly. Also, a single serving of this smoothie has 444 milligrams of potassium.
Pregnant: Each serving contains 52 milligrams of calcium, 48 micrograms of folate, and 1.6 milligrams of iron.

Strawberry Almond Shake *(FAST FIX)*

If the thick texture of a smoothie isn't to your liking, this blended drink has a smooth, frothy texture similar to that of a milkshake. Vary the fruit and add ingredients like wheat germ and bran to give the shake more fiber.

1 cup frozen unsweetened strawberries

1 cup plain soy milk

2 tablespoons sliced almonds

1 tablespoon ground flaxseed

1/4 teaspoon finely grated orange zest

3 ice cubes

Dash almond extract

2 fresh strawberries (optional)

1. Place frozen strawberries and next six ingredients (through extract) in a blender. Blend until smooth.

2. To serve, pour into glass. Garnish with fresh strawberry, if desired.

Yield: 2 servings; Serving: about 3/4 cup
Calories: 131; Protein: 5.9 g; Carbohydrate: 13.3 g; Fiber: 3.3 g; Sodium: 41 mg:
Fat: 6.8 g (Sat: 0.3, Mono: 2.4, Poly: 1.3 g, Trans: 0 g); Cholesterol 0 mg

General: Strawberries are on the recent government list of the top twenty most antioxidant-rich foods.
Diabetic: For carbohydrate counters, total is 13 grams. Equals 1/2 fruit exchange, 1/2 skim milk exchange, and 1 fat exchange.
Sodium-Restricted: No special considerations.
Pregnant: Contains 27 micrograms folate.

Mango Energy Blitz (*FAST FIX*)

With a small amount of caffeine from the brewed tea, and the natural energy from carrot juice and three kinds of fruits, this sweet drink can give a nutritious jump start to your day. Make the tea the night before so it will be chilled and ready to go in the morning. And try freezing the banana and mango in plastic freezer bags so that you can be ready to make this delicious beverage whenever you feel energy waning. Pure carrot juice can be found in health food stores.

1 teabag kiwi-pear green tea (such as Republic of Tea) or Earl Grey tea

1/2 cup boiling water

1 mango, peeled and chopped (about 1 cup)

1 banana, peeled and cut into sections

1 cup apricot nectar (such as R. W. Knudsen), chilled

1/2 cup carrot juice, chilled

1/8 teaspoon freshly grated nutmeg

1. Steep the teabag in boiling water for 3 minutes or according to package directions. Remove the teabag and put the tea in the refrigerator to chill.

2. Combine the mango, banana, and chilled tea in a blender or food processor and process until smooth. Add the remaining ingredients and pulse to mix. Pour into chilled glasses and serve.

Note: Leftovers will keep in the refrigerator for up to 24 hours. For a variation, consider adding ¼ cup toasted wheat germ for an extra dose of fiber.

Yield: 4 cups; Serving: 1 cup
Calories: 98; Protein: 0.7 g; Carbohydrate: 25.2 g; Fiber: 2 g; Sodium: 27 mg;
Fat 0.2 g (Sat: 0.06 g, Mono: 0.06 g, Poly: 0.05 g, Trans: 0 g); Cholesterol: 0 mg

General: Twelve milligrams of caffeine per serving. Hefty dose of vitamin A and beta-carotene. More than 25 percent of recommended amount of vitamin C.
Diabetic: For carbohydrate counters, total is 25 grams. Equals 1½ fruit exchanges.
Sodium-Restricted: By nature, fruits and vegetables are low in sodium. But when carrots are concentrated into juice, the sodium level does rise. If you are on a severely restricted sodium diet, consider omitting the carrot juice (which contains 61 milligrams of sodium) to bring down the sodium level. Also, 1 cup of this energy drink has 305 milligrams of potassium.
Pregnant: Although this drink contains only 12 milligrams of caffeine per serving, you might want to consider replacing the regular tea with either a decaffeinated tea or an herbal tea. Each serving contains 10 micrograms of folate.

BREADS AND GRAINS

Apple Crunch Oatmeal

Be sure to choose a sweet red apple rather than a tart variety like Granny Smith for this cereal. To save time in the morning, you can cook the spelt or wheat berries—kernels of wheat—the night before. Spelt and wheat berries are interchangeable in recipes, as both are just different strains of wheat. Either can be found in health food stores or via mail order.

    ½ cup spelt berries or soft wheat berries

    3½ cups water

    ½ teaspoon coarse salt

    1½ cups rolled oats

    2 large red apples (such as McIntosh or Rome), halved and cored

    1 teaspoon cinnamon

    ½ teaspoon vanilla extract

    2 tablespoons frozen unsweetened apple juice concentrate, thawed

Coarse salt to taste

4 tablespoons chopped walnuts, toasted

Brown sugar to taste (optional)

1. Add the spelt, water, and salt to a medium saucepan. Bring to a boil and simmer 12–15 minutes or until the berries are tender-crunchy. Return the mixture to a boil. Add the oats, stirring continuously to prevent lumps from forming. Reduce the heat to medium and cook until the oatmeal is thick and creamy, 6–8 minutes.

2. Grate the apples, including the skin, directly into the pan. (Alternatively, leave the apples whole and grate over a plate using a stand-up grater.) Stir in the cinnamon, vanilla, and juice concentrate. Taste for seasoning and add more salt, if needed. Spoon the oatmeal into each of 4 serving bowls and top each with 1 tablespoon toasted nuts and a sprinkling of brown sugar, if desired. Serve immediately.

Note: Steel-cut oats—Irish and Scotch oatmeals are made with these—can be substituted for the rolled oats; they take much longer to cook (about 40 minutes) but make a nuttier, creamier cereal. A small sprinkling of brown sugar makes a nice finish for this dish.

Yield: 4½ cups (6 servings); Serving: ¾ cup
Calories: 260; Protein: 8.63 g; Carbohydrate: 45 g; Fiber: 6.3 g; Sodium: 160 mg;
Fat 6.1 g (Sat: 0.76 g, Mono: 1.56 g, Poly: 2.95 g, Trans: 0 g); Cholesterol: 0 mg

General: No special considerations.
Diabetic: For carbohydrate counters, total is 45 grams. That may seem like a lot (3 starch exchanges), but there is no added sugar; most of the carbohydrate is in the form of whole grains (oats and spelt) and fruit. Add ½ fat exchange.
Sodium-Restricted: Most of the sodium comes from the salt that is cooked with the spelt. Omit that salt and the sodium level will drop considerably. Also, a single serving of this cereal has 328 milligrams of potassium.
Pregnant: Each serving of cereal contains 33 milligrams of calcium, 25 micrograms of folate, and 2.7 milligrams of iron.

Carrot–Wheat Germ Muffins

This light, moist, slightly sweet muffin is made even tastier by the addition of fresh-grated carrots, golden raisins, and chopped walnuts. Leftovers freeze well in zip-top bags; take them out one by one and reheat them in the oven or microwave for a fresh-baked flavor.

2 cups whole-wheat flour

1 cup toasted wheat germ

1 tablespoon baking powder

½ teaspoon coarse salt

2 eggs, lightly beaten

2 tablespoons vegetable oil

1 cup apple juice

$^1/_2$ cup frozen unsweetened apple juice concentrate, thawed

$^1/_3$ cup unsweetened applesauce

1 cup grated carrots

$^1/_2$ cup golden raisins, tightly packed

$^1/_3$ cup chopped walnuts

Vegetable cooking spray or canola oil

1. Preheat the oven to 375°F.

2. Combine the first four ingredients in a small mixing bowl; whisk well.

3. Combine the eggs and the next four ingredients in a large mixing bowl; beat well at medium speed of a mixer. Add the dry ingredients, stirring just until moist. Fold in the carrots, raisins, and walnuts; spoon the batter into muffin cups lightly coated with cooking spray or oil, filling the cups about two-thirds full. Bake at 375°F for 25–30 minutes or until a wooden pick inserted in the center comes out clean. Place the muffin tin on a wire rack and cool for 10 minutes; remove from the pan and cool completely on a wire rack.

Yield: 12; Serving: 1 muffin
Calories: 216; Protein: 7.4 g; Carbohydrate: 34 g; Fiber: 4.5 g; Sodium: 156 mg;
Fat 6.7 g (Sat: 0.88 g, Mono: 2.34 g, Poly: 2.91 g, Trans: 0.01 g); Cholesterol: 35 mg

General: These muffins carry nearly half a day's supply of vitamin E requirement in just one serving; they're also rich in vitamin A.
Diabetic: For carbohydrate counters, total is 34 grams. Equals 2 starch exchanges and 1 fat. No added sugars; fruit juice and fruit sugars are used to sweeten this muffin.
Sodium-Restricted: This muffin has less sodium than 2 slices of store-bought bread and most store-bought muffins. But you can omit the added salt to bring the sodium content down into the single digits. One muffin is packed with 391 milligrams of potassium.
Pregnant: Each muffin carries 28 milligrams of calcium, 50 micrograms of folate, and 2 milligrams of iron.

Banana-Apricot Nut Bread

A maranth, a tiny golden-yellow grain with lots of protein and calcium, adds a crunchy texture and wonderful speckled appearance to this quick bread. Be sure to leave the walnuts in fairly big pieces, as that makes for a spectacular-looking topping. And if you have a real sweet tooth, try spreading apple butter (the kind sweetened with just apples and apple juice) or an all-fruit spread onto slices.

1 cup apple juice

$^1/_2$ cup all-fruit apricot spread or jam

$^2/_3$ cup dried apricot pieces

$^1/_2$ cup amaranth

2 eggs, lightly beaten

$^1/_3$ cup canola oil

1 ripe banana, mashed (about $^1/_2$ cup)

2 tablespoons honey

2 cups whole-wheat flour

1 teaspoon baking powder

1 teaspoon cinnamon

$^1/_4$ teaspoon coarse salt

$^1/_4$ cup coarsely chopped walnuts or other nut

Vegetable cooking spray or canola oil

1. Bring the apple juice to a boil in a small saucepan. Remove from heat and add the apricot spread, apricots, and amaranth; let stand for 20 minutes.

2. Preheat the oven to 350°F.

3. Combine the eggs, oil, banana, and honey in a large mixing bowl; beat well on medium speed of a mixer. Add the apple juice mixture to the egg mixture, beating well. Combine the flour and the next three ingredients; whisk well. Add the dry ingredients to the egg–apple juice mixture, stirring just until moist. (Do not overmix.)

4. Spoon the batter into a 9- × 5-inch loaf pan lightly coated with cooking spray or oil. Bake at 350°F for 55–65 minutes or until a wooden pick inserted in the center comes out clean. Cool in the pan on a wire rack for 5 minutes; remove from the pan. Cool completely on a wire rack.

Yield: 1 loaf, 12 servings; Serving: 1 slice
Calories: 227; Protein: 5.87 g; Carbohydrate: 39 g; Fiber: 4.8 g; Sodium: 74 mg;
Fat 9.4 g (Sat: 1.05 g, Mono: 4.42 g, Poly: 3.30 g, Trans: 0.01 g); Cholesterol: 35 mg

General: One slice provides 20 percent of the recommended amount for vitamin E.
Diabetic: For carbohydrate counters, total is 39 grams. Equals 2 starch exchanges, 1 fat, and $^1/_2$ fruit. A small amount of honey is used to sweeten this bread, but the bulk of the sugar comes from fruit and fruit juice.
Sodium-Restricted: The sodium figures are without the added salt. There is no way to reduce the sodium further. Each slice is packed with 306 milligrams of potassium.
Pregnant: Each slice carries 33 milligrams of calcium, 21 micrograms of folate, and 2 milligrams of iron.

Hearty Wheat Berry–Oat Groat Bread

This bread is 100 percent whole grain, made with whole-wheat flour and both whole kernels of wheat (wheat berries) and oats (oat groats.) Sunflower seeds are thrown in to enhance the nuttiness of the whole grains. Keep in mind that whole-grain breads don't rise as high as breads made with all white flour. But the rich, wheaty flavor is superior. Look for wheat berries and oat groats in health food stores.

> 2 tablespoons sunflower seeds
>
> 2 tablespoons wheat berries
>
> 2 tablespoons oat groats
>
> 2 teaspoons active dry yeast
>
> 1¼ cups warm water (105°F to 115°F)
>
> 2 tablespoons molasses
>
> 1½ teaspoons coarse salt
>
> 2 tablespoons canola or other oil
>
> 2½–3 cups whole-wheat flour
>
> Vegetable cooking spray or canola oil

1. Place the first three ingredients in a dry nonstick skillet over medium heat and roast for 3–6 minutes or until lightly brown, stirring frequently to prevent scorching.

2. Combine the yeast and ½ cup warm water in a large bowl; let stand 5 minutes. Stir in the molasses and the next two ingredients. Add 2½ cups of wheat flour; stir to form a soft dough. Turn the dough out onto a lightly floured surface and knead until smooth and elastic (6–8 minutes), adding enough of the remaining flour, 1 tablespoon at a time, to prevent the dough from sticking to your hands. Knead the seeds, wheat berries, and oat groats into the dough until well dispersed, 1–2 minutes.

3. Place the dough in a large bowl lightly coated with cooking spray or oil, turning to coat the top. Cover and let rise in a warm place (85°F), free from drafts, 1–2 hours or until doubled in bulk. Punch the dough down; turn out onto a lightly floured surface and roll the dough into a 12- × 7-inch rectangle. Roll up the rectangle tightly, starting with the short edge; press firmly to eliminate air pockets; pinch the seam and ends to seal. Place the roll, seam side down, in an 8- × 5-inch nonstick loaf pan lightly coated with cooking spray or oil. Cover and let rise until the dough reaches the top of the pan, 50–60 minutes. Bake at

350°F for 45 minutes or until the loaf sounds hollow when tapped. Remove from the pan immediately; cool on a wire rack.

Bread Machine Instructions: Use bread machine yeast and a large-capacity bread machine. Follow manufacturer instructions for whole-wheat or specialty loafs.

Yield: 12 servings; Serving: 1 slice
Calories: 149; Protein: 5.1 g; Carbohydrate: 26 g; Fiber: 3.9 g; Sodium: 239 mg;
Fat 3.6 g (Sat: 0.32 g, Mono: 1.42 g, Poly: 0.95 g, Trans: 0.01 g); Cholesterol: 0 mg

General: Because it's 100 percent whole grain, this bread is not only rich in fiber, it also contains generous amounts of lots of the nutrients found in whole grains, such as vitamin E, zinc, iron, magnesium, and selenium.
Diabetic: For carbohydrate counters, total is 26 grams. Equals about 2 starch exchanges.
Sodium-Restricted: This bread is higher in sodium than a slice of store-bought bread, but that's mainly because it is so much more dense. Omit or cut down on the salt if you'd like to bring down the sodium level.
Pregnant: Each slice carries 24 milligrams of calcium, 29 micrograms of folate, and 1.7 milligrams of iron.

Olive Swirl Rolls

These simple-to-make rolls start with a premade frozen dough, a blend of whole wheat and white flour. It's not as high in fiber as a 100 percent whole-grain bread, but it still carries more fiber than a loaf made with all white flour. A small amount of Parmesan cheese makes a wonderful crunchy topping for the roll and contributes just over $^1/_2$ gram of fat per roll. You can omit the cheese, if necessary.

3 teaspoons olive oil, divided

$^1/_4$ cup chopped shallot or red onion

$1^1/_2$ tablespoons chopped fresh or $1^1/_2$ teaspoons dried basil

$^1/_2$ teaspoon dried oregano

$^1/_4$–$^1/_2$ teaspoon crushed red pepper flakes

1 (4.25-ounce) can black olives, drained and finely chopped (about $^3/_4$ cup)

$^3/_4$ cup bottled roasted red and yellow peppers, drained and coarsely chopped

2 teaspoons red wine vinegar

Coarse salt to taste

1 loaf frozen wheat bread dough (such as Rhodes), thawed per package directions

$^1/_4$ cup freshly grated Parmesan cheese, divided

Vegetable cooking spray or canola oil

1. Preheat the oven to 325°F.

2. Place a nonstick skillet over medium heat and add 2 teaspoons oil and the shallots. Cook for 2–3 minutes or until the shallots begin to soften. Stir in the next three ingredients; cook for 1 minute. Remove from the heat and stir in the olives, peppers, and vinegar. Taste for seasoning and add salt as needed.

3. Turn the dough onto a lightly floured surface and roll into a 12- × 9-inch rectangle. Spread the olive mixture over the dough, leaving a ¹/₂-inch border around the edges. Sprinkle 2 tablespoons of the cheese over the olive mixture. Roll the dough up lengthwise (like a carpet) and pinch the ends closed. Slice gently with a serrated knife into 1-inch-width rolls; place the rolls on a baking sheet lightly coated with cooking spray or oil. Brush the rolls with the remaining teaspoon of oil and cover with plastic wrap; let rise, away from drafts, for 30 minutes or until doubled in bulk.

4. Uncover the rolls and sprinkle with the remaining 2 tablespoons Parmesan cheese. Bake at 325°F for 20–25 minutes or until golden brown. Serve warm or at room temperature.

Note: These rolls freeze well.

Yield: 12; Serving: 1 roll
Calories: 144; Protein: 5.7 g; Carbohydrate: 20.6 g; Fiber: 1.8 g; Sodium: 326 mg;
Fat 4.9 g (Sat: 0.55 g, Mono: 2.01 g, Poly: 0.11 g, Trans: 0.01 g); Cholesterol: 1.6 mg

General: These pizza-style rolls carry as much fiber as many store-bought whole-wheat breads. They're rich in zinc and offer 25 percent of the requirement for vitamin C.
Diabetic: For carbohydrate counters, total is 21 grams. Equals 1 starch exchange, 1 vegetable, and 1 fat.
Sodium-Restricted: Olives are by far the biggest contributor of sodium. Omit the olives (920 milligrams sodium) and replace them with ¹/₂ cup sautéed mushrooms. Replace the oregano with rosemary and you'll have a swirl roll of a slightly different variation that is just as tasty and carries just the sodium found in a slice of the frozen bread dough.
Pregnant: No special considerations.

Multigrain Hotcakes with Warm Apple Syrup

These multigrain pancakes have a nutty flavor and crunchy texture due to toasted sunflower seeds and several whole grains—millet, barley, wheat. The addition of reduced-fat buttermilk makes for a light, tender texture, but you can substitute apple juice if necessary. Also, these pancakes cook perfectly well in a nonstick skillet without a drop of oil. But if you like a crispy edge on your hotcakes, add some oil to the griddle before cooking.

SYRUP

1½ cups frozen unsweetened apple juice concentrate, thawed

1 stick cinnamon or ¼ teaspoon ground cinnamon

2 whole cloves (optional)

⅓ cup unsweetened applesauce

HOTCAKES

2 tablespoons raw sunflower seeds

2 tablespoons millet

⅓ cup quick-cooking barley (such as Mother's)

1⅓ cups fat-free or reduced-fat buttermilk

2 eggs, lightly beaten

2 tablespoons canola oil

2 tablespoons frozen unsweetened apple juice concentrate, thawed

1 cup bran flakes cereal

½ cup whole-wheat flour

½ cup all-purpose flour

1½ teaspoons baking soda

1 teaspoon baking powder

½ teaspoon coarse salt

½ teaspoon cinnamon

¼ teaspoon freshly grated nutmeg

1. To make the syrup, place the juice concentrate, cinnamon stick, and cloves, if using, in a small saucepan over medium-high heat. Bring to a boil and simmer for 5–10 minutes or until the mixture is reduced by about a third. Remove the cinnamon stick and cloves with a slotted spoon. Stir in the applesauce. Reduce the heat to low and keep warm.

2. To make the pancakes, place a large nonstick skillet over medium to medium-high heat. Add the sunflower seeds and millet. Toast the seeds for 3–6 minutes or until lightly brown, stirring occasionally to prevent scorching. Remove from the heat and set aside. (You will use this same skillet to cook the hotcakes.)

3. Place the quick-cooking barley (do not use pearl barley) and buttermilk in a mixing bowl and let stand 30 minutes. Add the eggs, oil, juice concentrate, and bran flakes, mixing just until blended.

4. Combine the wheat and white flours, baking soda, and remaining ingredients in a medium mixing bowl. Whisk together until well blended. Add the buttermilk mixture to the flour mixture and stir just until moist.

5. Heat a large nonstick skillet or griddle over medium to medium-high heat. Pour $1/4$ cup batter into the skillet for each pancake (do not crowd) and cook for 2–3 minutes until tops bubble and edges look dry. Turn the pancakes and cook for 1–2 minutes more until the undersides are golden brown. Repeat with the remaining batter. Serve with Warm Apple Syrup.

Note: To keep pancakes warm, preheat oven to 200°. Place pancakes on nonstick baking sheet and cover loosely with foil. Keep in oven until ready to serve. Also, these pancakes freeze well. Pop them in the microwave or toaster to reheat.

Yield: 12 hotcakes, 1¹/8 cups syrup; Serving: 2 hotcakes and 3 tablespoons syrup
Calories: 282; Protein: 9 g; Carbohydrate: 43.7 g; Fiber: 4.4 g; Sodium: 502 mg;
Fat 8.9 g (Sat: 0.76 g, Mono: 1.56 g, Poly: 2.95 g, Trans: 0 g); Cholesterol: 0 mg

General: With an assortment of whole grains, it's no surprise these hotcakes are rich in fiber and vitamin E.
Diabetic: For carbohydrate counters, the total is 44 grams. That is a lot of carbohydrate, but it's mainly the complex or whole-grain (barley, bran, wheat, and millet) variety that is absorbed slowly into the blood sugar. Consider the 2 hotcakes as 2 starch exchanges plus 1 fat. Count the syrup as 1¹/2 fruits.
Sodium-Restricted: The sodium tab is high owing to baking soda, a leavening agent that is used when baking with acidic ingredients such as buttermilk. Switch to another liquid (skim milk, apple juice) and replace the baking soda with baking powder to lower the sodium levels.
Pregnant: Each serving contains 88 milligrams of calcium, 29 micrograms of folate, and 1.7 milligrams of iron.

ENTRÉES

Mediterranean Stuffed Breast of Chicken (FAST FIX)

The filling for these chicken breasts is simple to put together: canned artichoke hearts, bottled roasted peppers, and already crumbled feta cheese combined with some fresh basil and toasted pine nuts. Toast the pine nuts in a dry skillet on the stove; it will take just 2 or 3 minutes.

$1/4$ cup water-packed artichoke hearts, drained and finely chopped

1 (7-ounce) bottle roasted red peppers, drained and chopped

$1/2$ cup feta cheese (about 2 ounces), crumbled

2 tablespoons fresh basil, chopped

2 tablespoons pine nuts, toasted

2 teaspoons red wine vinegar

1^1/$_2$ tablespoons garlic olive oil, divided

4 (5-ounce) boneless, skinless chicken breasts

Coarse salt and freshly ground black pepper to taste

1. Combine the first six ingredients in a small bowl. Stir in 1 tablespoon garlic olive oil and set aside.

2. Using a thin, sharp knife (such as a boning knife), cut a 2-inch horizontal slit in the thickest part of each chicken breast, cutting to, but not through, the opposite side of the breast. Hold the knife blade parallel to the cutting board and guide the blade around inside the breast to create a pocket. Stuff ^{1}/$_4$ cup artichoke mixture into the pocket. Sprinkle the chicken with salt and pepper.

3. Heat ^{1}/$_2$ tablespoon garlic oil in a skillet over medium-high heat. Add the chicken and cook 5–6 minutes on each side or until the chicken is done.

Note: Don't be put off by the idea of cutting pockets into a chicken breast. If you start with a plump breast and use a sharp knife, the task is quite easy. If you accidentally cut through a side or bottom of the breast, a toothpick can help seal the pocket during cooking. Remove it before serving and no one will be the wiser.

Yield: 4 servings; Serving: 1 stuffed chicken breast
Calories: 261; Protein: 31 g; Carbohydrate: 4.5 g; Fiber: 0.8 g; Sodium: 283 mg;
Fat 12.6 g (Sat: 4.18 g, Mono: 5.75 g, Poly: 1.76 g, Trans: .050 g); Cholesterol: 82 mg

General: Loaded with zinc, this dish also contains generous amounts of other nutrients, including vitamin C, calcium, and iron.
Diabetic: For carbohydrate counters, the total is 5 grams. Equals 4 lean meat exchanges and 1 vegetable.
Sodium-Restricted: Sodium figures were calculated without added salt. The sodium in this dish comes mainly from canned convenience products (artichokes, red pepper). Omit the artichokes and roast your own red peppers to help cut the sodium.
Pregnant: No special considerations.

Tandoori Tuna (FAST FIX)

This spicy fish takes its flavor cues from India, where savory and sweet spices are blended and used on everything from meat to vegetables to seafood. The tuna is marinated briefly in the tandoori spice mixture and then cooked in a skillet. Fix some citrus-flavored couscous as a side dish.

4 (5-ounce) tuna steaks, about ^{1}/$_2$ inch thick

^{3}/$_4$ cup pineapple juice

1 tablespoon fresh lemon juice

1 tablespoon minced peeled fresh gingerroot

1 tablespoon minced fresh garlic

1 tablespoon ground coriander

1 tablespoon paprika

$^1/_2$ tablespoon ground cumin

1 teaspoon coarse salt

1 teaspoon cumin seeds

1 teaspoon chili garlic sauce

$^1/_4$ teaspoon cinnamon

$^1/_8$ teaspoon ground cloves

1 tablespoon canola or other oil

1. Combine the tuna and remaining ingredients in a large zip-top storage bag. Press the air out of the bag and seal; refrigerate for 15 minutes, turning once or twice.

2. Heat the oil in a large cast-iron or nonstick skillet over medium heat. Remove the tuna from the marinade; discard the marinade. Place the tuna in the hot skillet; cook for 4–5 minutes on each side or until done.

Note: Tuna can be grilled or broiled. Prepare grill or broiler rack. Brush with oil and cook as directed above. Look for the chili garlic sauce in the Asian section of most supermarkets.

Yield: 4 servings; Serving: 1 tuna steak
Calories: 195; Protein: 33 g; Carbohydrate: 2.5 g; Fiber: 0.3 g; Sodium: 67 mg;
Fat 4.9 g (Sat: 0.59 g, Mono: 2.30 g, Poly: 1.46 g, Trans: 0.01 g); Cholesterol: 64 mg

General: This dish provides small amounts of vitamin E and heart-healthy n-3 fats.
Diabetic: For carbohydrate counters, total is 2.5 grams. This small amount of carbohydrate comes from the ingredients used in the marinade; calculations are based on $^1/_4$ of marinade, since most of the marinade is discarded. Equals 5 very lean meat exchanges.
Sodium-Restricted: Sodium figures were calculated without added salt. A tiny amount of sodium is coming from the prepared chili garlic sauce. Omit that if you need to and substitute a small amount of cayenne pepper for the heat.
Pregnant: Contains 55 milligrams of calcium and 2.6 milligrams of iron.

Lemon-Oregano Grouper with Vegetables

When you use the French technique of oven-steaming single servings of fish, seasonings, and vegetables in individual packages, the reward is twofold: very little to clean up and lots of flavor. Any white fish, such as mahi-mahi, pollack, wahoo, or cod, will work in this recipe. Whole-wheat couscous makes a quick side dish for this fish; prepare it while the fish is cooking.

2 tablespoons olive oil, divided

2 small zucchini, julienned

1 cup fresh or frozen corn kernels

$^1/_4$ cup diced red pepper

$^1/_2$ teaspoon coarse salt

4 (5-ounce) grouper fillets, about 1 inch thick

Coarse salt and freshly ground black pepper to taste

2 teaspoons fresh lemon juice

2 tablespoons fresh oregano, coarsely chopped

4 paper-thin slices lemon, halved

1. Preheat the oven to 375°F.

2. Combine 1 tablespoon olive oil and the next four ingredients. Divide this vegetable mixture among four large pieces of aluminum foil, placing the vegetables in the center of each piece. Sprinkle each grouper fillet with salt and pepper and place the fish on top of the vegetables.

3. Combine the remaining tablespoon of olive oil, lemon juice, and oregano. Drizzle one-quarter of this mixture over each grouper fillet and top with 2 lemon-slice halves. Seal the package by rolling up the top and sides and bake at 375°F for 16–20 minutes or until the fish flakes easily with a fork. Place each foil package on a serving plate, open the package, and serve.

Yield: 4 servings; Serving: 1 grouper fillet with vegetables
Calories: 239; Protein: 30.4 g; Carbohydrate: 10 g; Fiber: 1.8 g; Sodium: 318 mg;
Fat 9 g (Sat: 1.36 g, Mono: 5.41 g, Poly: 1.34 g, Trans: 0.07 g); Cholesterol: 52 mg

General: One serving of this fish provides 50 percent of the requirement for vitamin C and a good laundry list of different minerals, including magnesium, iron, zinc, and phosphorus.
Diabetic: For carbohydrate counters, 10 grams. Equals 4 very lean meat exchanges, 2 vegetables, and 1 fat.
Sodium-Restricted: The bulk of the sodium comes from the salt added to vegetables. Omit the added salt and sodium will be reduced to under 20 milligrams.
Pregnant: No special considerations.

Chicken Enchilada Casserole

This casserole uses already prepared enchilada sauce (the Hatch brand is made with wheat flour instead of white), store-bought rotisserie chicken, and canned beans and chilies. If you can, buy the organic canned beans; they're worth the extra cost: better flavor, less salt, and a firm texture.

CASEROLE

2 tablespoons canola or olive oil, divided

2 cups chopped white or yellow onion (about 1 large)

2 garlic cloves, minced

1 cup thinly sliced green onion, divided

1 teaspoon dried oregano

$^1/_4$ cup fresh cilantro, finely chopped

2 cups skinless roasted chicken breast meat

1 cup bottled roasted red peppers, chopped

1 (4.5-ounce) can chopped green chilies, drained

2 tablespoons fresh lime juice

Coarse salt and freshly ground black pepper

1 (15-ounce) can enchilada sauce (such as Hatch)

1 (14.5-ounce) can diced tomatoes

$^1/_2$ cup defatted chicken stock or broth, preferably low-sodium

Vegetable cooking spray or canola oil

6 (6-inch) corn tortillas, torn or cut into thirds

1 (15-ounce) can black beans, rinsed and drained

TOPPING

$^1/_4$ cup shredded sharp cheddar cheese

4 tablespoons finely chopped black olives

Cilantro sprigs (optional)

1. Preheat the oven to 350°F.

2. To make the casserole, place a large skillet over medium to medium-high heat. Add the oil and onion; sauté for 5–8 minutes or until the onion is tender-crisp. Stir in the garlic, green onions, oregano, and cilantro; cook for 1 minute. Remove from the heat and add the chicken, roasted red peppers, chilies, and lime juice. Taste for seasoning and add salt and pepper, if desired.

3. Combine the enchilada sauce, tomatoes, and chicken stock in a bowl. Place $^1/_2$ cup of the sauce into the bottom of an 11- × 7-inch baking dish lightly coated with cooking spray or oil. Arrange 6 tortilla pieces over the sauce. Top with one-third of the onion-chicken mixture, one-third of the black beans, and $^3/_4$ cup sauce. Repeat layers, ending with the sauce. Bake at 350°F for 45–50 minutes or until bubbly. Remove from the oven and sprinkle with the cheese, 1 tablespoon at a time, making four diagonal rows across the casserole. Sprinkle 1

tablespoon of olives next to each row of cheese, following the same diagonal pattern. Let stand for 10 minutes before serving.

Yield: 6 servings; Serving: 1 (3.5-inch) square
Calories: 381; Protein: 23.8 g; Carbohydrate: 40.5 g; Fiber: 9.2 g; Sodium: 876 mg;
Fat 13.7 g (Sat: 2.45 g, Mono: 5.67 g, Poly: 2.85 g, Trans: 0.05 g); Cholesterol: 44 mg

General: One serving of this casserole provides a full day's supply of vitamin C and zinc, not to mention hefty amounts of vitamin E, calcium, iron, and fiber.
Diabetic: 41 grams for carbohydrate counters. Equals 2 lean meat exchanges, 2 breads, 2 vegetables, and ½ fat.
Sodium-Restricted: The canned convenience items (enchilada sauce, chilies, black beans, and tomatoes) provide the bulk of the sodium. Opt for salt-free canned tomatoes, fresh green chilies, and black beans cooked without salt and you can lower the sodium considerably.
Pregnant: Each serving contains 157 milligrams of calcium, 46 micrograms of folate, and 3.8 milligrams of iron.

Double Mushroom Meat Loaf

Dried and fresh mushrooms give this beef-and-turkey meat loaf a wonderful rich flavor. Be sure to use lean ground turkey and not ground breast of turkey in this loaf; the ground breast (all white meat) has very little fat and makes a dry loaf. Substitute lean ground turkey for the beef if you'd like.

> ½ ounce dried mixed mushroom blend (shiitake, oyster, porcini) or dried shiitakes
>
> 1 cup boiling water
>
> 1 pound 93 percent lean ground beef or lean ground round
>
> ½ pound lean ground turkey
>
> 1 cup chopped white or yellow onion
>
> ¼ cup chopped fresh parsley
>
> ½ cup diced button mushrooms (about 2 ounces)
>
> ¼ cup rolled oats
>
> 1 egg, lightly beaten
>
> 2½ tablespoons tomato paste
>
> ¾ teaspoon coarse salt
>
> 2 teaspoons dried basil
>
> 1 teaspoon dried oregano

1. Combine the dried mushrooms and water in a small bowl and let stand for 30 minutes or until the mushrooms are soft. Drain and finely chop the mush-

rooms, reserving the soaking liquid. Strain the soaking liquid through cheese-cloth or a fine sieve to remove the grit.

2. Preheat the oven to 325°F.

3. Combine the meat, turkey, rehydrated chopped mushrooms, 2 tablespoons of the reserved mushroom soaking liquid, and the remaining ingredients in a bowl and mix until well blended. Place the meat mixture into a nonstick 9- × 5-inch loaf pan and bake at 325°F for 45–50 minutes or until done.

Yield: 10 servings; Serving: 1 slice (about 3 ounces)
Calories: 161; Protein: 15.9 g; Carbohydrate: 7.0 g; Fiber: 1.6 g; Sodium: 254 mg;
Fat 7.6 g (Sat: 2.48 g, Mono: 2.79 g, Poly: 0.88 g, Trans: 0.04 g); Cholesterol: 56 mg

General: Nearly 3 milligrams of zinc and 2.4 milligrams of iron in a single slice.
Diabetic: For carbohydrate counters, total is 7 grams. Equals 2 lean meat exchanges and ½ starch exchange.
Sodium-Restricted: Sodium figures include added salt; omit salt to bring sodium level down. Also, 1 serving of this meat loaf has 356 milligrams of potassium.
Pregnant: Each serving contains 27 milligrams of calcium and 21 micrograms of folate.

BWT Wrap

The main ingredients in this quick-to-fix wrap are BWT: beef, watercress, and tomato. But roasted chicken will work nicely, too. Add some salad greens and a spunky horseradish cream dressing and you have the perfect light lunch or snack. Look for whole-wheat tortillas made without partially hydrogenated shortening in the health food store and some supermarkets. Flavored tortillas can also work here, although most seem to be made with small amounts of partially hydrogenated oils; check the ingredients label.

HORSERADISH CREAM

2 tablespoons canola or soybean oil mayonnaise

4 teaspoons prepared horseradish

½ teaspoon Dijon mustard

Freshly ground black pepper

WRAP

4 (8-inch) whole-wheat tortillas

½ pound lean deli roast beef, thinly sliced (about 8 slices)

½ small cucumber, cut into 24 paper-thin slices

16 sprigs of trimmed watercress or 1 cup fresh pea shoots

½ cup thinly sliced red onion

1 large beefsteak tomato, cut into 12 paper-thin slices

1. To prepare the horseradish cream, combine the first three ingredients in a small bowl. Add pepper to taste and set aside.

2. To prepare the wrap, place a tortilla on the cutting board or counter. Spread each tortilla with 1 tablespoon of horseradish cream. Place 2 slices of roast beef in the center of each wrap, extending the slices across the center to within 1/2 inch from the edge. (The edges need to be left free so that you can roll and wrap the sandwich.) Place 6 cucumber slices on top of the beef, then layer the red onions, 4 sprigs of watercress, and 3 slices of tomato. Roll the wraps, starting from the bottom, tucking in the sides as you go. Cut the wraps in half (on the diagonal if you like) and serve.

Note: Wraps can be made with just about any filling, even leftovers. For example, try wrapping leftovers of the Asparagus, Tofu, Shiitake, and Cashew Stir-Fry on page 281 with a prepackaged salad mix that includes shredded carrots and snow peas. Place strips of grilled chicken or leftover pork tenderloin with some Seven-Vegetable Slaw (page 301).

Yield: 4 wraps; Serving: 1 wrap
Calories: 219; Protein: 16.2 g; Carbohydrate: 27 g; Fiber: 3.9 g; Sodium: 848 mg;
Fat 4.2 g (Sat: 1.3 g, Mono: 4.0 g, Poly: 2.1 g, Trans: 0 g); Cholesterol: 30 mg

General: Nearly 3 milligrams each of minerals zinc and iron. Also provides half a day's supply of vitamin C and generous amounts of vitamins E and A.
Diabetic: Total of 28 grams for carbohydrate counters. Equals 2 very lean meat and 1 1/2 starch exchanges.
Sodium-Restricted: The bulk of the sodium comes from the deli roast beef. Some luncheon meats are made with less salt, but the best way to cut back on sodium is to cook your own roast beef without salt. You can also replace the beef with leftover baked chicken, turkey, or pork. The reduced-fat mayonnaise has 60 milligrams of sodium per tablespoon, so it's not contributing that much to the total.
Pregnant: You might want to follow the instructions above if you're retaining extra fluid. Otherwise, each serving contains 55 milligrams of calcium and 68 micrograms of folate.

Turkey Noodle Casserole

This casserole can easily be made with precooked turkey or leftovers from a holiday meal. Look for the 50 percent wheat noodles (a blend of whole-grain wheat and durum wheat) in health food stores or many large supermarkets. Their flavor is milder than some of the heartier whole-grain pastas and won't overpower the delicate flavors in this casserole.

CASSEROLE

3 tablespoons canola or olive oil

1 garlic clove, minced

1 cup diced celery

1 (8-ounce) package button mushrooms, sliced

$\frac{1}{3}$ cup oat or all-purpose flour

3 cups defatted turkey or chicken broth, preferably low-sodium

$1\frac{1}{2}$ tablespoons chopped fresh or $1\frac{1}{2}$ teaspoons dried thyme

$\frac{1}{2}$ tablespoon chopped fresh or $\frac{1}{2}$ teaspoon dried sage

Coarse salt and freshly ground black pepper to taste

$2\frac{1}{2}$ cups cooked white-meat turkey (about 10 ounces)

1 (10-ounce) package 50 percent wheat noodles (such as Eden Thick
   Kluski Noodles), cooked

Vegetable cooking spray or canola oil

TOPPING

12 slices sesame or plain melba toast, crushed

$\frac{1}{4}$ cup toasted wheat germ

2 tablespoons minced dried onion

1 tablespoon sesame seeds

3 tablespoons canola or olive oil

1. Preheat the oven to 350°F.

2. Place a large nonstick skillet over medium-high heat. Add 1 teaspoon oil and the garlic. Sauté for 30 seconds and add the celery. Continue cooking for 4–5 minutes or until the celery begins to soften. Remove the celery from the pan and add 2 teaspoons oil and the mushrooms; cook for 3–4 minutes or until the mushrooms start to brown and have given up their liquid.

3. Remove the vegetables from the pan and add 2 tablespoons oil to the pan. Stir in the flour and cook for 1 minute. Reduce the heat to medium and gradually add the turkey broth; cook for 8–10 minutes or until thickened, stirring frequently as the mixture thickens. Stir in the thyme and sage, and salt and pepper to taste. Remove from the heat and add the turkey, mushroom mixture, and cooked noodles. Place the mixture in a 9- × 13-inch baking dish lightly coated with cooking spray or oil.

4. Combine the crushed melba toast, wheat germ, dried onion, sesame seeds, and oil; sprinkle the mixture over the casserole and bake at 350° for 25–30 minutes or until bubbly.

Note: For even better flavor, consider buying a skinless turkey breast and cooking it in a bath of water (about 6 cups), fresh herbs, and a splash of white wine. Once the turkey is cooked, reduce the cooking liquid by half and you will have the 3 cups of broth needed for this recipe.

Yield: 8 servings; Serving: about 1½ cups
Calories: 439; Protein: 31.9 g; Carbohydrate: 44 g; Fiber: 5.5 g; Sodium: 367 mg;
Fat 15.2 g (Sat: 1.22 g, Mono: 7.67 g, Poly: 4.31 g, Trans: 0.04 g); Cholesterol: 53 mg

General: Rich in vitamin E and a host of minerals, including iron and zinc.
Diabetic: For carbohydrate counters, total is 44 grams. Equals 3½ lean meat exchanges and 3 starches.
Sodium-Restricted: The canned broth contributes the bulk of sodium to this dish. Switch to low-sodium canned broth or cook turkey and broth from scratch to reduce the sodium. The melba toast contains only 30 milligrams of sodium per slice. But if your sodium is severely limited, you could omit the toast and increase the wheat germ.
Pregnant: Each serving contains 45 milligrams of calcium, 43 micrograms of folate, and 2.6 milligrams of iron.

Pad Thai–Style Fried Rice

One of the most popular menu choices at a Thai restaurant is a noodle dish with Thai spices, shrimp, eggs, and Thai rice noodles. Here's a version of that popular dish made with brown rice, which is easier to find and higher in fiber than the rice noodles. The secret to making a great fried rice is to cook the rice the night before and to use a little bit less liquid than is called for on the package instructions. Rice that's cooked a bit on the "dry" side won't become mushy when stir-fried.

PEANUT SAUCE

2 tablespoons fish sauce or tamari soy sauce

2 tablespoons defatted chicken stock or broth, preferably low-sodium

1 tablespoon ketchup sweetened with fruit juice, or plain ketchup

1 tablespoon natural-style peanut butter

1 tablespoon fresh lime juice

FRIED RICE

3 tablespoons roasted peanut oil or canola oil, divided

2 eggs, lightly beaten

½ cup shredded carrots

2 large garlic cloves, minced

1 teaspoon minced peeled fresh gingerroot

1 cup thinly sliced green onion

½ cup diced red pepper

¼ teaspoon crushed red pepper flakes

4 cups cooked brown rice, chilled

½ pound precooked peeled medium shrimp

10 fresh Thai or regular basil leaves, chopped

¼ cup fresh cilantro, minced

½ cup fresh bean sprouts (optional)

Chopped peanuts (optional)

1. To prepare the peanut sauce, mix together the first five ingredients in a small bowl. Set aside.

2. To prepare the fried rice, place a large nonstick skillet over medium-high heat. Add 1 teaspoon oil and the eggs, stirring to scramble loosely; cook until done, 1–2 minutes. Remove the eggs to a plate. Add 2 teaspoons oil to the skillet with the carrots; cook for 2–3 minutes or until the carrots begin to soften. Remove from the pan. Add the remaining 2 tablespoons oil to the skillet with the garlic, gingerroot, green onion, red pepper, and crushed red pepper flakes. Cook for 1–2 minutes or until the vegetables begin to soften. Reduce the heat to low and add the cooked rice. Cook for 1–2 minutes; stir in the eggs, shrimp, basil, cilantro, and peanut sauce; cook until heated through. Taste for seasoning and add salt if needed. Garnish with the bean sprouts and chopped peanuts, if desired. Serve immediately.

Note: Look for the fish sauce or tamari soy sauce in the Asian section of most supermarkets.

Yield: 6 servings; Serving: About 1 cup
Calories: 303; Protein: 14.9 g; Carbohydrate: 35 g; Fiber: 3.9 g; Sodium: 634 mg;
Fat 11.5 g (Sat: 2.11 g, Mono: 4.89 g, Poly: 3.26 g, Trans: 0 g); Cholesterol: 145 mg

General: This rice dish is rich in antioxidants, including vitamin E, vitamin C, beta-carotene, and sele-nium.
Diabetic: For carbohydrate counters, total is 35 grams. Equals 1 high-fat meat exchange, 2 starch, 1 veg-etable, and ½ fat.
Sodium-Restricted: Most of the sodium is coming from the convenience products (ketchup, chicken broth, peanut butter) used to make the peanut sauce. You can omit the peanut sauce if you'd like and have a more traditional fried rice dish. There will still be plenty of flavor from the herbs and other seasonings.
Pregnant: No special considerations.

Grilled Salmon Steaks with Papaya-Mint Salsa

Salmon is perfectly great just plain off the grill. But this tart-sweet fruit salsa complements the richness of the fatty fish. Make the salsa earlier in the day to allow the flavors to blend. Be sure to cut down on the amount of jalapeño or leave it out altogether if you don't like hot peppers.

SALSA

¾ cup peeled chopped papaya

¼ cup chopped yellow pepper

$^{1}/_{4}$ cup thinly sliced green onion

1 tablespoon chopped pimiento

1 tablespoon fresh mint, chopped

1 tablespoon rice wine vinegar

1 tablespoon fresh lime juice

1 teaspoon grated peeled fresh gingerroot

1 teaspoon minced seeded jalapeño pepper

SALMON

Vegetable cooking spray or oil

4 (5-ounce) salmon steaks or fillets, about 1–1$^{1}/_{4}$ inches thick

Coarse salt and freshly ground black pepper to taste

1. Combine the first nine ingredients in a small bowl. Cover and chill for at least 30 minutes to allow the flavors to blend.

2. Prepare the grill or broiler. Lightly coat the grill or broiler pan with cooking spray or oil to prevent the fish from sticking. Sprinkle both sides of the fish with salt and pepper. Grill or broil the fish 5 minutes on each side or until done. Top the salmon with the salsa and serve.

Yield: 4 servings; Serving: 1 salmon fillet and $^{1}/_{4}$ cup salsa
Calories: 281; Protein: 28.8 g; Carbohydrate: 4.9 g; Fiber: 0.9 g; Sodium: 86 mg;
Fat 15.6 g (Sat: 3.1 g, Mono: 5.5 g, Poly: 5.6 g, Trans: 0 g); Cholesterol: 84 mg

General: The oils from fatty fish are good for the heart. One serving of the salsa provides more than 80 percent of the recommended amount of vitamin C.
Diabetic: For carbohydrate counters, total is 5 grams. Equals 4 lean fat meat exchanges, 1 vegetable, and 1 fat.
Sodium-Restricted: The sodium figures are without added salt. They can't be lowered. One serving has 636 milligrams of potassium.
Pregnant: Fatty fish like salmon are rich in n-3 fats, particularly the type of n-3 fat (DHA) that aids in early brain development of infants. Each serving contains 34 milligrams of calcium and 57 micrograms of folate.

Pork Tenderloin with Pistachio-Gremolata Crust *(FAST FIX)*

Typically served with osso buco, gremolata is a mixture of garlic, lemon, and fresh parsley. Here we've added some pistachios and bread crumbs to the mix to build in extra flavor and a little crunch to the crust. A little of the gremolata is then mixed into canned white beans to offer a simple side dish to the pork.

2 garlic cloves, minced

1$^{1}/_{2}$ tablespoons finely grated lemon rind (zest of 1–2 lemons)

$^3/_4$ cup fresh parsley leaves

3 tablespoons pistachio nuts, shelled

1 (1-ounce) slice hearty whole-wheat bread

$^1/_2$ teaspoon coarse salt

1 tablespoon olive oil

1 (1-pound) pork tenderloin

1 egg white, lightly beaten

Vegetable cooking spray or olive oil

1 (15-ounce) can white beans, rinsed and drained

1 tablespoon red wine vinegar

1 tablespoon defatted chicken stock or broth, preferably low-sodium

Parsley sprigs (optional)

1. Preheat the oven to 350°F.

2. Combine the first six ingredients in a food processor and process until crumbly. Add the oil and pulse to mix. Divide the mixture in half and set both portions aside.

3. Trim the fat from the pork. Dip the pork in the egg white; dredge in one-half of the reserved gremolata–bread crumb mixture. Place the pork on a nonstick baking sheet lightly coated with cooking spray or oil. Bake at 350°F for 20–25 minutes or until a meat thermometer registers 160°F. Cover with foil and let rest 5 minutes.

4. Warm the beans on the stove or in the microwave. Stir the vinegar, chicken broth, and remaining gremolata into the beans. Taste for seasoning and add salt if needed. Slice the pork and serve over the white beans. Garnish with parsley sprigs, if desired.

Note: Be sure to use a good-quality, firm-textured canned bean for this dish, as the mushy texture of some products makes for a less than attractive presentation. In general, organic varieties tend to be firmer textured.

Yield: 4 servings; Serving: 3 slices tenderloin and $^1/_2$ cup beans
Calories: 298; Protein: 30.6 g; Carbohydrate: 19.4 g; Fiber: 5.9 g; Sodium: 649 mg;
Fat 13 g (Sat: 2.98 g, Mono: 7.25 g, Poly: 1.42 g, Trans: 0.06 g); Cholesterol: 75 mg

General: Provides nearly one-third of the requirement for iron. Rich in zinc.
Diabetic: For carbohydrate counters, total is 19 grams. Equals 4 lean meat exchanges and 1 starch exchange. Omit the beans and you'll have just 4 meats.
Sodium-Restricted: Pork tenderloin, like other meats, is very low in sodium. The sodium in this dish is due mainly to the added salt, which can easily be omitted, and the canned beans.
Pregnant: Contains 88 milligrams of calcium and 39 micrograms of folate.

Spicy Shrimp and Peanut Noodle Salad

Typically, this Asian noodle salad is made with soba (buckwheat) noodles. Here we've substituted whole-wheat spaghetti noodles for a little extra fiber. The change is hardly noticeable, since the flavors in the spicy peanut sauce are the most predominant. Don't be put off by the ingredient list; most of the items are seasonings that can be quickly measured and mixed together for the sauce. To save time, buy precooked shrimp and precut veggies so the only cooking you'll be doing is boiling a few noodles.

PEANUT SAUCE

2 garlic cloves, minced

2 teaspoons minced peeled fresh gingerroot

3 tablespoons natural chunky-style peanut butter

2 tablespoons tamari soy sauce

2 tablespoons rice wine vinegar

2 tablespoons water

2 tablespoons sesame oil

1–2 teaspoons chili garlic sauce

SALAD

1 pound peeled cooked medium shrimp

1 cup julienned red pepper

1 cup shredded carrots

1/4 pound snow peas, trimmed and cut in half

1 cup sliced green onion

1/4 cup fresh cilantro, chopped

4 cups cooked whole-wheat spaghetti or soba (buckwheat) noodles

Chopped peanuts (optional)

1. Whisk together the first eight ingredients in a small bowl and set aside.

2. Combine the shrimp and remaining ingredients (except for the noodles) in a large serving bowl. Add the noodles and peanut sauce and toss gently to mix. Sprinkle with chopped peanuts, if desired. Serve at room temperature.

Note: The salad is versatile: switch to chicken or pork instead of shrimp or just leave the meat out altogether for a vegetarian noodle dish. Look for the chili garlic sauce in the Asian section of most supermarkets. Brand names vary, but the basic ingredients are similar from sauce to sauce.

Yield: 6 servings; Serving: 1½ cups
Calories: 337; Protein: 27.7 g; Carbohydrate: 33.7 g; Fiber: 6.8 g; Sodium: 545 mg;
Fat 10.9 g (Sat: 1.68 g, Mono: 4.17 g, Poly: 4.05 g, Trans: 0 g); Cholesterol: 144 mg

General: One serving delivers more than 75 percent of the recommended amount of vitamin C. Also rich in two other antioxidants: beta-carotene and vitamin E.
Diabetic: For carbohydrate counters, total is 34 grams. Equals 3 lean meat exchanges, 2 starch, and ½ vegetable.
Sodium-Restricted: The bulk of the sodium here comes from the soy sauce. If you switch to low-sodium tamari soy sauce or low-sodium soy sauce, sodium levels will drop. Also, 1 serving of this salad has 456 milligrams of potassium.
Pregnant: You might want to switch to low-sodium soy sauce if you're retaining water. Each serving contains 86 milligrams of calcium, 34 micrograms of folate, and 4 milligrams of iron.

California Chicken Salad (FAST FIX)

This cool summer salad is very versatile; substitute whole-wheat couscous for the bulgur if you'd like a milder flavor, and vary the greens (arugula instead of spinach). Leave out the chicken for a vegetarian meal.

LEMON-BASIL VINAIGRETTE

1 tablespoon chopped fresh or 1 teaspoon dried basil

¼ cup extra-virgin olive oil

⅓ cup fresh lemon juice

¼ teaspoon garlic powder

Coarse salt and freshly ground black pepper to taste

SALAD

1 cup bulgur

1 cup boiling water

2 cups chopped fresh spinach

1 cup roasted chicken, shredded (about 4 ounces)

1 medium avocado, peeled and chopped (about 1 cup)

¼ cup thinly sliced green onion

¼ cup fresh parsley, chopped

12 Kalamata olives, pitted and quartered

1. Whisk together the first five ingredients in a small bowl to make the vinaigrette.

2. Place the bulgur in a large bowl and cover with boiling water. Let stand for 30 minutes or until the liquid is completely absorbed. Stir in the spinach and remaining ingredients. Add the vinaigrette and toss gently. Serve at room temperature.

Yield: 8 cups, 5 servings; Serving: about 1½ cups
Calories: 355; Protein: 19.7 g; Carbohydrate: 34 g; Fiber: 10.6 g; Sodium: 51 mg;
Fat 17.2 g (Sat: 3.19 g, Mono: 7.42 g, Poly: 1.66 g, Trans: 0.08 g); Cholesterol: 38 mg

General: This salad is rich in a trio of antioxidant vitamins: A, E, and C.
Diabetic: For carbohydrate counters, total is 34 grams. Equals 2 medium-fat meat exchanges, 2 breads, 1 vegetable, and ½ fat.
Sodium-Restricted: The sodium figures are calculated without added salt (in the vinaigrette). Add salt as allowed in your diet.
Pregnant: Each serving contains 38 milligrams of calcium, 42 micrograms of folate, and 2 milligrams of iron.

VEGETARIAN ENTRÉES

Veggie Burgers

Serve these burgers with the Spicy Sweet Potato Fries (page 308) for a colorful and satisfying meal. The secret to making burgers that don't crumble is twofold. First, you'll need to chill the vegetable mixture so it will hold its shape. Next, pan-fry the patties in hot oil so that the outside crust becomes crispy.

½ cup bulgur

½ cup boiling water

2 tablespoons olive or canola oil, divided

3 garlic cloves, minced

½ cup minced red onion

1½ teaspoons ground cumin

1 teaspoon dried oregano

2 tablespoons chopped walnuts

½ cup chopped fresh spinach

1 (15-ounce) can black beans, drained

2 tablespoons dry sherry or white wine vinegar

Coarse salt and freshly ground black pepper to taste

1. Place the bulgur in a small bowl. Add the boiling water and let stand 20–25 minutes.

2. Heat 2 teaspoons oil in a nonstick skillet over medium heat. Add the garlic and sauté for 1 minute. Stir in the red onion and sauté for 4–5 minutes or until the onion begins to soften. Stir in the cumin, oregano, and walnuts; cook 45 seconds. Add the spinach and cook 30 seconds or until the spinach is wilted.

3. Combine the beans and vinegar in a medium bowl. Mash well with a fork. Stir in the bulgur and onion-spinach mixture and mix until well blended. Taste the mixture for seasoning and add salt and pepper if desired. Cover and place the bowl in the refrigerator for at least 1 hour.

4. Heat the remaining 4 teaspoons of oil in a large nonstick skillet. Remove the bean mixture from the refrigerator and quickly shape the mixture into 6 equal patties. Place the patties in a skillet and cook for 3 minutes on each side or until hot.

Yield: 6 burgers; Serving: 1 burger
Calories: 158: Protein 5.9 g; Carbohydrate: 20 g; Fiber: 6.3 g; Sodium: 223 mg;
Fat 6.8 g (Sat: 0.78 g, Mono: 3.69 g, Poly: 1.70 g, Trans: 0.05 g); Cholesterol: 0 mg

General: No special considerations.
Diabetic: For carbohydrate counters, total is 20 grams. Equals 1 starch exchange, 1 vegetable, and 1 fat.
Sodium-Restricted: Figures are without added salt. The high sodium tab comes from the canned black beans. Rinsing the beans will help drop sodium levels a bit, but for a significant cut, you'll need to cook the beans from scratch.
Pregnant: If you're retaining water, you may want to follow the instructions above.

Mediterranean Vegetable Salad

The chickpeas (garbanzo beans) help boost the protein of this all-vegetable salad and make it satisfying for a main dish. Consider adding whole-grain pasta to create a pasta salad. Or serve the salad over couscous or bulgur for a more filling meal.

VINAIGRETTE

1/2 cup fresh basil leaves, chopped

1/4 cup balsamic vinegar

1 1/2 tablespoons Dijon mustard

2 teaspoons grated lemon rind

Coarse salt and freshly ground black pepper to taste

3 tablespoons extra-virgin olive oil

SALAD

12 ounces trimmed portobello mushrooms, sliced 1/4-inch thick

1 cup water-packed artichoke hearts, quartered

1 small red onion, cut into thin rings

1 medium yellow squash, cut lengthwise (about 2 cups)

1 cup julienned red pepper

1 (15-ounce) can chickpeas, rinsed and drained

1. To prepare the vinaigrette, combine the first six ingredients in a small bowl. Whisk in the oil.

2. Combine the mushrooms and the next five ingredients in a medium bowl. Pour the vinaigrette over the mushroom mixture; toss gently to coat. Cover and chill for at least 2 hours to give the vegetables time to marinate. Serve chilled or at room temperature.

Yield: 6 cups, 4 servings; Serving: 1½ cups
Calories: 316; Protein: 11.3 g; Carbohydrate: 41 g; Fiber: 12.5 g; Sodium: 1026 mg;
Fat 13.8 g (Sat: 1.6 g, Mono: 9.12 g, Poly: 2.60 g, Trans: 0 g); Cholesterol: 0 mg

General: Contains more than a third of the recommended amount of iron, with small amounts of calcium, zinc, and vitamin E.
Diabetic: For carbohydrate counters, total is 41 grams. Equals 2 starch exchanges, 2 vegetables, 1½ fats, and ½ high-fat meat.
Sodium-Restricted: Figures are without added salt. The high sodium tab comes from the canned chickpeas and the canned artichoke hearts. Rinsing these canned products will help drop sodium levels, but for a significant cut, you'll need to cook the chickpeas from scratch.
Pregnant: If you're retaining water, you may want to follow the instructions above.

Asparagus, Tofu, Shiitake, and Cashew Stir-Fry (FAST FIX)

Roasted peanut oil has an intensely nutty flavor that adds something special to this stir-fry. It can be found in most large supermarkets or health food stores. Tamari soy sauce is a special variety that has a more concentrated soy flavor. It can be found in most supermarkets in both regular and low-sodium varieties. Consider cooking up a larger batch of the brown rice and then saving leftovers for the Pad Thai–Style Fried Rice on page 273.

¼ cup raw cashews

2 tablespoons roasted peanut oil or canola oil

½ tablespoon minced peeled fresh ginger

2 garlic cloves, minced

½ pound thin fresh asparagus, trimmed and cut on the diagonal into 3-inch lengths

½ cup shiitake mushrooms (about 4 ounces), sliced

1 (16-ounce) package firm or extra-firm water-packed tofu, drained and cut into 1-inch cubes

½ cup vegetable stock or broth, divided

2 tablespoons tamari soy sauce

1 tablespoon rice wine vinegar

1 tablespoon cornstarch

2²/₃ cups hot cooked brown or brown basmati rice

1. Place a large wok or nonstick skillet over medium-high heat and add the cashews and 1 teaspoon of roasted peanut oil. Stir-fry for 2–3 minutes or until nuts are lightly browned, stirring occasionally to prevent scorching. Remove nuts from pan and set aside.

2. Add 2 teaspoons of oil to the pan with the ginger and garlic and stir-fry for 45 seconds. Add the asparagus and stir-fry for 3–4 minutes or until tender-crisp. Remove the asparagus mixture to a plate and keep warm. Repeat the procedure with the mushrooms and 1 teaspoon of oil and stir-fry for 2–3 minutes. Remove the mushrooms to the plate with the asparagus and keep warm. Add 2 teaspoons of oil to the pan and stir-fry the tofu for 3–4 minutes until the cubes are lightly browned. Remove the tofu to the plate with the vegetables and keep warm. Add 6 tablespoons of the broth, the soy sauce, and the vinegar to the pan; cook over medium-low heat for 2–3 minutes or until hot. Stir together the remaining 2 tablespoons of broth and the cornstarch. Add to the pan and cook for 1 minute or until the mixture thickens. Return the tofu and vegetables to the pan and toss gently in the sauce to reheat. Serve over cooked brown rice.

Yield: 4 servings; Serving: 1¹/₃ cups stir-fry mixture, ²/₃ cup brown rice
Calories: 420; Protein: 19.1 g; Carbohydrate: 49 g; Fiber: 7.2 g; Sodium: 604 mg;
Fat 17.04 g (Sat: 2.87 g, Mono: 6.96 g, Poly: 6.08 g, Trans: 0 g); Cholesterol: 0 mg

General: No special considerations. If you'd like to cut the calories in this dish, you can switch to reduced-fat or "lite" tofu. Its delicate texture makes it a bit more difficult to stir-fry, but if you're careful, it will work.
Diabetic: For carbohydrate counters, total is 49 grams. Since tofu is high in protein like meat but also rich in carbohydrate (soybeans are a legume), the exchanges are trickier to calculate. This dish roughly equals 2 high-fat meats, 2 starches, and 1 "other" carbohydrate.
Sodium-Restricted: By nature, stir-fry dishes are high in sodium owing to the liberal use of soy sauce and broth. To lower the sodium levels, buy the low-sodium variety of tamari or plain soy sauce and use a salt-free stock.
Pregnant: If you buy the tofu processed with calcium, each serving contains 241 milligrams of calcium. Also contains 49 micrograms of folate and 4.1 milligrams of iron.

Pesto Corn Spaghetti (FAST FIX)

Pesto and pasta are always a perfect pair. But this time the pasta is a whole-grain one made with corn. And the match is extraordinary flavor-wise. But there's one little problem. Corn pasta is very delicate and tends to break apart easily; it's best cooked a few minutes less than the package instructs. Even so, the noodles tend to break into smaller pieces. If that doesn't suit you, opt for the sturdier whole-wheat spaghetti noodle with this recipe.

4 cups hot cooked corn spaghetti or whole-wheat spaghetti

BASIL-ALMOND PESTO

3 cups firmly packed basil leaves

1 garlic clove, minced (about 1 teaspoon)

2 tablespoons almonds

$\frac{1}{4}$ teaspoon grated lemon rind

3 tablespoons olive oil

$\frac{1}{4}$ cup defatted chicken stock or broth, preferably low-sodium

Coarse salt and freshly ground black pepper to taste

1. Place the basil and the next three ingredients into a food processor and blend to mix. Slowly add the olive oil to the mixture until it forms a paste. Add the chicken broth, 1 tablespoon at a time, until the paste is moist. Taste for seasoning and add salt and pepper as desired.

2. Gently toss the hot spaghetti noodles with the pesto and serve immediately.

Note: If the pesto isn't moist enough to mix with the noodles, add more chicken broth or olive oil to moisten. Keep in mind that the pesto can be made in advance and kept for several days in the refrigerator. Place it in a small ramekin and drizzle a little olive oil over the top; cover tightly with foil.

Yield: 4 cups; Serving: 1 cup
Calories: 355; Protein: 0.89 g; Carbohydrate: 26 g; Fiber: 7.5 g; Sodium: 42 mg;
Fat 17 g (Sat: 2.15 g, Mono: 11.66 g, Poly: 2.21 g, Trans: 0.14 g); Cholesterol: 0 mg

General: A small serving of this dish is very filling, owing mainly to the fact that corn pasta has 5 grams of fiber in a 1-cup of serving; most regular pasta contains none.
Diabetic: For carbohydrate counters, total is 26 grams. Equals 2 bread exchanges and 2½ fats.
Sodium-Restricted: Figures for sodium are calculated without added salt. The major contribution to the sodium in this dish is the small amount of reduced-sodium chicken broth used in the pesto recipe. Use salt-free chicken stock instead.
Pregnant: No special considerations.

Portobello and Caramelized Onion Pizza

Too often pizzas are smothered with cheese, usually a bland mozzarella, and the flavors of vegetables and delicate toppings are muted. Here the vegetables dominate, a pairing of savory-sweet caramelized onions and rich, meaty-flavored portobello mushrooms. A small sprinkling of Asiago cheese holds everything together. The crust is made from part wheat and part white flour with a few whole grains thrown in for texture. Buy those grains (oat groats, flaxseed) at any health food store.

WHOLE-WHEAT PIZZA CRUST

2 teaspoons active dry yeast

1 cup warm water (105°F–115°F)

2 tablespoons olive oil

1 teaspoon coarse salt

1¼ cups all-purpose flour

²/₃ cup whole-wheat flour

¼ cup oat groats, toasted

2 tablespoons flaxseed, ground, or 3 tablespoons flaxseed meal

TOPPINGS

2 tablespoons olive oil, divided

2 cups sliced white or yellow onion

Coarse salt and freshly ground black pepper to taste

1 (6-ounce) package sliced portobello mushrooms, cut into quarters

1 (4-ounce) package sliced mushrooms

1 large garlic clove, minced

2 tablespoons fresh parsley, chopped

1 tablespoon fresh thyme leaves

1 tablespoon sherry vinegar

Cornmeal for dusting

2 tablespoons freshly grated Asiago or Parmesan cheese

1. To prepare the crust, dissolve the yeast in warm water in a mixing bowl; let stand 5 minutes. Add the oil, salt, 1 cup of all-purpose flour, and remaining crust ingredients; stir until a soft dough forms. Turn the dough out onto a lightly floured surface. Knead until smooth and elastic (8–10 minutes), adding enough of the remaining all-purpose flour, 1 tablespoon at a time, to prevent the dough from sticking to your hands. The dough will feel slightly tacky.

2. Place the dough in a large bowl coated lightly with cooking spray or oil, turning once to coat the top. Cover with plastic wrap and let rise in a warm place (85°F), free from drafts, for 30 minutes or until doubled in size.

3. To prepare the toppings, heat 1 tablespoon oil in a large nonstick skillet over medium heat. Add the onions and cook for 5 minutes, stirring occasionally to prevent scorching. Add salt and pepper to taste. Reduce the heat to low and cook for 20 minutes or until the onions are soft and golden. Remove the onions to a plate and keep warm. Add the remaining tablespoon of oil to the skillet and turn the heat to medium high. Add the mushrooms and sauté for 5–8 minutes or until the mushrooms are nicely browned. Remove from the heat and stir in the next four ingredients.

4. Preheat the oven to 450°F; insert the pizza stone if you are using one.

5. Punch the dough down; cover and let rest 5 minutes. Roll the dough into a 12-inch circle on a floured surface. Place the dough on a pizza peel or baking sheet sprinkled with cornmeal. Crimp the edges of the dough with your fingers to form a rim. Cover and let rise for 10 minutes.

6. Spread the caramelized onions over the pizza crust, leaving a $^1/_2$-inch border; top with the mushroom mixture. Sprinkle with the cheese. Bake at 450°F (on either a pizza stone or baking sheet) for 10 minutes or until the crust is brown. Remove the pizza to the cutting board and cut into 6 slices.

Note: Toast oat groats just as you would any nut; place oat groats on a small baking sheet and toast in oven at 350°F for 16–20 minutes or until lightly browned, checking periodically to make sure they don't scorch. Remove from oven and cool. Flaxseed can be ground in a clean coffee grinder or purchased already ground.

Yield: 6 slices; Serving: 1 slice
Calories: 296; Protein: 8.7 g; Carbohydrate: 42 g; Fiber: 4.7 g; Sodium: 326 mg;
Fat 11.6 g (Sat: 1.72 g, Mono: 6.89 g, Poly: 1.19 g, Trans: 0.09 g); Cholesterol: 2 mg

General: One slice contains 20 percent of the requirement for vitamin E as well as generous amounts of many different minerals, including iron, zinc, selenium, and magnesium.
Diabetic: For carbohydrate counters, total is 42 grams. Equals 3 starch exchanges, 2$^1/_2$ vegetable, and 1$^1/_2$ fats.
Sodium-Restricted: The amount of cheese is so small that it isn't making much contribution to the sodium level. The bulk of the sodium comes via the salt added to the crust. Leave that salt out and the sodium levels will decline significantly.
Pregnant: Each slice contains 97 micrograms of folate.

Onion-Crusted Tofu-Steak Sandwich

Pan-fried tofu steaks make a delicious and quick sandwich filling. Splurge with a nice whole-grain bakery bun and top with a buttery lettuce such as Boston, a thick slice of fresh tomato, and a quick flavored mayonnaise spread that's created from store-bought mayonnaise. The Seven-Vegetable Slaw on page 301 makes a nice accompaniment for this sandwich. In fact, you can omit the aioli and top the tofu with slaw for another version of this sandwich.

LEMON-CILANTRO AIOLI

$\frac{1}{3}$ cup canola or soybean oil mayonnaise

2 tablespoons fresh cilantro, minced

1 small garlic clove, minced

1 teaspoon sesame oil

$\frac{1}{4}$ teaspoon grated lemon rind

SANDWICH

1 (16-ounce) package extra-firm tofu, cut crosswise into 12 slices

$\frac{1}{4}$ cup oat or all-purpose flour

$\frac{1}{4}$ cup minced dried onion

2 tablespoons sesame seeds

$\frac{1}{2}$ teaspoon paprika

Coarse salt and freshly ground black pepper to taste

1 large egg, lightly beaten

2 tablespoons water

2 tablespoons roasted peanut oil or canola oil

6 whole-grain sandwich buns

$1\frac{1}{2}$ cups shredded butterhead (Boston/Bibb) lettuce

6 ($\frac{1}{2}$-inch thick) slices ripe yellow or red tomato

1. Combine the first five ingredients in a small bowl and set aside to let the flavors blend.

2. Place the tofu slices on double thickness of paper towels and let sit for 5 minutes.

3. Combine the next six ingredients (flour through pepper) in a shallow bowl. Place the egg in another shallow bowl and whisk in the water. Dip the tofu slices into the egg mixture and then dredge one at a time in the flour mixture.

4. Heat 1 tablespoon oil in a large nonstick skillet over medium heat. Add 6 tofu slices and sauté for 2–3 minutes on each side or until lightly browned. Remove from the pan. Repeat with the remaining oil and tofu. Place 2 tofu slices on the bottom half of a bun. Top with $\frac{1}{4}$ cup lettuce and a tomato slice. Spread 1 tablespoon aioli on each top bun half and place the bun over the tomato. Serve immediately.

Note: Tofu packed in water makes the best tofu "steak." The texture is firmer, which makes it much easier to work with when breading and dipping. You can certainly use the silken or reduced-fat tofu in this recipe; you'll just need to be more careful since its delicate nature causes it to break apart more easily.

Yield: 6 sandwiches; Serving: 1 sandwich
Calories: 420; Protein: 20.3 g; Carbohydrate: 33.7 g; Fiber: 6 g; Sodium: 344 mg;
Fat 18.1 g (Sat: 3.1 g, Mono: 9.9 g, Poly: 8.1 g, Trans: 0 g); Cholesterol: 40 mg

General: Tofu, which is made from soybeans, is more than 50 percent fat by weight, which explains why this sandwich carries a lot of fat. But keep in mind it's a good kind of fat that's healthy to the heart and body. However, if you're looking for a lower-calorie version of this sandwich, you can switch to the reduced-fat or "lite" tofu, keeping in mind that it is much more delicate to handle.
Diabetic: For carbohydrate counters, total is 34 grams. Equals 2 medium-fat meat exchanges, 2 starch, and 1½ fat.
Sodium-Restricted: The sodium figures are without added salt. The lion's share of sodium comes from two ingredients—the bun and the mayonnaise. Buy a salt-free sandwich bun and that will reduce the sodium levels considerably. The reduced-fat canola oil mayonnaise contributes only 60 milligrams of sodium per tablespoon.
Pregnant: Some tofus are processed with calcium; others aren't. If you use the former, this sandwich will contribute more than half a day's supply of this bone-strengthening mineral. The sandwich also provides more than 10 milligrams of iron.

Roasted Walnut & Brown Rice Loaf

Brown rice comes in all different colors. And Lundberg brown rice blends, since they include so many colors and varieties, give a nice appearance to this meatless loaf. To make the bread crumbs, place a slice of leftover bread into a food processor and pulse until crumbly.

1 cup brown rice blend or brown rice

2 cups mushroom broth (such as Pacific) or vegetable broth

½ cup (½ ounce) dried porcini or shiitake mushroom pieces, diced

3 tablespoons olive oil, divided

1 teaspoon salt, divided

2 cups chopped walnuts

1 cup finely chopped onion

¼ cup finely chopped celery

2 cloves garlic, minced

1 cup fresh whole grain bread crumbs

¼ cup chopped fresh parsley

2 teaspoons chopped fresh or ½ teaspoon dried thyme

3 eggs, lightly beaten

Preheat oven to 375°F.

1. Combine rice, broth, mushrooms, 1 tablespoon of oil, and $^{1}/_{2}$ teaspoon salt in a large saucepan. Bring mixture to a boil; cover and simmer 45 minutes or until rice is tender. Place rice in large bowl and let cool.

2. Place walnuts on a baking sheet and roast at 375°F for 3–5 minutes or until they begin to brown lightly. Watch carefully to make sure nuts do not burn. Remove from oven and finely chop.

3. Pour remaining 2 tablespoons oil into a large nonstick skillet and warm over medium heat. Add onions and celery and sauté for 5–7 minutes or until tender. Stir in remaining $^{1}/_{2}$ teaspoon salt and garlic and cook 1 minute. Remove from heat and stir in bread crumbs, parsley, and thyme. Add bread crumb mixture to cooled rice. Stir in eggs and pat mixture into an 8- × 8-inch loaf pan coated with a small amount of olive oil. Bake at 375°F for 40–50 minutes or until loaf is firm. Remove from oven and let cool in pan for 10 minutes before slicing.

Yield: 1 loaf, 12 slices; Serving: 1 slice
Calories: 266; Protein: 7.3 g; Carbohydrate: 20.3 g; Fiber: 3 g; Sodium: 234 mg;
Fat: 18.4 g (Sat: 2.20 g, Mono: 5.03 g, Poly: 10.17 g, Trans 0 g); Cholesterol 53 mg

General: Walnuts are a good plant source of omega-3 fats.
Diabetic: For carbohydrate counters, total is 20 grams. Equals 1 bread/starch exchange, $^{1}/_{2}$ lean meat exchange, 1 vegetable exchange, and 3 fat exchanges.
Sodium-Restricted: Most of the sodium comes from the added salt; cut down on it or replace it with a salt substitute.
Pregnant: Contains 38 micrograms folate and 2 milligrams of iron.

Winter Squash with Pecan Stuffing

Carnival squash are the same shape and size as the acorn variety, but the skin is an attractive speckled green or speckled orange color. If you can't find it, use acorn or any variety of winter squash.

    2 (14-ounce) carnival or acorn squash
    1$^{1}/_{2}$ tablespoons olive oil, divided
    1 cup coarsely chopped yellow or white onion
    1 teaspoon coarse salt, divided
    1 cup cooked brown rice
    $^{1}/_{2}$ cup chopped pecans, toasted
    2 tablespoons roasted sunflower seeds

¹/₄ cup dried cherries

¹/₄ cup dried currants

3 tablespoons chopped fresh parsley

2 teaspoons finely chopped fresh sage

¹/₄ teaspoon fresh ground pepper

1. Preheat oven to 375°F.

2. Cut squash in half from stem to tip and scoop out seeds; brush cut side lightly with 1 teaspoon of oil and place, cut side down, onto baking sheet. Bake at 375°F for 30–35 minutes or until squash is wrinkled and soft. Scoop out most of squash flesh, leaving a thin border next to skin; mash with fork.

3. Heat remaining oil in a large nonstick skillet over medium heat. Add onion and cook 4–5 minutes until it begins to soften. Stir in ¹/₂ teaspoon salt. Add rice and cook 3–4 minutes or until warmed through. Stir in squash, ¹/₂ teaspoon salt, and remaining ingredients and cook for 4–6 minutes.

4. To serve, spoon squash-rice mixture into squash halves, pressing down with the back of the spoon to pack tightly. Serve immediately.

Yield: 4 servings; Serving: 1 stuffed squash half
Calories: 379; Protein: 6.2 g; Carbohydrate: 52.3 g; Fiber: 7.8 g; Sodium: 482 mg;
Fat: 18.5 g (Sat: 2 g, Mono: 10.4, Poly: 5.3 g, Trans: 0 g; Cholesterol: 0 mg

General: This dish is rich in antioxidants, particularly vitamin E and beta-carotene.
Diabetic: For carbohydrate counters, total is 53 grams. Equals 1 bread/starch exchange, 1 fruit exchange, 4 vegetable exchanges, and 3 ¹/₂ fat exchanges.
Sodium-Restricted: Contains nearly 1 gram of potassium, a mineral important to healthy blood pressure.
Pregnant: Contains 61 micrograms folate and nearly 3 milligrams of iron.

SOUPS AND STEWS

Curried Winter Squash Soup (FAST FIX)

This version of winter squash soup is a snap to make. Start with frozen winter squash and add some new flavors—apple and curry—to make a delicious but quick entrée. Serve with a crusty whole-grain bread and a mixed green salad for a complete cold-weather meal. If you don't have any homemade stock on hand, opt for reduced-sodium canned broth or reduced-sodium powdered stock; regular canned or powdered stocks are extremely salty. It's much better to start with a lower-sodium stock and add salt to taste.

2 tablespoons olive oil

2 cups coarsely chopped onion

1–2 teaspoons minced peeled fresh gingerroot

1 tablespoon curry powder

2¹/₂ cups defatted chicken stock or broth, preferably low-sodium

1 cup apple cider or apple juice

2 (14-ounce) boxes frozen mashed winter squash, thawed

¹/₄ cup unsweetened applesauce

Coarse salt to taste

1. Place a large soup pot or Dutch oven over medium heat. Add the oil and onion; sauté for 12–18 minutes or until the onion has softened. Stir in the ginger and curry and cook for 1 minute, stirring constantly. Add the broth, apple cider, winter squash, and applesauce. Bring the soup to a boil, reduce the heat, and simmer for 5–10 minutes to blend the flavors.

2. Place a small amount of the soup in a blender or food processor, and carefully purée on low speed, leaving the center part of the cover off so that steam can escape. Continue puréeing the soup in small batches until the mixture is smooth. Return the soup to the pot and keep warm until ready to serve. Taste for seasoning and add salt as desired.

Note: Soup will be thick. If you like a thinner soup, add more chicken stock.

Yield: 6 cups; Serving: 1¹/₂ cups
Calories: 192; Protein: 4.8 g; Carbohydrate: 32 g; Fiber: 5.7 g; Sodium: 391 mg;
Fat 6.9 g (Sat: 0.93 g, Mono: 7.83 g, Poly: 0.61 g, Trans: 0.07 g); Cholesterol: 0 mg

General: This soup is an excellent source of fiber and vitamin A.
Diabetic: Equals 1¹/₂ bread exchanges, 1 vegetable, and 1 fat. Cook the onions in a nonstick pot with vegetable cooking spray if you want to omit the fat serving.
Sodium-Restricted: Sodium figures are calculated without added salt and using reduced-sodium chicken stock. To reduce sodium further, you'll need to use a salt-free stock.
Pregnant: No special considerations.

Chipotle Chicken Chili

Substitute 2 (15-ounce) cans of any variety of cooked legume—black bean, soybean, red kidney bean—for the dried beans if you're short on time. But do try the anasazi bean version at least once; it will be worth the extra effort. This ancient bean variety has a beautiful speckled appearance and a hint of sweetness not found in other dried beans. Chipotle peppers in adobo sauce are large, dried, and smoked jalapeño peppers rehydrated in a tomato-vinegar-based sauce. They lend a wonderful smoky flavor and a small amount of heat to this chili. You'll find them in the Mexican food section of the supermarket. Leave out the chicken if you'd like a vegetarian chili.

- 1¹/₂ cups dried anasazi beans, soaked overnight
- 1 cup dried white kidney beans (cannellini), soaked overnight
- 2 tablespoons canola oil
- 2 garlic cloves, chopped
- 1 bay leaf
- 1 tablespoon paprika
- 1 tablespoon chili powder
- 1 tablespoon dried oregano
- 1 teaspoon cumin seed
- 1 teaspoon ground cumin
- 2 cups coarsely chopped white onion
- 2 cups coarsely chopped green pepper
- 4 cups water
- 1 chipotle pepper in adobo sauce, finely chopped
- 1 (14.5-ounce) can diced tomatoes
- 1 (28-ounce) can whole tomatoes, chopped with liquid
- 1 cup cooked or canned hominy, drained
- 8 raw chicken tenders (about 12 ounces), cut into 2-inch pieces
- ¹/₄ cup fresh cilantro, chopped
- Coarse salt to taste
- Chopped white onion and chopped fresh cilantro, mixed together (optional)

1. Soak the beans overnight. (Or use the quick-soak method: Place the beans in a stockpot and cover with water. Bring the mixture to a boil; boil for 1 minute. Remove from the heat and let stand 1 hour. Drain the beans and proceed to step 2.)

2. Heat the canola oil in a large soup pot or Dutch oven over medium heat. Add the garlic and the next six ingredients (bay leaf through cumin). Sauté for 1 minute. Stir in the onion and green pepper; sauté for 3–5 minutes. Add the beans, water, and chipotle pepper. Bring the mixture to a boil; reduce the heat and simmer for 60–75 minutes or until the beans are soft but still somewhat

firm. Add the diced and chopped tomatoes and their liquid. Stir in the hominy, chicken, and cilantro and simmer uncovered for 15–20 minutes or until the chicken is cooked. Add salt to taste and garnish with a mixture of chopped raw onion and cilantro, if desired.

Note: Leftovers will freeze well; freeze chili without chopped raw onion–cilantro garnish.

Yield: 9 servings; Serving: 1½ cups
Calories: 309; Protein: 22.4 g; Carbohydrate: 46.3 g; Fiber: 13.8 g; Sodium: 315 mg;
Fat 4.9 g (Sat: 0.47 g, Mono: 3.67 g, Poly: 1.38 g, Trans: 0.01 g); Cholesterol: 22 mg

General: This chili is rich in vitamin A, beta-carotene, iron, and zinc. One serving also offers a full day's supply of vitamin C.
Diabetic: Equals 1½ lean meat exchanges, 2½ bread, and 1 vegetable. If you need more meat servings at the meal, consider adding more chicken or a small amount of reduced-fat cheese.
Sodium-Restricted: The sodium figure is without added salt. Switch to salt-free canned tomatoes to lower the sodium level further.
Pregnant: Each serving contains 140 milligrams of calcium and 5 milligrams of iron.

Garlicky Six-Bean Soup

For garlic lovers, this soup has a double punch of garlic. Garlic is cooked with the beans and then stirred in raw just before serving. Omit the raw garlic if you're not keen on the pungent flavor. Creating your own mix of six different bean types makes for a unique and attractive soup. But if you'd rather buy one of those prepackaged bean soup mixes, that will work just fine.

2½ cups assorted dried beans (lima, black, cranberry, red, anasazi, northern, or red or yellow lentils)

2 tablespoons olive or canola oil

2 cups chopped white or yellow onion

1 cup chopped fennel or celery

1 cup chopped carrot

4 garlic cloves, minced

2 bay leaves

1 tablespoon chopped fresh or 1 teaspoon dried thyme

½ teaspoon freshly ground black pepper

2 tablespoons soy sauce

¼ cup tomato paste

4 cups vegetable stock, preferably low-sodium

Coarse salt to taste

2 garlic cloves, minced

1. Soak the beans overnight. (Or use the quick-soak method: Place the beans in a stockpot and cover with water. Bring the mixture to a boil; boil for 1 minute. Remove from the heat and let stand 1 hour. Drain the beans and proceed to step 2.)

2. Heat the oil in a large soup pot or Dutch oven over medium-high heat. Add the next five ingredients (onion through bay leaves) and sauté for 5 minutes, stirring frequently. Add the thyme and pepper; cook for 2 minutes. Stir in the soy sauce and tomato paste. Add the beans and vegetable stock. Bring to a boil, cover, and simmer until the beans are soft, about 1½ hours. Taste for seasoning and add salt and more pepper if desired. Stir in the raw garlic and serve.

Note: This soup freezes well.

Yield: 11½ cups, 7 servings; Serving: 1½ cups
Calories: 286; Protein: 16.2 g; Carbohydrate: 47 g; Fiber: 15 g; Sodium: 970 mg;
Fat 5.2 g (Sat: 0.62 g, Mono: 2.88 g, Poly: 0.50 g, Trans: 0.04 g); Cholesterol: 0 mg

General: One serving of this soup provides about half your day's fiber requirement and one-third of the iron. And beans—which are high in everything from protein to folic acid—are an excellent substitute for meat.
Diabetic: Equals 1 lean meat exchange and 3 bread. Add chicken or reduced-fat cheese if you need a little more meat.
Sodium-Restricted: The bulk of the sodium from this dish comes from the soy sauce and canned vegetable broth. To lower the sodium levels, buy low-sodium tamari or plain soy sauce and use a salt-free vegetable stock or water.
Pregnant: Consider the low-sodium soy sauce and salt-free stock if you're retaining water. Each serving contains 119 milligrams of calcium, 125 micrograms of folate, and 4.9 milligrams of iron.

Simple Seafood Stew

Buy the prepeeled and deveined raw shrimp to save time. Serve leftovers over fresh spinach linguine for a different meal.

2 tablespoons olive oil

1 cup diced white or yellow onion

½ cup diced fennel or celery

2 garlic cloves, minced

½ teaspoon crushed red pepper

1 bay leaf

½ cup dry white wine

1 (28-ounce) can Italian tomatoes, chopped with liquid

1 cup water

½ cup fresh or frozen corn kernels

¼ cup fresh parsley, finely chopped

½ pound raw medium shrimp, peeled and deveined

⅓ pound cod or pollock, cut into 2-inch pieces

⅓ pound bay scallops

Coarse salt to taste

Chopped fresh parsley (optional)

1. Heat the oil in a large nonstick skillet over medium heat. Add the onion and fennel and sauté for 8–10 minutes or until the vegetables soften. Stir in the garlic, red pepper, and bay leaf and sauté for 1 minute. Add the wine and cook for 1–2 minutes. Stir in the tomatoes, water, and corn. Bring to a boil, reduce the heat, and simmer covered for 10–12 minutes or until the corn is cooked. Uncover and add the shrimp, parsley, and cod and cook gently for 2 minutes. Stir in the scallops and cook for 1–2 minutes or until all of the seafood is opaque. Remove the bay leaf and add salt to taste; ladle the soup into shallow bowls. Garnish with parsley, if desired.

Yield: 4 servings (6 cups); Serving: 1½ cups
Calories: 287; Protein: 28.5 g; Carbohydrate: 22 g; Fiber: 4.2 g; Sodium: 475 mg;
Fat 9.1 g (Sat: 1.3 g, Mono: 5.4 g, Poly: 1.5 g, Trans: 0.07 g); Cholesterol: 115 mg

General: With all the seafood, this stew is rich in trace minerals, everything from selenium to magnesium to boron. It's also high in vitamins A and E and provides nearly three-fourths of the recommended amount of vitamin C.
Diabetic: For carbohydrate counters, count 22 grams. Equals 3½ lean fat meat exchanges, 1½ vegetable, and 1 bread.
Sodium-Restricted: Omit added salt and use salt-free canned tomatoes to bring sodium level down. One serving contains 1,211 milligrams of potassium.
Pregnant: Each serving contains 127 milligrams of calcium, 60 micrograms of folate, and 3.4 milligrams of iron.

Wheat Berry & Lentil Soup

Start this soup early in the day since the wheat berries take about 45 minutes to cook. Or consider cooking several cups of wheat berries to have on hand. That way you can slip them into this soup, hot cereal, or casseroles at the last minute.

1 cup wheat berries

$^3/_4$ teaspoon coarse salt, divided

9 cups water

2 tablespoons olive oil

1$^1/_2$ cups chopped onion

1 cup diced carrot

$^3/_4$ cup diced celery

2 garlic cloves, minced

1 cup dried French green or other lentils

2 cups vegetable broth

1 tablespoon tomato paste

1 tablespoon soy sauce

3 thyme sprigs

1 bay leaf

$^1/_4$ teaspoon freshly ground pepper

4 cups baby leaf spinach

1. Place wheat berries in a large Dutch oven or saucepan. Add $^1/_4$ teaspoon salt and 4 cups water; bring to a boil. Cover and simmer for 45–50 minutes or until tender. Drain.

2. Warm oil in a large Dutch oven or large saucepan over medium heat. Add onion, carrot, and celery and sauté for 6–8 minutes or until they begin to become tender. Stir in garlic and $^1/_4$ teaspoon salt and cook 1 minute.

3. Add lentils, remaining 5 cups water, broth, tomato paste, soy sauce, thyme, and bay leaf to pan. Raise heat to high and bring to a boil. Reduce heat and simmer for 15 minutes. Stir in remaining $^1/_4$ teaspoon salt, pepper, and spinach and cook for 2–3 minutes or until spinach is wilted. Stir in wheat berries and cook until warmed through, about 1–2 minutes.

Yield: 6 servings; Serving: about 1$^1/_2$ cups   •
Calories: 283; Protein: 12.4 g; Carbohydrate: 50 g; Fiber: 10.6 g; Sodium: 706 mg;
Fat: 5.2 g (Sat: 0.73 g, Mono: 3.40 g, Poly: 0.73 g, Trans: 0 g); Cholesterol 0 mg

General: At 11 grams of fiber per serving, this soup contributes close to half the daily requirement for fiber. It's also rich in beta-carotene.
Diabetic: For carbohydrate counters, total is 50 grams. Equals 2$^1/_2$ bread/starch exchanges, 1 vegetable exchange, and 1 fat exchange.
Sodium-Restricted: Consider cutting back on the added salt and using a salt-free vegetable broth to help cut sodium levels. Each serving contains over 665 milligrams of potassium.
Pregnant: Contains 66 micrograms folate and 4 milligrams of iron.

White Bean, Chicken, & Spinach Soup

Try this quick but hearty version of chicken soup for days when you're feeling a little under the weather. Instead of refined white noodles, it's chock-full of white beans and spinach, two antioxidant-rich vegetables.

1 tablespoon olive oil

1 small onion, chopped

1 stalk celery, chopped

1 large carrot, peeled and chopped

2 bay leaves

3 cups reduced-sodium chicken broth

2 cups water

12 ounces chicken tenders, chopped

1 (15-ounce) can small white beans, drained

1 cup tightly packed baby spinach leaves

3 tablespoons finely chopped fresh oregano

$1/4$ cup finely chopped fresh parsley

2 tablespoons lemon juice

$1/4$ teaspoon salt

$1/2$ teaspoon freshly ground pepper

1. Place a large saucepan over medium heat, add oil, and heat until hot. Stir in onion, celery, and carrot and sauté for 6–8 minutes or until they begin to soften. Stir in bay leaves and sauté for 1 minute.

2. Add chicken broth and water and bring mixture to a boil. Reduce heat and stir in chicken and beans. Simmer gently for 3–4 minutes or until chicken is tender. Stir in spinach and remove from heat. Let stand 2–3 minutes or until spinach wilts. Stir in oregano, parsley, lemon juice, salt, and pepper. Serve immediately.

Yield: 4 servings; Serving: about 1½ cups
Calories: 200; Protein: 26.6 g; Carbohydrate: 15.9 g; Fiber: 4.3 g; Sodium: 871 mg;
Fat: 4.9 g (Sat 0.76 g, Mono: 2.77 g, Poly: 0.63 g, Trans: 0 g); Cholesterol 49 mg

General: This soup is rich in the antioxidants, particularly beta-carotene.
Diabetic: For carbohydrate counters, total is 16 grams. Equals ½ bread/starch exchange, 3 very lean meat/protein exchanges, 1 vegetable exchange, and 1 fat exchange.
Sodium-Restricted: The higher sodium level is due mainly to canned chicken broth and canned beans. Try Pacific brand chicken broth and organic canned beans for lower sodium counts. Or try cooking these two ingredients from scratch.
Pregnant: Contains 33 micrograms folate and 2 grams iron.

SALADS AND SIDES

Roasted Winter Vegetable Medley

Tossed with a garlicky bread crumb topping, this colorful assortment of root vegetables and winter squash makes a nice side dish for a holiday meal. Or use it as a hearty main course for a vegetarian supper. Chop vegetables in large irregular chunks, about 2 inches in length, for the best appearance.

BREAD CRUMB TOPPING

$1/4$ cup walnuts, toasted

1 (1-ounce) slice whole-wheat peasant-style bread

2 garlic cloves, minced

2 tablespoons fresh parsley leaves

$1/2$ teaspoon coarse salt

ROASTED VEGETABLES

2 cups parsnips, peeled and coarsely chopped (about 4)

4 cups butternut squash, peeled and coarsely chopped (about 1 large)

3 cups carrots, peeled and coarsely chopped (about 6)

1 dozen large shallots, peeled

$1 1/2$ tablespoons olive or canola oil

Coarse salt and freshly ground black pepper to taste

1. Preheat the oven to 400°F.

2. Combine the first four ingredients and coarse salt, if you are using, in a food processor; process until well blended.

3. Toss the parsnips and the next four ingredients together and place in a large baking dish. Bake at 400°F for 40–45 minutes or until the vegetables are tender and nicely browned. Remove from the oven and toss the vegetables with the walnut–bread crumb mixture. Taste for seasoning and add salt and pepper as desired. Serve immediately.

Yield: 7 cups (14 servings); Serving: $1/2$ cup
Calories: 105; Protein: 2.2 g; Carbohydrate: 18.3 g; Fiber: 3.5 g; Sodium: 132 mg;
Fat 3.3 g (Sat: 0.27 g, Mono: 1.22 g, Poly: 1.43 g, Trans: 0.05 g); Cholesterol: 0 mg

General: One serving provides nearly one-third of the day's vitamin C requirement and a hefty dose of vitamin A, most of it in the form of the antioxidant powerhouse beta-carotene.
Diabetic: For carbohydrate counters, total is 18 grams. Equals 1 starch exchange and $1/2$ fat.

Sodium-Restricted: Sodium profile was calculated with ³/₄ teaspoon added salt. To lower sodium, omit or cut down on the salt. Each serving contains 451 milligrams of potassium.
Pregnant: Each serving contains 41 micrograms of folate and 1 milligram of iron.

Wild Rice–Quinoa Pilaf

Quinoa (keen-WAH), high in protein and other nutrients, is being dubbed by some as a supergrain. But once you see it and taste it for the first time, the nutty flavor and pearly appearance are what you'll remember most. Here quinoa is paired with wild rice for a dark, rich-colored pilaf. To save time, cook the wild rice the night before, following the package instructions. Resist the temptation to use instant wild rice if possible; it doesn't look or taste quite as good as the regular variety, nor does it deliver quite as many nutrients.

1 tablespoon canola oil

¹/₃ cup finely chopped onion

¹/₃ cup finely chopped celery

¹/₄ cup pistachio nuts or almonds, chopped

1 cup quinoa, rinsed and drained

3 cups defatted chicken stock or vegetable broth, preferably low-sodium

1 cup cooked wild rice

Coarse salt and freshly ground black pepper to taste

1. Place the oil in a saucepan over medium heat. Add the onion and celery and sauté for 5–6 minutes or until the vegetables begin to soften. Stir in the nuts and quinoa and cook for 1–2 minutes. Add the chicken broth and bring to a boil; reduce the heat to low, cover, and simmer for 18–20 minutes. Stir in the wild rice, cover, and continue cooking for 2–3 minutes or until the mixture is hot. Taste for seasoning and add salt and pepper as desired.

Yield: 5 cups; Serving: ¹/₂ cup
Calories: 165; Protein: 6.2 g; Carbohydrate: 26 g; Fiber: 2.6 g; Sodium: 228 mg;
Fat 4.8 g (Sat: 0.51 g, Mono: 2.62 g, Poly: 1.26 g, Trans: 0 g); Cholesterol: 0 mg

General: Not only does this nutty-flavored side dish have more fiber than a traditional rice pilaf, it's loaded with small amounts of all the minerals that make whole grains so healthy, everything from calcium to magnesium to iron.
Diabetic: For carbohydrate counters, totals 26 grams. Equals 2 bread exchanges.
Sodium-Restricted: Switch to low-sodium canned broth or make some chicken stock from scratch to lower the sodium levels.
Pregnant: Contains small amounts of key nutrients: 2 milligrams of iron and 28 micrograms of folate.

Roasted Corn Tabbouleh

A popular Lebanese salad made with cracked wheat (bulgur), tabbouleh is definitely for parsley lovers. This version cuts down a bit on the parsley and adds fresh pan-roasted corn for a new flavor twist.

1 cup bulgur

1 cup boiling water

6 teaspoons olive oil, divided

1½ cups fresh corn kernels (about 2 ears)

1 cup chopped, seeded tomato

½ cup thinly sliced green onion

½ cup fresh parsley, chopped

2 tablespoons white wine vinegar

Coarse salt and freshly ground black pepper to taste

Extra-virgin olive oil (optional)

1. Place the bulgur in a medium bowl. Add the boiling water and let stand 30 minutes or until the liquid is completely absorbed.

2. Place 1 teaspoon of the oil in a nonstick skillet over medium-high heat. Add the corn kernels and pan roast for 8–10 minutes or until brown, stirring occasionally to prevent scorching.

3. Add the tomato, green onion, and parsley to the bulgur. Mix the remaining 5 teaspoons of oil and the vinegar, salt, and pepper together and pour over the bulgur mixture. Toss gently and serve. Drizzle with a small amount of extra-virgin olive oil just prior to serving, if desired.

Yield: 5 cups; Serving: ½ cup
Calories: 100; Protein: 2.7 g; Carbohydrate: 16.7 g; Fiber: 3.7 g; Sodium: 10 mg;
Fat 3.2 g (Sat: 0.45 g, Mono: 2.11 g, Poly: 0.46 g, Trans: 0 g); Cholesterol: 0 mg

General: With nearly 4 grams of fiber in ½ cup, this salad has more fiber than 2 slices of whole-wheat bread. Consider doubling up on the servings and adding some chicken or pork to make this a satisfying main dish.
Diabetic: For carbohydrate counters, the total is 17 grams. Equals 1 starch exchange and ½ fat.
Sodium-Restricted: Sodium figures are without added salt. Consider adding a small amount of salt as your diet allows.
Pregnant: No special considerations.

Wild Mushroom–Barley Risotto

Pearl barley makes a great stand-in for arborio rice. The whole grain has a similar chewiness and swells gradually as it cooks, just like short-grain rice. Even better, it's not as labor-intensive to cook. Periodic stirring is all that's necessary. Here the nutty flavor of the barley is complemented by the rich, almost meaty taste of dried porcini mushrooms. You'll find these mushrooms in the produce section or on the canned-vegetable aisle of most supermarkets.

> 1/4 cup dried porcini mushrooms (about 1/2 ounce)
>
> 1 1/2 cups boiling water
>
> 2 cups chicken stock or broth, preferably low-sodium
>
> 2 tablespoons olive oil
>
> 1/4 cup minced shallot or red onion
>
> 1 cup pearl barley
>
> 1 1/2 teaspoons chopped fresh or 1/2 teaspoon dried thyme
>
> Coarse salt and freshly ground black pepper to taste

1. Combine the dried mushrooms and boiling water in a small bowl and let stand for 30 minutes or until the mushrooms are soft. Let cool slightly and remove the mushrooms from the liquid with a slotted spoon. Chop the mushrooms and set aside. Strain the soaking liquid through cheesecloth (to remove any grit that came with the dried mushrooms) into a small saucepan. Add the chicken broth and chopped mushrooms; bring to a boil. Reduce the heat and keep the liquid cooking at a simmer on a back burner.

2. Place the oil in a large saucepan over medium heat. Add the shallots and sauté for 3–4 minutes or until the shallots have softened. Stir in the barley and sauté for 1 minute. Stir in 1/2 cup of the mushroom-broth mixture and cook at a simmer until the liquid is absorbed, stirring occasionally. Continue adding the hot broth 1/2 cup at a time until the barley is tender, about 30–35 minutes. Stir in the thyme. Taste for seasoning and add salt and pepper as desired.

Note: Fresh or dried rosemary can be substituted for the thyme.

Yield: 3 cups, 6 servings; Serving: 1/2 cup
Calories: 188; Protein: 6.3 g; Carbohydrate: 30 g; Fiber: 6.2 g; Sodium: 213 mg;
Fat 5.1 g (Sat: 0.72 g, Mono: 3.48 g, Poly: 0.66 g, Trans: 0.05 g); Cholesterol: 0 mg

General: With over 6 grams of fiber in 1/2 cup, this side dish makes a huge contribution to daily fiber quotas. It's also a good source of iron and contains small amounts of vitamin E. Consider doubling the serving and making this risotto a main dish.

Diabetic: For carbohydrate counters, total is 30 grams. Equals 2 starch exchanges and ½ fat.
Sodium-Restricted: Sodium figures come mainly from the reduced-sodium chicken broth. Consider making your own chicken stock without added salt or using a salt-free stock.
Pregnant: No special considerations.

Seven-Vegetable Slaw *(FAST FIX)*

Start with one of the prepackaged vegetable slaw mixes and add more vegetables to make it tastier and more unique. Here we've added red pepper, zucchini, and the less familiar fennel, a crunchy vegetable with a mild anise flavor. If you don't like the flavor of anise, substitute celery.

1 (16-ounce) package preshredded broccoli slaw or cabbage slaw

1 cup shredded carrots

1 cup thinly sliced fennel or celery

1 large red pepper, julienned (about 1 cup)

2 small zucchini, julienned (about 2 cups)

½ cup canola or soybean oil mayonnaise

¼ cup fresh-squeezed orange juice

½ teaspoon grated orange rind

1 teaspoon celery seed

Coarse salt and freshly ground black pepper to taste

1. Combine the first five ingredients in a large bowl and toss to mix.

2. Combine the mayonnaise and the next five ingredients and stir until blended. Pour dressing over the slaw and toss gently.

Note: For a spunkier slaw, omit the celery seed, orange juice, and rind from the dressing; add prepared horseradish to taste.

Yield: 8 cups, 16 servings; Serving: ½ cup
Calories: 71; Protein: 1.9 g; Carbohydrate: 7.2 g; Fiber: 2.6 g; Sodium: 60 mg;
Fat 2.1 g (Sat: 0.4 g, Mono: 0.4 g, Poly: 1.3 g, Trans: 0 g); Cholesterol: 2 mg

General: One serving provides a full day's supply of vitamin C as well as large amounts of vitamin A and potassium.
Diabetic: For carbohydrate counters, total is 8 grams. Equals 2 vegetable exchanges.
Sodium-Restricted: The sodium in this salad comes via the reduced-fat mayonnaise. If the level is too high, consider making a vinaigrette-style dressing for the vegetables.
Pregnant: Contains 46 micrograms of folate.

Pear and Mixed Green Salad

A simple but elegant salad dressed with a lemon-shallot vinaigrette. Add some toasted walnuts or a little bit of blue cheese for special occasions—a little of either one of these higher-fat items can go a long way. But make sure to include at least one strong-flavored green such as arugula or endive. They make a nice match for the sweet pear.

3 tablespoons extra-virgin olive oil, divided

1 tablespoon minced shallot or red onion

1¹/₂ tablespoons fresh lemon juice

¹/₂ tablespoon water

Coarse salt to taste

4 cups mixed salad greens

2 cups frisée, endive, or arugula

2 unpeeled Bosc pears, cored and sliced lengthwise into 12 sections

Freshly ground black pepper to taste

1. Place 1 teaspoon oil in a small nonstick skillet over medium heat. Add the shallots and sauté for 2–3 minutes or until the shallots have softened. Remove from the heat and cool. Combine the shallots, lemon juice, water, and salt; whisk to blend. Slowly add the remaining olive oil and continue whisking until well blended.

2. Combine the salad greens and frisée in a large bowl; add the vinaigrette and toss gently so that the greens are well coated with the dressing. Add the pears and toss gently to mix. Season with pepper to taste, and serve.

Note: Prepare the vinaigrette in advance, but leave the greens undressed and the pears unsliced until just before serving. That way the greens will stay crisp and the pears won't discolor. Alternatively, toss the pears with the vinaigrette and keep refrigerated; the acid in the lemon juice will help keep pears from turning brown. Toss with greens just prior to serving.

Yield: 8 cups; Serving: 2 cups
Calories: 176; Protein: 1.8 g; Carbohydrate: 20.1 g; Fiber: 4.9 g; Sodium: 15 mg;
Fat 11.1 g (Sat: 1.52 g, Mono: 8.18 g, Poly: 1.13 g, Trans: 0 g); Cholesterol: 0 mg

General: This salad is rich in vitamin E and contains generous amounts of fiber. The fat level is high for a single serving, but it's mainly unsaturated fat, the kind that is healthy to the heart and body.
Diabetic: For carbohydrate counters, total is 20 grams. Equals 2 fat exchanges, 1 vegetable, and 1 fruit.
Sodium-Restricted: The sodium figures are calculated without added salt. Add a small amount of salt to the vinaigrette as allowed within your diet prescription.
Pregnant: Each serving contains 89 micrograms of folate, most of it from the leafy greens.

Greek Salad

This salad tastes great either with or without the feta cheese. Serve it as a side salad at dinner. Or consider adding some grilled chicken to make it a substantial main dish.

VINAIGRETTE

3 tablespoons extra-virgin olive oil

2 tablespoons red wine vinegar

1 tablespoon fresh lemon juice

Coarse salt and freshly ground black pepper to taste

SALAD

3 cups chopped romaine lettuce (about 8 leaves)

1 cup sliced radishes (about 3 ounces)

1 large yellow pepper, julienned (about 1 cup)

1 cup diced cucumber

1/2 cup thinly sliced red onion

1/2 cup fresh mint, chopped

1/3 cup pitted Kalamata olives, cut or torn into large pieces

Feta cheese, crumbled (optional)

1. To prepare the vinaigrette, whisk together the oil, vinegar, lemon juice, salt, and pepper in a small bowl.

2. To prepare the salad, combine the remaining ingredients in a large salad bowl; toss to mix. Just prior to serving, add the vinaigrette and toss gently to coat.

Yield: 6 cups; Serving: 1½ cups
Calories: 160; Protein: 2 g; Carbohydrate: 9.7 g; Fiber: 2.7 g; Sodium: 167 mg;
Fat 13.4 g (Sat: 1.83 g, Mono: 10.0 g, Poly: 1.40 g, Trans: 0 g); Cholesterol: 0 mg

General: This salad is rich in vitamin E, owing mainly to the oil used in the dressing.
Diabetic: For carbohydrate counters, total is 10 grams. Equals 2 vegetable exchanges and 2½ fats.
Sodium-Restricted: The sodium figures are tabulated without added salt. It's the olives that contribute the sodium to this dish. Leave them out and the sodium level will plummet.
Pregnant: Each serving of salad contains 93 micrograms of folate or close to 25 percent of the daily requirement.

Tex-Mex Wheat Berry Salad with Tomatillo Vinaigrette

Wheat berries, whole kernels of the wheat grain, cook up tender-crunchy and make a great substitute for pasta in summer salads. They have a beautiful light brown color that complements the bright colors of the raw vegetables. Take this salad on a picnic; wheat berries won't absorb the vinaigrette and go soft and mushy like cooked pasta.

TOMATILLO VINAIGRETTE

1 cup fresh tomatillos, chopped (about 5 large)

2 tablespoons fresh lime juice

3 tablespoons olive oil

1 tablespoon white wine vinegar

2 teaspoons minced seeded jalapeño pepper

Coarse salt to taste

SALAD

1 cup soft wheat berries or spelt berries

5 cups water

$1/4$ teaspoon coarse salt

1 large yellow pepper, julienned (about 1 cup)

1 cup pear or cherry tomato halves

1 medium avocado, chopped (about 1 cup)

5 cups mixed greens or shredded romaine lettuce

2 tablespoons pine nuts, toasted (optional)

1. Whisk together the tomatillos, lime juice, oil, vinegar, jalapeño, and salt.

2. Place the wheat berries, water, and salt in a large saucepan over high heat. Cover and bring to a boil. Reduce the heat and simmer for 15–20 minutes or until wheat berries are tender-crunchy. Remove from the heat. Cool in the liquid. Drain and place in a medium bowl. Add the yellow pepper and the remaining ingredients. Pour half of the vinaigrette mixture into the wheat berry mixture and toss gently.

3. Place the mixed greens in a large bowl and toss with the remaining vinaigrette. To serve, place 1 cup of greens onto each of five plates. Top each with 1 cup of the wheat berry mixture and garnish with pine nuts, if desired.

Note: It's fine to make the wheat berry part of this salad ahead of time. But wait to toss the greens with the vinaigrette just prior to serving so they stay crisp.

Yield: 5 servings; Serving: 1 cup wheat berry salad, 1 cup mixed greens
Calories: 255; Protein: 6.1 g; Carbohydrate: 35 g; Fiber: 3.1 g; Sodium: 115 mg;
Fat 12.7 g (Sat: 1.66 g, Mono: 7.97 g, Poly: 1.34 g, Trans: 0.08 g); Cholesterol: 0 mg

General: No special considerations.
Diabetic: For carbohydrate counters, total is 35 grams. Equals ¹/₂ high-fat meat exchange, 1¹/₂ starch, 1 veg-
etable, and 1 fat. You can add grilled chicken, shrimp, or a vegetarian meat substitute to this substantial
side dish to boost protein and make it a main course.
Sodium-Restricted: Omit the salt used to cook the wheat berries if you need to reduce sodium levels further.
Skip the salt in the vinaigrette.
Pregnant: No special considerations.

Tempeh Salad with Pita & Pine Nuts

The addition of tempeh, nuts, and pita makes this Greek-style salad a main course rather than a side dish. If the weather is good, consider grilling the pita bread and tempeh to add a wonderful smoky flavor to the dish.

        2 tablespoons oil, divided

        2 (2-ounce) whole-wheat pita breads

        1 (8-ounce) package five-grain tempeh

        4 Roma tomatoes, seeded and diced (about 2 cups)

        2 small peeled cucumbers, seeded and diced (about 2 cups)

        ¹/₃ cup thinly sliced red onion

        ¹/₄ cup diced green bell pepper

        ¹/₂ cup pine nuts, toasted

        2 tablespoons chopped fresh basil

        2 tablespoons fresh oregano leaves

        1 tablespoon fresh lemon juice

        ¹/₄ teaspoon Dijon mustard

        ¹/₂ teaspoon coarse salt

        ¹/₄ teaspoon freshly ground pepper

1. Preheat broiler or prepare grill.

2. Brush ¹/₂ teaspoon oil on pita bread and broil or grill for 2 minutes per side or until it begins to brown. Cool and cut each bread into 8 wedges or triangles.

3. Place 1¹/₂ teaspoons oil in a large nonstick skillet over medium high heat. Add tempeh and sauté for 3–4 minutes or until nicely browned.

4. Combine tomatoes, cucumber, tempeh, pita, red onion, bell pepper, pine nuts, basil, and oregano in a large bowl; toss gently to mix.

5. Combine lemon juice and mustard in a small bowl. Whisk to blend. Gradually stir in remaining oil and salt and pepper. Pour vinaigrette over cucumber mixture. Toss gently to blend and serve.

Yield: 4 servings; Serving: 1½ cups
Calories: 372; Protein: 14.8 g; Carbohydrate: 39.6 g; Fiber: 10.7 g; Sodium: 428 mg;
Fat: 19 g (Sat: 2.3 g, Mono: 6.8 g, Poly: 4.1 g, Trans: 0 g); Cholesterol 0 mg

General: With close to 11 grams of fiber per serving, this salad provides nearly half of the recommended daily amount of fiber.
Diabetic: For carbohydrate counters, total is 40 grams. Equals 1 bread/starch exchange, 1 vegetable exchange, and 2½ fat exchanges.
Sodium-Restricted: Most of the sodium comes from the salt that is added to the vinaigrette. Take it out or replace it with a salt substitute if needed.
Pregnant: Contains small amounts of key nutrients: 39 micrograms of folate and 2 milligrams of iron.

Pistachio-Apricot Bulgur Salad (FAST FIX)

Since bulgur cooks so quickly, this salad is a snap to put together. To add even more pistachio flavor, try using pistachio oil in place of olive oil. Look for the rich green oil in specialty grocery stores or order it online.

1 cup fine- or medium-grain bulgur

½ cup chopped dried apricots

1 cup boiling water

1 cup chopped fresh parsley

3 tablespoons finely chopped fresh mint

½ cup shelled chopped pistachios

⅓ cup olive oil or pistachio oil

3 tablespoons orange juice or white wine vinegar

¼ cup minced red onion

2 tablespoons thinly sliced green onion

¾ teaspoon coarse salt

¼ teaspoon fresh ground pepper

1. Combine bulgur and apricots in a bowl. Add boiling water and let stand 30 minutes or until liquid is absorbed. Add remaining ingredients and toss gently to mix.

Yield: 6 servings cups; Serving: ¾ cup
Calories: 267; Protein: 6.1 g; Carbohydrate: 31.6 g; Fiber: 6.8 g; Sodium: 247 mg;
Fat: 14.2 g (Sat: 1.87 g, Mono: 9.21 g, Poly: 2.49 g, Trans: 0 g); Cholesterol 0 mg

General: Fruit, nuts, and wheat give this salad a good dose of fiber, about one-third of the recommended amount.
Diabetic: For carbohydrate counters, total is 32 grams. Equals 1 bread/starch exchange, ½ fruit exchange, and 2½ fat exchanges.
Sodium-Restricted: Salt contributes the bulk of sodium to this dish. Leave it out if needed.
Pregnant: Contains 35 micrograms folate and 2.6 milligrams of iron.

Dijon-Herb Carrots

Vegetables don't have to be dripping with butter to taste great. Here we've paired olive oil with some fresh herbs and Dijon mustard for an elegant-looking and flavorful sauce.

 1 cup fresh parsley leaves, loosely packed

 6 large leaves of fresh basil

 1 garlic clove, minced

 1 tablespoon water

 2 teaspoons Dijon mustard

 Coarse salt to taste

 1 tablespoon olive oil

 4 cups carrots, sliced thickly on the diagonal

1. Place the parsley, basil, garlic, water, mustard, and salt in a food processor and blend. Add the oil and blend until it forms a thick sauce. Alternatively, mince the parsley and basil. Combine the herbs, garlic, water, mustard, and salt in a small bowl. Whisk in the oil until well blended.

2. Steam the carrots in a large saucepan until tender, about 8–10 minutes. Toss carrots gently with the sauce and serve.

Yield: 4 cups; Serving: ½ cup
Calories: 46; Protein: 1.0 g; Carbohydrate: 6.9 g; Fiber: 2 g; Sodium: 57 mg;
Fat 2 g (Sat: 0.26 g, Mono: 0.13 g, Poly: 0.23 g, Trans: 0.02 g); Cholesterol: 0 mg

General: A single serving supplies well more than the recommended amount of vitamin A.
Diabetic: For carbohydrate counters, total is 7 grams. Equals 1 vegetable serving and ½ fat. Double or triple the serving if you need more vegetables at a meal. You'll still have only 1–1½ fat exchanges.
Sodium-Restricted: The sodium figures are calculated without added salt. Dijon mustard is providing most of the sodium for this dish. It doesn't come in a low-sodium variety, so you'll need to omit it if this sodium level is too high for your diet.
Pregnant: No special considerations.

Spicy Sweet Potato Fries

Sweet potatoes have a lot more going for them nutritionally than white potatoes. Sweets are rich in beta-carotene, vitamin C, fiber, and a whole host of other nutrients. Try a small amount of these sweet-and-spicy "oven" fries with the Veggie Burgers on page 279. Make the fries ahead of time if you need to, then reheat them under the broiler for 1–2 minutes to get them crisp.

> 1 large sweet potato, cut into thin matchstick pieces (about 3¹/₂ cups)
>
> 1 tablespoon olive or canola oil
>
> ¹/₂ teaspoon freshly ground black pepper
>
> ¹/₄ teaspoon chili powder
>
> ¹/₄ teaspoon ground cumin
>
> ¹/₄ teaspoon paprika
>
> Coarse salt to taste
>
> Vegetable cooking spray or oil

1. Preheat the oven to 450°F.

2. Place the sweet potato pieces into a bowl and drizzle with the oil; toss gently to coat. Combine the next four ingredients and the salt, if using, and sprinkle over the sweet potatoes; toss gently to coat. Place the sweet potatoes on a large baking sheet lightly coated with oil or vegetable spray. Bake at 450°F for 12–15 minutes or until the ends begin to crisp. Remove from the oven and serve.

Yield: 3¹/₂ cups; Serving: ¹/₂ cup
Calories: 52; Protein: 0.6 g; Carbohydrate: 8 g; Fiber: 1.1 g; Sodium: 5 mg;
Fat 2.1 g (Sat: 0.28 g, Mono: 1.45 g, Poly: 0.21 g, Trans: 0.02 g); Cholesterol: 0 mg

General: More than a day's supply of vitamin A in 1 serving.
Diabetic: For carbohydrate counters, total is 8 grams. Double the serving to 1 cup and you will have 1 starch exchange and 1 fat.
Sodium-Restricted: Sodium figures are calculated without added salt. Add salt as allowed with your diet. If you use ¹/₂ teaspoon of salt for the whole batch of fries, a single serving will contain 176 grams of sodium.
Pregnant: No special considerations.

Wilted Spinach with Nuts & Golden Raisins *(FAST FIX)*

Buy the prewashed baby spinach leaves and this colorful side dish will come together quickly. To save time and cleanup, toast the pine nuts in the same skillet used for cooking the spinach.

2 teaspoons olive oil

$^1/_4$ cup thinly sliced red onion

1 clove garlic, thinly sliced

$^1/_4$ teaspoon coarse salt

2 (6-ounce) packages baby leaf spinach

2 tablespoons golden raisins

2 tablespoons pine nuts, toasted

Dash fresh ground pepper

1. Heat oil in a large nonstick skillet over medium low heat. Add red onion and sauté 5–6 minutes or until tender. Stir in garlic and cook 1 minute. Add salt, spinach, and raisins and cook for 3–4 minutes or until spinach begins to wilt. Remove from heat and stir in pine nuts and pepper. Serve immediately.

Yield: 4 servings; Serving: about $^3/_4$ cup
Calories: 89; Protein: 3.3 g; Carbohydrate: 9 g; Fiber: 2.4 g; Sodium: 186 mg;
Fat: 5.5 g (Sat: 0.57 g, Mono: 2.47 g, Poly: 1.83 g, Trans: 0 g); Cholesterol 0 mg

General: Spinach is rich in antioxidants, particularly beta-carotene and vitamin E.
Diabetic: For carbohydrate counters, total is 9 grams. Equals 1 vegetable exchange and 1 fat exchange.
Sodium-Restricted: The added salt can be left out or replaced with salt substitute.
Pregnant: Contains 170 micrograms of folate and nearly 3 milligrams of iron.

Lemony Kale with Toasted Almonds (FAST FIX)

Since kale requires a longer cooking time than many greens, it's boiled here and then combined with oil and seasonings. Any variety of kale will work, although the dark green, curly-leafed dinosaur kale looks spectacular.

2 bunches kale, about 12 ounces

$^1/_4$ cup sliced almonds

2 teaspoons olive oil

1 teaspoon fresh grated lemon zest

$^1/_2$ teaspoon salt

$^1/_4$ teaspoon freshly ground pepper

1. Remove tough inner stem from kale and coarsely chop leaves. Bring water to a boil in a large Dutch oven. Add kale and boil gently for 10 minutes or until tender. Drain well, pressing excess water out of kale using the back of a spoon.

2. Place almonds in a skillet over medium heat and cook, stirring constantly for 1–2 minutes or until they begin to brown lightly. Add nuts and remaining ingredients to kale and serve.

Yield: 4 servings; Serving: 1 cup
Calories: 82; Protein: 3 g; Carbohydrate: 6.5 g; Fiber: 1.7 g; Sodium: 258 mg;
Fat: 5.6 g (Sat: 0.59 g, Mono: 3.57 g, Poly: 1.13 g, Trans: 0 g); Cholesterol 0 mg

General: Kale is extremely rich in antioxidants, both beta-carotene and vitamin E.
Diabetic: For carbohydrate counters, total is 7 grams. Equals 1 vegetable exchange and 1 fat exchange.
Sodium-Restricted: The added salt is contributing most of the sodium. Cut down or omit and consider adding a splash of lemon juice to boost flavor.
Pregnant: No special considerations.

DESSERTS

Easy Peach, Pineapple, and Apricot Crisp

Using frozen and precut fresh and dried fruits lets you put together this crisp in a hurry. The topping is a quick mix of oats, pecans, and wheat germ for crunch. A little pineapple juice concentrate provides sweetness.

FILLING

1 (16-ounce) package frozen unsweetened peach slices, cut into chunks

2 cups fresh precut pineapple tidbits

1/2 cup dried unsweetened apricot pieces

1/4 cup frozen unsweetened pineapple juice concentrate, thawed

1/4 cup oat flour

1/2 teaspoon cinnamon

1/8 teaspoon freshly grated nutmeg

1/4 teaspoon coarse salt

Vegetable cooking spray or canola oil

TOPPING

1/3 cup oat flour

1/3 cup oats

1/4 cup toasted wheat germ

3 tablespoons canola oil

2 tablespoons chopped pecans

2 tablespoons frozen unsweetened pineapple juice concentrate, thawed

1/8 teaspoon salt

1. Preheat the oven to 375°F.

2. Combine the first eight ingredients in a medium bowl and toss gently to combine. Place the fruit mixture into an 11- × 7-inch baking dish lightly coated with vegetable spray or canola oil.

3. Combine the oat flour and next six ingredients in a small bowl. Sprinkle the topping mixture over the fruit and bake at 375°F for 30–35 minutes or until mixture is bubbly.

Yield: 8 servings; Serving: about 3/4 cup
Calories: 212; Protein: 4.3 g; Carbohydrate: 34 g; Fiber: 4.9 g; Sodium: 90 mg;
Fat 7.7 g (Sat: 0.59 g, Mono: 0.40 g, Poly: 2.23 g, Trans: 0.01 g); Cholesterol: 0 mg

General: Provides more than 30 percent of the recommended amount for vitamin E.
Diabetic: For carbohydrate counters, total is 34 grams. Equals 1 fruit exchange, 1 starch, 1 1/2 fats. No added sugars.
Sodium-Restricted: Omit salt in filling and in topping to reduce sodium. Contains 454 milligrams of potassium.
Pregnant: No special considerations.

Cinnamon Applesauce

Try varying your mix of apples to include both sweet and tart varieties (McIntosh, Gala, Granny Smith) to give this applesauce a nice depth of flavor.

8 large apples (about 2 1/2 pounds), peeled, cored, and cut into large chunks

1 cup apple juice

1 tablespoon fresh lemon juice

1 teaspoon cinnamon

1/8 teaspoon freshly grated nutmeg

1. Place the apples, apple juice, and lemon juice into a large pot. Bring the mixture to a boil, reduce the heat, and simmer uncovered for 35–40 minutes or until the apples are soft.

2. Remove the pan from the heat and stir in the cinnamon and nutmeg. (The mixture will be slightly soupy.) Mash the apples with a fork or potato masher

until desired consistency. Alternatively, push through a sieve for a smoother texture.

Yield: 3¹/₂ cups; Serving: ¹/₂ cup
Calories: 103; Protein: 0.89 g; Carbohydrate: 28 g; Fiber: 2 g; Sodium: 1 mg;
Fat 0.7 g (Sat: 0.07 g, Mono: 0.08 g, Poly: 0.23 g, Trans: 0 g); Cholesterol: 0 mg

General: Even without the skin, apples provide a healthy dose of fiber, most of it the soluble variety that studies show can help lower blood cholesterol levels.
Diabetic: For carbohydrate counters, total is 28 grams. Equals 2 fruit exchanges. No added sugar.
Sodium-Restricted: Recipe is low in sodium.
Pregnant: No special considerations.

Orange Juice Sorbet

This sorbet has a refreshing sweet-tart flavor rather than the overpowering sugary taste found in many commercial sorbets. Be sure to use fresh-squeezed orange juice for the best flavor. Serve it with sliced fresh strawberries for a special dessert.

> 1 quart of fresh-squeezed orange juice
>
> 2 tablespoons Cointreau or other orange liqueur
>
> ¹/₄ teaspoon lemon extract
>
> Sliced fresh strawberries (optional)

1. Place the first three ingredients in an ice-cream freezer and freeze according to the manufacturer's instructions. Alternatively, combine the ingredients and pour the mixture into three large ice-cube trays; freeze until firm or overnight. Remove from the freezer and let stand at room temperature for 5–10 minutes until the cubes begin to thaw and soften. Place the cubes into a blender or food processor and blend until smooth. Serve immediately with sliced strawberries, if desired.

Note: Leftovers can be returned to the freezer and reblended in a food processor as needed. The sorbet texture actually becomes smoother with a second freezing and blending.

Yield: 4 cups; Serving: ¹/₂ cup
Calories: 69; Protein: 0.9 g; Carbohydrate: 14.5 g; Fiber: 0.3 g; Sodium: 1.5 mg;
Fat 0.3 g (Sat: 0.03 g, Mono: 0.05 g, Poly: 0.05 g, Trans: 0 g); Cholesterol: 0 mg

General: One serving supplies 100 percent of the recommended amount of vitamin C.
Diabetic: For carbohydrate counters, total is 15 grams. Equals 1 fruit exchange. No added sugar.
Sodium-Restricted: Recipe is low in sodium. Provides 249 milligrams of potassium.
Pregnant: Contains 38 micrograms of folate.

Spiced Poached Pears

Anjou or Comice pears are the best for poaching. Choose fruit that is ripe but firm. Cardamom is a sweet-spicy seasoning used frequently in desserts served in India. It adds a unique flavor to the pear syrup, but you can omit it if you like.

PEARS

4 large Anjou pears, peeled and cored

1 cup dry white wine

$^1/_2$ cup water

$^1/_2$ cup white grape juice

1 tablespoon honey

1 teaspoon vanilla extract

1 cardamom pod or $^1/_8$ teaspoon ground cardamom

2 whole cloves

Pinch freshly grated nutmeg

TOPPING

2 tablespoons slivered almonds, toasted

2 tablespoons pistachio nuts, toasted

1. Slice $^1/_4$ inch from the bottom of each pear so it will sit flat.

2. Combine the next eight ingredients (wine through nutmeg) in a medium saucepan; bring to a boil. Add the pears; reduce the heat and simmer covered for 12–15 minutes or until the pears are tender. Remove the pears from the cooking liquid with a slotted spoon. Turn the heat to medium-high and bring the cooking liquid to a boil; cook for 10–15 minutes or until the liquid is reduced by half and the mixture becomes syrupy. Strain the syrup through a sieve into a bowl or large measuring cup, discarding the solids. Cover and chill.

3. Place the nuts into a mini–food processor and pulse until the mixture is coarse and crumbly. Alternatively, finely chop the nuts by hand; combine and set aside.

4. Cut each pear in half and then slice each half lengthwise from top to bottom into 5 sections, leaving the top and stem intact. Place 2 pear halves on a small dessert plate and fan the sections so that the pear lies flat (the pear will still be connected at the stem). Spoon $^1/_4$ cup of the syrup over the pear and sprinkle with 1 tablespoon of the nut mixture.

Yield: 4 servings; Serving: 2 pear halves with nuts and syrup
Calories: 220; Protein: 2.7 g; Carbohydrate: 42 g; Fiber: 5.9 g; Sodium: 4 mg;
Fat 5 g (Sat: 0.47 g, Mono: 2.86 g, Poly: 0.95 g, Trans: 0 g); Cholesterol: 0 mg

General: One serving has nearly a full day's supply of the requirement for vitamin C and a hefty dose of vitamin E.
Diabetic: For carbohydrate counters, total is 42 grams. Equals 2 fruit exchanges, 1 other carbohydrate, and 1 fat.
Sodium-Restricted: One serving carries 360 milligrams of potassium.
Pregnant: Most of the alcohol cooks off while the pears are poaching. But you might want to omit the wine and increase the grape juice to make a completely alcohol-free dessert.

Rum-Glazed Pineapple *(FAST FIX)*

To save time, buy an already peeled and cored pineapple.

> ⅛ teaspoon freshly grated nutmeg
>
> ¼ cup frozen unsweetened pineapple juice concentrate, thawed
>
> ½ cup fresh-squeezed orange juice
>
> 2 tablespoons rum or ⅛ teaspoon rum extract
>
> 1 fresh pineapple, peeled, cored, and cut lengthwise into 12 wedges (about 2 pounds)
>
> Grated orange rind (optional)

1. Combine the first three ingredients and place in a small saucepan over high heat. Bring to a boil and simmer for 8–10 minutes or until the mixture becomes syrupy. Remove from the heat and stir in the rum. Cover to keep warm.

2. Place a large nonstick skillet over medium-high heat. Add 6 pineapple wedges (do not crowd) and cook for 3–4 minutes or until the pineapple begins to brown around the edges, turning once. Remove the pineapple from the pan and place on a serving plate; repeat with the remaining wedges. Pour the rum sauce over the pineapple and serve. Garnish with a sprinkling of freshly grated orange rind, if desired.

Yield: 12 wedges; Serving: 2 wedges
Calories: 119; Protein: 0.9 g; Carbohydrate: 27 g; Fiber: 2 g; Sodium: 2 mg;
Fat: 0.8 g (Sat: 0.07 g, Mono: 0.09 g, Poly: 0.24 g, Trans: 0 g); Cholesterol: 0 mg

General: One serving provides about two-thirds the recommended amount of vitamin C.
Diabetic: For carbohydrate counters, total is 27 grams. Equals 2 fruit exchanges (1 juice, 1 solid fruit). No added sugar.
Sodium-Restricted: Recipe is low in sodium.

Pregnant: Since the rum is not cooked in this recipe, you will be getting a tiny amount of alcohol (1 teaspoon) per serving. Consider using extract instead.

Apple-Cherry Crumb Pie

Filling a whole-wheat piecrust with fruit and nut toppings makes for a healthful special occasion or holiday dessert. Using a combination of tart and sweet apples can give more depth to flavor. Look for premade whole-wheat crusts in whole-food supermarkets. One of the better brands, called *Mother Nature's Goodies*, is both sugar-free and trans-fat-free.

> 2 peeled, cored small Granny Smith apples, thinly sliced into wedges, about 14 ounces
>
> 2 peeled, cored Rome apples, thinly sliced into wedges, about 12 ounces
>
> $1/2$ tablespoon fresh lemon juice
>
> $1/3$ cup dried cherries
>
> 5 tablespoons whole-wheat flour, divided
>
> $1/2$ teaspoon cinnamon
>
> 2 tablespoons honey
>
> 1 (9-inch) prepared whole-wheat pastry crust
>
> $1/3$ cup sliced almonds
>
> $1/4$ cup rolled oats
>
> 2 tablespoons canola oil
>
> 1 tablespoon brown sugar
>
> $1/8$ teaspoon salt

1. Preheat oven to 350°F.

2. Combine apples and lemon juice in a large bowl and toss to coat. Add cherries, 1 tablespoon flour, and cinnamon; toss gently to mix. Place half of apples in prepared crust; drizzle evenly with 1 tablespoon honey. Repeat layers.

3. Combine almonds, oats, remaining $1/4$ cup flour, oil, brown sugar, and salt in a small bowl. Mix with fork until well blended. Sprinkle nut mixture evenly over top of apples and bake at 350°F for 50–55 minutes or until apples are tender.

Yield: 8 servings; Serving: 1 wedge
Calories: 271; Protein: 4.2 g; Carbohydrate: 39.6 g; Fiber: 6.8 g; Sodium: 149 mg;
Fat: 11.8 g (Sat: 1.47 g, Mono: 3.38 g, Poly: 1.62 g, Trans: 0 g); Cholesterol 0 mg

General: Fruit and a whole-wheat crust give this dessert a generous amount of fiber, more than double the fiber of traditional apple pie.
Diabetic: For carbohydrate counters, total is 40 grams. Equals ¹/₂ bread/starch exchange, 1 fruit exchange, and 1 fat exchange.
Sodium-Restricted: Omit added salt to lower sodium levels.
Pregnant: No special considerations.

Oatmeal-Raisin & Nut Cookies

O ats and whole-wheat pastry flour gives these cookies a wonderfully chewy texture. For added crunch there's both sunflower seeds and nuts. And for sweetness, we've cut down on the sugar of traditional cookie recipes and let dried fruits add some natural sweetness.

$^1/_2$ cup canola oil

$^1/_3$ cup brown sugar

2 tablespoons honey

1 large egg

1 teaspoon vanilla extract

2 cups rolled oats

$^3/_4$ cup whole-wheat pastry flour

$^3/_4$ teaspoon cinnamon

1 teaspoon baking powder

$^1/_8$ teaspoon salt

$^1/_2$ cup raisins

3 tablespoons coarsely chopped pecans

3 tablespoons blanched slivered almonds

1. Preheat oven to 350°F.

2. Combine first three ingredients in a large bowl and beat at medium speed with a mixer to blend. Stir in egg and vanilla extract.

3. Spoon oats into a small bowl. Add flour, cinnamon, baking powder, and salt, stirring well with a whisk. Add oat and flour mixture to oil mixture; beat well. Stir in raisins, pecans, and almonds. Place dough in refrigerator for 30 minutes to chill.

4. Spoon heaping tablespoons of dough onto a nonstick cookie sheet and flatten gently with fingers. Bake at 350°F for 10–12 minutes or until lightly

browned. Let cookies cool on sheet for 2 minutes. Transfer to wire racks and cool completely.

Yield: 36 cookies.
Calories: 79; Protein: 1.4 g; Carbohydrate: 9.2 g; Fiber: 1 g; Sodium: 33 mg;
Fat: 4.3 g (Sat: 0.38 g, Mono: 2.38 g, Poly: 1.24 g, Trans: 0 g); Cholesterol 6 mg

General: Using canola oil instead of butter or shortening keeps these cookies low in saturated fat and trans-fat-free.
Diabetic: For carbohydrate counters, total is 9 grams. Equals 1/2 bread/starch exchange and 1 fat exchange.
Sodium-Restricted: Sodium is low, but salt can be omitted to lower it even further.
Pregnant: No special considerations.

Sweet Spiced Couscous

In Tunisia, home cooks make a breakfast meal of farka, a cooked couscous studded with dates and nuts and sweetened with sugar. This version is sweetened naturally with fruit juice and dried dates and makes a nice light dessert. Since it's traditionally served with milk, try it with a splash of soy milk if you'd like.

> 1/4 cup chopped raw cashews
>
> 1/4 cup slivered blanched almonds
>
> 2 tablespoons chopped hazelnuts
>
> 1 1/2 cups apple juice
>
> 1 cup whole-wheat couscous
>
> 1 1/2 tablespoons hazelnut or canola oil
>
> 3/4 cup pitted chopped dates
>
> Soy milk (optional)

1. Place nuts in a large nonstick skillet over medium high heat and cook 3–4 minutes, stirring frequently until they begin to lightly brown. Remove from heat.

2. Place apple juice in a small saucepan and bring to a boil. Stir in couscous and cook 1 minute. Remove from heat and let stand five minutes. Stir in oil, dates, and nuts. Spoon into bowls and serve with a splash of soy milk, if desired.

Yield: 6 servings; Serving: 2/3 cup
Calories: 268; Protein: 5.6 g; Carbohydrate: 41.8 g; Fiber: 5.1 g; Sodium: 23 mg;
Fat: 10.4 g (Sat: 0.99 g, Mono: 6.85 g, Poly: 1.52 g, Trans: 0 g); Cholesterol 0 mg

General: This dessert contains about one-fifth the recommended dose of fiber.
Diabetic: For carbohydrate counters, total is 42 grams. Equals 1 bread/starch exchange, 1½ fruit exchanges, and 2 fat exchanges.
Sodium-Restricted: No special considerations.
Pregnant: Contains nearly 2 milligrams of iron.

Credits

MyPyramid on page 12 is from the U.S. Department of Agriculture and the U.S. Department of Health and Human Services.

The New Healthy Eating Pyramid on pages 13 and 209 is illustrated by Christopher Bing and Heather Foley.

The Food Guide Pyramid on page 17 is from the U.S. Department of Agriculture and the U.S. Department of Health and Human Services.

The graph on page 36 is adapted from Willett, W.C., et al., *New England Journal of Medicine*, vol. 341, no. 6 (August 5, 1999): p. 430.

The tables on page 38, courtesy of Harvard Health Publications, are adapted from the National Heart, Lung, and Blood Institute's "Body Mass Index Table," http://www.nhlbi.nih.gov/guidelines/obesity/bmi_tbl.htm.

The chart on page 40, courtesy of Harvard Health Publications, is adapted from the National Heart, Lung, and Blood Institute's "Body Mass Index Table," http://www.nhlbi.nih.gov/guidelines/obesity/bmi_tbl.htm.

The illustration on page 44 is from "Metabolic Syndrome: Putting the Heart in Harm's Way," *Harvard Heart Letter,* vol. 12, no. 9 (May 2002): p. 2.

The illustration on page 65 is from "Low Carb vs. Low Fat," *Harvard Health Letter,* vol. 29, no. 10 (August 2004): p. 4.

The illustration on page 75 was adapted from U.S. Department of Agriculture data.

The graph on page 77 is adapted from *Nutritional Epidemiology* by Walter Willett, p. 419.

The graph on page 80 is adapted from deLorgeril et al., *Circulation,* vol. 99, no. 6 (February 16, 1999): p. 781.

The illustration on page 82 is from the U.S. Food and Drug Administration.

The illustration on page 96 is adapted from "The Skinny on Olestra," *HealthNews,* vol. 2, no. 4 (March 5,1996): p. 2.

The illustration on page 103 is from Harvard Health Publications.

The illustration on page 111 is from "Heart Gains from Whole Grains," *Harvard Heart Letter,* vol. 13, no. 3 (November 2002): p. 3.

The illustration on page 112 was adapted from Salmeron, J., et al., *JAMA,* vol. 277, no. 6 (February 12, 1997): p. 476.

The graph on page 163 is adapted from Hegsted, D. M., *Journal of Nutrition,* vol. 116, no. 11 (November 1986): p. 2317.

The illustration on page 188 is adapted from *Nutritional Epidemiology* by Walter Willett, p. 451.

Further Reading

CHAPTER 1

Dietary Guidelines for Americans 2005. Washington, D.C.: U.S. Department of Agriculture, 2005. http://www.healthierus.gov/dietaryguidelines

The Healthy Eating Index (Report CNPP-1). Washington, D.C.: Center for Nutrition Policy and Promotion, U.S. Department of Agriculture, 1995. http://www.nal.usda.gov/fnic/HEI/hlthyeat.pdf

McCullough, M. L., et al. "Adherence to the Dietary Guidelines for Americans and Risk of Major Chronic Disease in Men." *American Journal of Clinical Nutrition* 72 (2000): 1223–31.

———. "Adherence to the Dietary Guidelines for Americans and Risk of Major Chronic Disease in Women." *American Journal of Clinical Nutrition* 72 (2000): 1214–22.

———. "Diet Quality and Major Chronic Disease Risk in Men and Women: Moving Toward Improved Dietary Guidance." *American Journal of Clinical Nutrition* 76 (2002): 1261–71.

CHAPTER 2

Willett, W. *Nutritional Epidemiology*, second edition. New York: Oxford University Press, 1998.

CHAPTER 3

Baik, I., et al. "Adiposity and Mortality in Men." *American Journal of Epidemiology* 152 (2000): 264–71.

Calle, E. E., et al. "Overweight, Obesity, and Mortality from Cancer in a Prospectively Studied Cohort of U.S. Adults." *New England Journal of Medicine* 348 (2003): 1625–38.

Dansinger, M. L., et al. "Comparison of the Atkins, Ornish, Weight Watchers, and Zone Diets for Weight Loss and Heart Disease Risk Reduction: A Randomized Trial." *JAMA* 293 (2005): 43–53.

Hedley, A. A., et al. "Prevalence of Overweight and Obesity Among US Children, Adolescents, and Adults, 1999–2002." *JAMA* 291 (2004): 2847–50.

Ludwig, D. S., et al. "High Glycemic Index Foods, Overeating, and Obesity." *Pediatrics* 103 (1999): E261–66.

McManus, K., et al. "A Randomized Controlled Trial of a Moderate-fat, Low-energy Diet Compared with a Low-fat, Low-energy Diet for Weight Loss in Overweight Adults." *International Journal of Obesity and Related Metabolic Disorders* 25 (2001): 1503–11.

Nestle, M., and M. Jacobson. "Halting the Obesity Epidemic: A Public Health Policy Approach." *Public Health Reports* 115 (2000): 12–24.

Stevens, J., et al. "The Effect of Age on the Association Between Body-Mass Index and Mortality." *New England Journal of Medicine* 338 (1998): 1–7.

Willett, W. C., and R. L. Leibel. "Dietary Fat Is Not a Major Determinant of Body Fat." *American Journal of Medicine* 113, Suppl 9B (2002): 47S-59S.

Willett, W. C., et al. "Guidelines for Healthy Weight." *New England Journal of Medicine* 341 (1999): 427–34.

CHAPTER 4

Albert, C. M., et al. "Blood Levels of Long-Chain n-3 Fatty Acids and the Risk of Sudden Death." *New England Journal of Medicine* 346 (2002): 1113–18.

American Heart Association. *2005 Heart and Stroke Statistical Update.* Dallas, Tex.: American Heart Association, 2005.

Baylin, A., et al. "Adipose Tissue Alpha-linolenic Acid and Nonfatal Acute Myocardial Infarction in Costa Rica." *Circulation* 107 (2003): 1586–91.

Deckelbaum, R. J., et al. "Summary of a Scientific Conference on Preventive Nutrition: Pediatrics to Geriatrics." *Circulation* 100 (1999): 450–56.

deLorgeril, M., et al. "Mediterranean Alpha-linolenic Acid-rich Diet in Secondary Prevention of Coronary Heart Disease." *Lancet* 343 (1994): 1454–59.

———. "Mediterranean Diet, Traditional Risk Factors, and the Rate of Cardiovascular Complications after Myocardial Infarction: Final Report of the Lyon Diet Heart Study." *Circulation* 99 (1999): 779–85.

Gruppo Italiano per lo Studio della Sopravvivenza nell'Infarto Miocardico. "Dietary Supplementation with N-3 Polyunsaturated Fatty Acids and Vitamin E after Myocardial Infarction: Results of the GISSI-Prevenzione Trial." *Lancet* 354 (1999): 447–55.

Holmes, M. D., et al. "Association of Dietary Intake of Fat and Fatty Acids with Risk of Breast Cancer." *Journal of the American Medical Association* 281 (1999): 914–20.

Horrobin, D. F. "Essential Fatty Acid Metabolism and Its Modification in Atopic Eczema." *American Journal of Clinical Nutrition* 71 (2000): 367s–72s.

Hu, F. B., et al. "A Prospective Study of Egg Consumption and Risk of Cardiovascular Disease in Men and Women." *Journal of the American Medical Association* 281 (1999): 1387–94.

———. "Diet, Lifestyle, and the Risk of Type 2 Diabetes Mellitus in Women." *New England Journal of Medicine* 345 (2001): 790–97.

Knopp, R. H., et al. "Long-term Cholesterol-lowering Effects of Four Fat-restricted Diets in Hypercholesterolemic and Combined Hyperlipidemic Men: The Dietary Alternatives Study." *Journal of the American Medical Association* 278 (1997): 1509–15.

Mensink, R. P., and M. B. Katan. "Effect of Dietary Trans Fatty Acids on High-density and Low-density Lipoprotein Cholesterol Levels in Healthy Subjects." *New England Journal of Medicine* 323 (1990): 439–45.

———. "Effect of Monounsaturated Fatty Acids Versus Complex Carbohydrates on High-density Lipoproteins in Healthy Men and Women." *Lancet* 1 (1987): 122–25.

Mozaffarian, D., et al. "Dietary Intake of Trans Fatty Acids and Systemic Inflammation in Women." *American Journal of Clinical Nutrition* 79 (2004): 606–12.

Salmeron, J., et al. "Dietary Fat Intake and Risk of Type 2 Diabetes in Women." *American Journal of Clinical Nutrition* 73 (2001): 1019–26.

CHAPTER 5

Aldoori, W. H., et al. "A Prospective Study of Dietary Fiber Types and Symptomatic Diverticular Disease in Men." *Journal of Nutrition* 128 (1998): 714–19.

Block, G. "Foods Contributing to Energy Intake in the US: Data from NHANES III and NHANES 1999–2000." *Journal of Food Composition and Analysis* 17 (2004): 439–47.

Brand-Miller, J. C. "Glycemic Load and Chronic Disease." *Nutrition Reviews* 61 (2003): S49–S55.

Harris, M. I., et al. "Prevalence of Diabetes, Impaired Fasting Glucose, and Impaired Glucose Tolerance in U.S. Adults." The Third National Health and Nutrition Examination Survey, 1988–1994. *Diabetes Care* 21 (1998): 518–24.

Hu, F. B. "Plant-based Foods and Prevention of Cardiovascular Disease: An Overview." *American Journal of Clinical Nutrition* 78 (suppl) (2003): 544-51.

Jacobs, D. R., Jr., et al. "Whole-Grain Intake and Cancer: An Expanded Review and Meta-analysis." *Nutrition and Cancer* 30 (1998): 85–96.

King, H., et al. "Global Burden of Diabetes, 1995–2025: Prevalence, Numerical Estimates, and Projections." *Diabetes Care* 21 (1998): 1414–31.

Liu, S., et al. "A Prospective Study of Dietary Glycemic Load, Carbohydrate Intake and Risk of Coronary Heart Disease in U.S. Women." *American Journal of Clinical Nutrition* 71 (2000): 1455–61.

Ludwig, D. S. "The Glycemic Index: Physiological Mechanisms Relating to Obesity, Diabetes, and Cardiovascular Disease." *JAMA* 287 (2002): 2414–23.

Schulze, M. B., et al. "Glycemic Index, Glycemic Load, and Dietary Fiber Intake and Incidence of Type 2 Diabetes in Younger and Middle-aged Women." *American Journal of Clinical Nutrition* 80 (2004): 348–56.

Slavin, J. "Why Whole Grains Are Protective: Biological Mechanisms." *Proceedings of the Nutrition Society* 62 (2003): 129–34.

Sweeney, M. "Constipation: Diagnosis and Treatment." *Home Care Provider* 2 (1997): 250–55.

CHAPTER 6

Anderson, J. W., et al. "Meta-analysis of the Effects of Soy Protein Intake on Serum Lipids." *New England Journal of Medicine* 333 (1995): 276–82.

Feskanich, D., et al. "Protein Consumption and Bone Fractures in Women." *American Journal of Epidemiology* 143 (1996): 472–79.

Fung, T. T., et al. "Dietary Patterns, Meat Intake, and the Risk of Type 2 Diabetes in Women." *Archives of Internal Medicine* 164 (2004): 2235–40.

Giovannucci, E., et al. "Alcohol, Low-Methionine-Low-Folate Diets, and Risk of Colon Cancer in Men." *Journal of the National Cancer Institute* 87 (1995): 265–73.

Hu, F. B., et al. "Dietary Fat Intake and the Risk of Coronary Heart Disease in Women." *New England Journal of Medicine* 337 (1997): 1491–99.

———. "Frequent Nut Consumption and Risk of Coronary Heart Disease in Women: Prospective Cohort Study." *British Medical Journal* 317(7169) (1998): 1341–45.

———. "Dietary Protein and Risk of Ischemic Heart Disease in Women." *American Journal of Clinical Nutrition* 70 (1999): 221–27.

Iocono, G., et al. "Intolerance of Cow's Milk and Chronic Constipation in Children." *New England Journal of Medicine* 339 (1998): 1100–104.

Key, T. J., et al. "Soya Foods and Breast Cancer Risk: A Prospective Study in Hiroshima and Nagasaki." *British Journal of Cancer* 81 (1999): 1248–56.

McMichael-Phillips, D. F., et al. "Effects of Soy-Protein Supplementation on Epithelial Proliferation in the Histologically Normal Human Breast." *American Journal of Clinical Nutrition* 68 (suppl) (1998): 1431–36.

Mills, P. K., et al. "Animal Product Consumption and Subsequent Fatal Breast Cancer Among Seventh-Day Adventists." *American Journal of Epidemiology* 127 (1988): 440–53.

Murkies, A. L., et al. "Dietary Flour Supplementation Decreases Post-menopausal Hot Flushes: Effect of Soy and Wheat." *Maturitas* 21 (1995): 189–95.

Washburn, S., et al. "Effect of Soy Protein Supplementation on Serum Lipoproteins, Blood Pressure, and Menopausal Symptoms in Perimenopausal Women." *Menopause* 6 (1999): 7–13.

White, L. R., et al. "Brain Aging and Midlife Tofu Consumption." *Journal of the American College of Nutrition* 19 (2000): 242–55.

Wolfe, B. M., and L. A. Piche. "Replacement of Carbohydrate by Protein in a Conventional-Fat Diet Reduces Triglyceride Concentrations in Healthy Normolipidemic Subjects." *Clinical and Investigative Medicine* 22 (1999): 140–48.

Yamamoto, S., et al. "Soy, Isoflavones, and Breast Cancer Risk in Japan." *Journal of the National Cancer Institute* 95 (2003): 906–13.

Yuan, J. M., et al. "Diet and Breast Cancer in Shanghai and Tianjin, China." *British Journal of Cancer* 71 (1995): 1353–58.

CHAPTER 7

Appel, L. J., et al. "A Clinical Trial of the Effects of Dietary Patterns on Blood Pressure." *New England Journal of Medicine* 336 (1997): 1117–24.

Carr, A. C., and B. Frei. "Toward a New Recommended Dietary Allowance for Vitamin C Based on Antioxidant and Health Effects in Humans." *American Journal of Clinical Nutrition* 69 (1999): 1086–107.

Chasan-Taber, L., et al. "A Prospective Study of Vitamin Supplement Intake and Cataract Extraction Among U.S. Women." *Epidemiology* 10 (1999): 679–84.

Chobanian, A. V., et al. "The Seventh Report of the Joint National Committee on Prevention, Detection, Evaluation, and Treatment of High Blood Pressure: the JNC 7 Report." *JAMA* 289 (2003): 2560–72.

Fuchs, C. S., et al. "Dietary Fiber and the Risk of Colorectal Cancer and Adenoma in Women." *New England Journal of Medicine* 340 (1999): 169–76.

Giovannucci, E. "Tomatoes, Tomato-based Products, Lycopene, and Cancer: Review of the Epidemiologic Literature." *Journal of the National Cancer Institute* 91 (1999): 317–31.

Giovannucci, E., et al. "Calcium and Fructose Intake in Relation to Risk of Prostate Cancer." *Cancer Research* 58 (1998): 442–47.

Heimendinger, J., and M. A. Van Duyn. "Dietary Behavior Change: The Challenge of Recasting the Role of Fruit and Vegetables in the American Diet." *American Journal of Clinical Nutrition* 61 (suppl) (1995): 1397–401.

Hung, H. C., et al. "Fruit and Vegetable Intake and Risk of Major Chronic Disease." *Journal of the National Cancer Institute* 96 (2004): 1577–84.

Krebs-Smith, S. M. "U.S. Adults' Fruit and Vegetable Intakes, 1989 to 1991: A Revised Baseline for the Healthy People 2000 Objective." *American Journal of Public Health* 85 (1995): 1623–29.

Michels, K. B., et al. "Prospective Study of Fruit and Vegetable Consumption and Incidence of Colorectal Cancers." *Journal of the National Cancer Institute* 92 (2000): 1740–52.

Serdula, M. K., et al. "Fruit and Vegetable Intake Among Adults in 16 States: Results of a Brief Telephone Survey." *American Journal of Public Health* 85 (1995): 236–39.

"The Sixth Report of the Joint National Committee on Prevention, Detection, Evaluation, and Treatment of High Blood Pressure." *Archives of Internal Medicine* 157 (1997): 2413–46.

U.S. Supreme Court. *Nix v. Hedden.* FindLaw. http://laws.findlaw.com/US/149/304.html

Vainio, H., and F. Bianchini. *Fruit and Vegetables—IARC Handbooks of Cancer Prevention* (Vol. 8). Lyon, France: International Agency for Research on Cancer, 2005.

Willett, W. C. "Goals for Nutrition in the Year 2000." *CA: A Cancer Journal for Clinicians* 49 (1999): 331–52.

World Cancer Research Fund. *Food, Nutrition and Cancer.* Washington, D.C.: American Institute for Cancer Research, 1997.

Chapter 8

Curhan, G. C., et al. "Prospective Study of Beverage Use and the Risk of Kidney Stones." *American Journal of Epidemiology* 143 (1999): 240–47.

Leitzmann, M. F., et al. "Coffee Intake Is Associated with Lower Risk of Symptomatic Gallstone Disease in Women." *Gastroenterology* 123 (2002): 1823–30.

"Liquid Candy." Center for Science in the Public Interest. http://www.cspinet.org/sodapop/liquid_candy.htm

Mukamal, K. J., et al. "Roles of Drinking Pattern and Type of Alcohol Consumed in Coronary Heart Disease in Men." *New England Journal of Medicine* 348 (2003): 109–18.

Salazar-Martinez, E., et al. "Coffee Consumption and Risk for Type 2 Diabetes Mellitus." *Annals of Internal Medicine* 140 (2004): 1–8.

Schulze, M. B., et al. "Sugar-sweetened Beverages, Weight Gain, and Incidence of Type 2 Diabetes in Young and Middle-aged Women." *JAMA* 292 (2004): 927–34.

Valtin, H. " 'Drink At Least Eight Glasses of Water a Day.' Really? Is There Scientific Evidence for '8 x 8'?" *American Journal of Physiology—Regulatory, Integrative and Comparative Physiology* 283 (2002): R993–1004.

Weisburger, J. H. "Second International Scientific Symposium on Tea and Human Health: An Introduction." *Proceedings of the Society for Experimental Biology and Medicine* 220 (1999): 193–94.

Willett, W. C., et al. "Coffee Consumption and Coronary Heart Disease in Women. A Ten-year Follow-up." *JAMA* 275 (1996): 458–62.

CHAPTER 9

Bischoff-Ferrari, H. A., et al. "Positive Association Between 25-Hydroxy Vitamin D Levels and Bone Mineral Density: A Population-based Study of Younger and Older Adults." *American Journal of Medicine* 116 (2004): 634–39.

Chan, J. M., et al. "Dairy Products, Calcium, and Prostate Cancer Risk in the Physicians' Health Study." *American Journal of Clinical Nutrition* 74 (2001): 549–54.

Cho, E., et al. "Dairy Foods, Calcium, and Colorectal Cancer: A Pooled Analysis of 10 Cohort Studies." *Journal of the National Cancer Institute* 96 (2004): 1015–22.

Cummings, S. R., et al. "Risk Factors for Hip Fracture in White Women." *New England Journal of Medicine* 332 (1995): 767–73.

Eastell, R. "Treatment of Postmenopausal Osteoporosis." *New England Journal of Medicine* 338 (1998): 736–46.

Feskanich, D., et al. "Vitamin K Intake and Hip Fractures in Women: A Prospective Study." *American Journal of Clinical Nutrition* 69 (1999): 74–79.

———. "Walking and Leisure-Time Activity and Risk of Hip Fracture in Postmenopausal Women." *JAMA* 288 (2002): 2300–6.

———. "Calcium, Vitamin D, Milk Consumption, and Hip Fractures: A Prospective Study Among Postmenopausal Women." *American Journal of Clinical Nutrition* 77 (2003): 504–11.

Giovannucci, E. "Calcium and Fructose Intake in Relation to Risk of Prostate Cancer." *Cancer Research* 58 (1998): 442–47.

———. "Epidemiologic Characteristics of Prostate Cancer." *Cancer* 75 (suppl) (1995): 1766–77.

Kleerekoper, M. "The Role of Fluoride in the Prevention of Osteoporosis." *Endocrinology and Metabolism Clinics of North America* 27 (1998): 441–52.

"Lactose intolerance." NIDDK. http://digestive.niddk.nih.gov/ddiseases/pubs/lactoseintolerance/

Looker, A. C., et al. "Dietary Calcium and Hip Fracture Risk: The NHANES I Epidemiologic Follow-up Study." *Osteoporosis International* 3 (1993): 177–84.

Michaelsson, K., et al. "Diet and Hip Fracture Risk—A Case-Control Study." *International Journal of Epidemiology* 24 (1995): 771–82.

"Osteoporosis: Fast Facts." National Osteoporosis Foundation. http://www.nof.org/osteoporosis/diseasefacts.htm

Owusu, W., et al. "Calcium Intake and the Incidence of Forearm and Hip Fractures among Men." *Journal of Nutrition* 127 (1997): 1782–87.

Ringe, J. D., et al. "Avoidance of Vertebral Fractures in Men with Idiopathic Osteoporosis by a Three Year Therapy with Calcium and Low-dose Intermittent Monofluorophosphate." *Osteoporosis International* 8 (1998): 47–52.

Suarez, F. L., et al. "A Comparison of Symptoms after the Consumption of Milk or Lactose-hydrolyzed Milk by People with Self-reported Severe Lactose Intolerance." *New England Journal of Medicine* 333 (1995): 1–4.

Thomas, M. K., et al. "Hypovitaminosis D in Medical Inpatients." *New England Journal of Medicine* 338 (1998): 777–83.

Utiger, R. D. "The Need for More Vitamin D." *New England Journal of Medicine* 338 (1998): 828–29.

"WHI—Clinical Trial and Observational Study." National Heart, Lung, and Blood Institute. http://www.nhlbi.nih.gov/whi/ctos.htm

Wickham, C. A. C., et al. "Dietary Calcium, Physical Activity, and Risk of Hip Fracture: A Prospective Study." *British Medical Journal* 299 (1989): 889–92.

CHAPTER 10

Ames, B. N. "Cancer Prevention and Diet: Help from Single Nucleotide Polymorphisms." *Proceedings of the National Academy of Sciences of the United States of America* 96 (1999): 12216–18.

Ames, B. N., et al. "The Causes and Prevention of Cancer." *Proceedings of the National Academy of Sciences of the United States of America* 92 (1995): 5258–65.

Ascherio, A., et al. "Vitamin E Intake and Risk of Amyotrophic Lateral Sclerosis." *Annals of Neurology* 57 (2005): 104–10.

Ascherio, A., and W. C. Willett. "Are Body Iron Stores Related to the Risk of Coronary Heart Disease?" *New England Journal of Medicine* 330 (1994): 1152–54.

Baik, H. W., and R. M. Russell. "Vitamin B12 Deficiency in the Elderly." *Annual Review of Nutrition* 19 (1999): 357–77.

Beckman, K. B., and B. N. Ames. "The Free Radical Theory of Aging Matures." *Physiological Reviews* 78 (1998): 547–81.

Booth, S. L., et al. "Food Sources and Dietary Intakes of Vitamin K-1 (Phylloquinone) in the American Diet: Data from the FDA Total Diet Study." *Journal of the American Dietetic Association* 96 (1996): 149–54.

Botto, L. D., et al. "Neural-tube Defects." New England Journal of Medicine 341 (1999): 1509–19.

Bressler, N. M., et al. "Potential Public Health Impact of Age-Related Eye Disease Study Results: AREDS Report No. 11." *Archives of Ophthalmology* 121 (2003): 1621–24.

Brown, L., et al. "A Prospective Study of Carotenoid Intake and Risk of Cataract Extraction in U.S. Men." *American Journal of Clinical Nutrition* 70 (1999): 517–24.

Campbell, M. J., and H. P. Koeffler. "Toward Therapeutic Intervention of Cancer by Vitamin D Compounds." *Journal of the National Cancer Institute* 89 (1997): 182–85.

Carr, A. C., and B. Frei. "Toward a New Recommended Dietary Allowance for Vitamin C Based on Antioxidant and Health Effects in Humans." *American Journal of Clinical Nutrition* 69 (1999): 1086–107.

Chasan-Taber, L., et al. "A Prospective Study of Vitamin Supplement Intake and Cataract Extraction Among U.S. Women." *Epidemiology* 10 (1999): 679–84.

Clark, L. C., et al. "Effects of Selenium Supplementation for Cancer Prevention in Patients with Carcinoma of the Skin: A Randomized Controlled Trial." Nutritional Prevention of Cancer Study Group. *Journal of the American Medical Association* 276 (1996): 1957–63.

Clarke, R., et al. "Hyperhomocysteinemia: An Independent Risk Factor for Vascular Disease." *New England Journal of Medicine* 324 (1991): 1149–55.

Federal Register. "Food Standards: Amendment of Standards of Identity for Enriched Grain Products to Require Addition of Folic Acid. Final Rule." Washington, D.C.: Food and Drug Administration, 5 March 1996: 8781–97.

Feskanich, D., et al. "Plasma Vitamin D Metabolites and Risk of Colorectal Cancer in Women." *Cancer Epidemiology, Biomarkers and Prevention* 13 (2004): 1502–8.

———. "Vitamin K Intake and Hip Fractures in Women: A Prospective Study." *American Journal of Clinical Nutrition* 69 (1999): 74–79.

Gennari, F. J. "Hypokalemia." *New England Journal of Medicine* 339 (1998): 451–58.

Grodstein, F., et al. "A Large Randomized Trial of Beta-carotene Supplements and Cognitive Function." *Neurobiology of Aging* 25, Supplement 2 (2004): 54.

Gruppo Italiano per lo Studio della Sopravvivenza nell'Infarto Miocardico. "Dietary Supplementation with N-3 Polyunsaturated Fatty Acids and Vitamin E after Myocardial Infraction: Results of the GISSI-Prevenzione Trial." *Lancet* 354 (1999): 447–55.

Harvard Health Publications. *Vitamins and Minerals.* Boston, Mass.: Harvard Medical School, 2003.

Hercberg, S., et al. "The SU.VI.MAX Study: A Randomized, Placebo-controlled Trial of the Health Effects of Antioxidant Vitamins and Minerals." *Archives of Internal Medicine* 164 (2004): 2335–42.

Institute of Medicine. *Dietary Reference Intakes for Calcium, Phosphorous, Magnesium, Vitamin D, and Fluoride.* Washington, D.C.: National Academy Press, 1997. http://www.nap.edu/books/0309063507/html

———. *Dietary Reference Intakes for Thiamin, Riboflavin, Niacin, Vitamin B6, Folate, Vitamin B12,*

Pantothenic Acid, Biotin, and Choline. Washington, D.C.: National Academy Press, 1999.
http://www.nap.edu/books/0309065542/html

———. *Dietary Reference Intakes for Vitamin C, Vitamin E, Selenium, and Carotenoids.* Washington, D.C.: National Academy Press, 2000. http://www.nap.edu/books/0309069351/html

———. *Dietary Reference Intakes for Energy, Carbohydrate, Fiber, Fat, Fatty Acids, Cholesterol, Protein, and Amino Acids (Macronutrients).* Washington, D.C.: National Academy Press, 2002.
http://www.nap.edu/books/0309085373/html

———. *Dietary Reference Intakes for Vitamin A, Vitamin K, Arsenic, Boron, Chromium, Copper, Iodine, Iron, Manganese, Molybdenum, Nickel, Silicon, Vanadium, and Zinc.* Washington, D.C.: National Academy Press, 2002. http://www.nap.edu/books/0309072794/html

———. *Dietary Reference Intakes for Water, Potassium, Sodium, Chloride, and Sulfate.* Washington, D.C.: National Academy Press, 2004. http://www.nap.edu/books/0309091691/html

Jackson, J. L., et al. "A Meta-analysis of Zinc Salts Lozenges and the Common Cold." *Archives of Internal Medicine* 157 (1997): 2373–76.

Jacobson, M. D., et al. "Vitamin B6 (Pyridoxine) Therapy for Carpal Tunnel Syndrome." *Hand Clinics* 12 (1996): 253–57.

Jacques, P. F. "The Potential Preventive Effects of Vitamins for Cataract and Age-related Macular Degeneration." *International Journal for Vitamin and Nutrition Research* 69 (1999): 198–205.

Jacques, P. F., et al. "The Effect of Folic Acid Fortification on Plasma Folate and Total Homocysteine Concentrations." *New England Journal of Medicine* 340 (1999): 1449–54.

Kim, Y. I. "Folate and Cancer Prevention: A New Medical Application of Folate Beyond Hyperhomocysteinemia and Neural Tube Defects." *Nutrition Review* 57 (1999): 314–21.

Knekt, P., et al. "Antioxidant Vitamins and Coronary Heart Disease Risk: A Pooled Analysis of 9 Cohorts." *American Journal of Clinical Nutrition* 80 (2004): 1508–20.

Larkin, M. "Kilmer McCully: Pioneer of the Homocysteine Theory." *Lancet* 352 (1998): 1364.

LeBoff, M. S., et al. "Occult Vitamin D Deficiency in Postmenopausal U.S. Women with Acute Hip Fracture." *Journal of the American Medical Association* 281 (1999): 1505–11.

Malinow, M. R., et al. "Reduction of Plasma Homocyst(e)ine Levels by Breakfast Cereal Fortified with Folic Acid in Patients with Coronary Heart Disease." *New England Journal of Medicine* 338 (1998): 1009–15.

Massaro, E. J., and J. M. Rogers. *Folate and Human Development.* Totowa, N.J.: Humana Press, 2002.

Miller, E. R., 3rd, et al. "Meta-analysis: High-dosage Vitamin E Supplementation May Increase All-cause Mortality." *Annals of Internal Medicine* 142 (2005): 37–46.

Rimm, E. B., et al. "Folate and Vitamin B6 from Diet and Supplements in Relation to Risk of Coronary Heart Disease Among Women." *Journal of the American Medical Association* 279 (1998): 359–64.

Rohan, T. E., et al. "Dietary Folate Consumption and Breast Cancer Risk." *Journal of the National Cancer Institute* 92 (2000): 266–69.

Shankar, A. H., and A. S. Prasad. "Zinc and Immune Function: The Biological Basis of Altered Resistance to Infection." *American Journal of Clinical Nutrition* 68 (suppl) (1998): 447–63.

Sommerburg, O., et al. "Fruits and Vegetables That Are Sources for Lutein and Zeaxanthin: The Macular Pigment in Human Eyes." *British Journal of Ophthalmology* 82 (1998): 907–10.

Stampfer, M. J., et al. "A Prospective Study of Plasma Homocyst(e)ine and Risk of Myocardial Infarction in U.S. Physicians." *Journal of the American Medical Association* 268 (1992): 877–81.

Thomas, M. K., et al. "Hypovitaminosis D in Medical Inpatients." *New England Journal of Medicine* 338 (1998): 777–83.

Tucker, K. L., et al. "Dietary Intake Pattern Relates to Plasma Folate and Homocysteine Concentrations in the Framingham Heart Study." *Journal of Nutrition* 126 (1996): 3025–31.

Wyatt, K. M., et al. "Efficacy of Vitamin B-6 in the Treatment of Premenstrual Syndrome: Systematic Review." *British Medical Journal* 318 (1999): 1375–81.

Yusuf, S., et al. "Vitamin E Supplementation and Cardiovascular Events in High-risk Patients." The Heart Outcomes Prevention Evaluation Study Investigators. *New England Journal of Medicine* 342 (2000): 154–60.

Zhang, S., et al. "A Prospective Study of Folate Intake and the Risk of Breast Cancer." *Journal of the American Medical Association* 281 (1999): 1632–37.

Chapter 11 Summary

Drewnowski, A. "Obesity and the Food Environment: Dietary Energy Density and Diet Costs." *American Journal of Preventive Medicine* 27 (2004): 154–62.

Frazão, E. "High Costs of Poor Eating Patterns in the United States." In: Frazão E, ed. *America's Eating Habits: Changes & Consequences.* Washington, D.C.: Economic Research Service, U.S. Department of Agriculture, 1999. http://www.ers.usda.gov/publications/aib750

Keys, A. *Seven Countries: A Multivariate Analysis of Death and Coronary Heart Disease.* Cambridge, Mass.: Harvard University Press, 1980.

Keys, A. B., and M. Keys. *How to Eat Well and Stay Well the Mediterranean Way.* Garden City, N.Y.: Doubleday, 1975.

Reed, J., et al. *How Much Do Americans Pay for Fruits and Vegetables?* Washington, D.C.: Economic Research Service, U.S. Department of Agriculture, 2004. http://www.ers.usda.gov/publications/aib790

Trichopoulou, A., et al. "Adherence to a Mediterranean Diet and Survival in a Greek Population." *New England Journal of Medicine* 348 (2003): 2599–608.

Willett, W. C., et al. "Mediterranean Diet Pyramid: A Cultural Model for Healthy Eating." *American Journal of Clinical Nutrition* 61 (suppl) (1995): 1402–6.

General Index

bisphosphonates, 170–71
bladder cancer, 141, 147
blood clots, 55, 113, 122, 137, 154, 178
    dietary fats and, 70, 71, 72, 82, 87
    vitamin E and, 186
    vitamin K and, 172, 194
    zinc and, 202
blood pressure, *see* high blood-pressure
    (hypertension)
blood sugar, 19, 44, *see also* glucose;
    glycemic index
    carbohydrates and, 23, 69, 99, 100,
        101, 103–4
    fiber and, 142–43
    low-carbohydrate diets and, 47, 60
    protein and, 125
Bob's Red Mill, 237–38
body mass index (BMI), 35, 37–41
bone, 181–82, 192, *see also* osteoporosis
    calcium alternatives and, 168–72
    calcium and, 159–65, 168, 173
    coffee and, 153
    density of, 164, 194
    fractures of, 18–19, 162–63, 164–65,
        168, 171–72, 182, 194
    protein and, 60, 61, 126, 131
    remodeling, 161, 181
    remodeling space, 164
brain cancer, 193
bran, 115, 233
breast cancer, 30, 109, 120, 151, 183,
    193
    alcohol and, 154–55, 156, 157
    dietary fats and, 90–91
    exercise and, 50
    folic acid and, 190
    hormone replacement therapy and,
        170
    milk and, 167, 168
    soy and, 128–29, 130–31
    weight and, 22, 35
Brigham and Women's Hospital, 49
British Medical Journal, 189
buckwheat, 230

bulgur, 230–31
butter, 27, 28, 73, 84, 225

caffeine, 151–52, 197
calcium, 18–19, 26, 158–73, 192, 204
    alternatives to, 168–72
    benefits of, 159–62
    daily requirements for, 158, 162–65,
        195
    dark side of, 165–68
    protein and, 60, 126, 131, 172
    sources of, 159, 195
    in specific foods, 160–61
calcium supplements, 159, 162, 165, 171,
    173, 194, 195
caloric density, *see* energy density
calories, 41–42, 45–49, 64
    defined, 45
    diet types and, 46–49
    exercise and, 50–51
    on food labels, 224
    keeping track of, 56
    in menu selections, 239
    in milk, 167
    MyPyramid on, 20–21
    in typical restaurant meal, 43
Canada, 158
cancer, 19, 148, 151, 209
    alcohol and, 154–55, 156, 157
    antioxidants and, 179–80
    bladder, 141, 147
    brain, 193
    breast *(see* breast cancer)
    calcium and, 162
    carotenoids and, 183
    cervical, 183
    colon *(see* colon cancer)
    dietary fats and, 80, 90–92
    endometrial, 22, 35
    esophageal, 141
    exercise and, 50
    folic acid and, 190
    gallbladder, 113
    glycemic load and, 109

trans fats (*cont.*)
   percentage in common oils and fats, 94
   sources and properties of, 71, 74
   in typical processed foods, 83
   USDA Pyramid on, 15
triglycerides, 127, 143, 149
   in the bloodstream, 72, 73
   carbohydrates and, 23, 78, 100, 104
   dietary fats and, 82
   low-carbohydrate diets and, 65
   protein and, 120
   structure of, 70
triticale, 235
tryptophan, 189
twin studies, 42

umbels (Umbelliferae), 135
Union of Concerned Scientists, 125
United Kingdom, 153, 158
United States Pharmacopeia (USP), 204
University of California, Berkeley, 177
University of Toronto, 105
University of Washington, 78
unsaturated fats, 22, 68–69, 70, 79–80, 81, 85, 93–95, *see also* monounsaturated fats; polyunsaturated fats

vegan diet, 189
vegetables and fruits, 132–45
   color variety in, 135–36, 144–45
   cost of, 216
   defined, 133–34
   disease prevention with, 136–41
   families of, 134–36
   Healthy Eating Pyramid on, 23
   limitations of guidelines, 136
   shopping for, 236–37
   supplements compared with, 133
vegetable shortening, 74, 81, 92, 93, 220, 225
vegetarian diet, 21, 23, 118, 129, 189, 202

VISP (Vitamin Intervention for Stroke Prevention) trial, 187–88
vitamin(s), 174–207
   common deficiencies, 203
   defined, 176
   fat-soluble, 176
   Healthy Eating Pyramid on, 24
   recommended daily intake, 205–7
   selecting, 203–4
   USDA Pyramid failure to address, 19
   in vegetables and fruits, 143–44
   water-soluble, 176
vitamin A, 97, 159, 171, 173, 176, 194, 204
   properties and functions of, 181–82
   recommended intake of, 181
vitamin B_6, 24, 186–89, 203
vitamin B_{12}, 24, 186–88, 189–90, 203
vitamin C, 145, 150, 176, 177, 180
   functions and properties of, 183–84
   recommended intake of, 184
vitamin D, 24, 97, 143, 159, 161, 165, 168, 169, 171–72, 173, 195, 203
   functions and properties of, 192–94
   in multivitamins, 204
   recommended intake of, 171
   sources of, 171, 192
   vitamin A blocking of, 182, 194
vitamin E, 27, 97, 113, 177, 178, 180, 201, 203
   functions and properties of, 184–86
   in multivitamins, 204
vitamin K, 97, 161, 169, 172, 173, 194–95
Volumetrics diet, 62–63, 65

waist-to-hip ratio, 43, 45
walking, 52–53
warfarin (Coumadin), 172
water, 148
Web sites:
   Harvard Health Publications, 37
   MyPyramid, 20

Recipe Index

wild mushroom–barley risotto,
    300–301
wild rice–quinoa pilaf, 298
wilted spinach with nuts & golden
    raisins, 308–9

winter squash soup, curried, 289–90
winter squash with pecan stuffing,
    288–89
winter vegetable medley, roasted,
    297–98